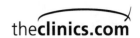

ENDOCRINOLOGY AND METABOLISM CLINICS OF NORTH AMERICA

Pituitary Disorders

GUEST EDITOR
Ariel L. Barkan, MD

CONSULTING EDITOR
Derek LeRoith, MD, PhD

March 2008 • Volume 37 • Number 1

SAUNDERS

An Imprint of Elsevier, Inc.
PHILADELPHIA   LONDON   TORONTO   MONTREAL   SYDNEY   TOKYO

W.B. SAUNDERS COMPANY
A Division of Elsevier Inc.

1600 John F. Kennedy Boulevard • Suite 1800 • Philadelphia, Pennsylvania 19103-2899

http://www.theclinics.com

ENDOCRINOLOGY AND METABOLISM	Volume 37, Number 1
CLINICS OF NORTH AMERICA	ISSN 0889-8529
March 2008	ISBN-13: 978-1-4160-5858-8
Editor: Rachel Glover	ISBN-10: 1-4160-5858-3

The ideas and opinions expressed in *Endocrinology and Metabolism Clinics of North America* do not necessarily reflect those of the Publisher. The Publisher does not assume any responsibility for any injury and/or damage to persons or property arising out of or related to any use of the material contained in this periodical. The reader is advised to check the appropriate medical literature and the product information currently provided by the manufacturer of each drug to be administered to verify the dosage, the method and duration of administration, or contraindications. It is the responsibility of the treating physician or other health care professional, relying on independent experience and knowledge of the patient, to determine drug dosages and the best treatment for the patient. Mention of any product in this issue should not be construed as endorsement by the contributors, editors, or the Publisher of the product or manufacturers' claims.

Endocrinology and Metabolism Clinics of North America (ISSN 0889-8529) is published quarterly by Elsevier Inc., 360 Park Avenue South, New York, NY 10010-1710. Months of publication are March, June, September, and December. Business and editorial offices: 1600 John F. Kennedy Boulevard, Suite 1800, Philadelphia, PA 19103-2899. Customer Service Office: 6277 Sea Harbor Drive, Orlando, FL 32887-4800. Periodicals postage paid at New York, NY and additional mailing offices. Subscription prices are USD 220 per year for US individuals, USD 364 per year for US institutions, USD 113 per year for US students and residents, USD 276 per year for Canadian individuals, USD 437 per year for Canadian institutions, USD 301 per year for international individuals, USD 437 per year for international institutions and USD 157 per year for Canadian and foreign students/residents. To receive student/resident rate, orders must be accompanied by name of affiliated institution, date of term, and the *signature* of program/residency coordinator on institution letterhead. Orders will be billed at individual rate until proof of status is received. Foreign air speed delivery is included in all *Clinics* subscription prices. All prices are subject to change without notice. POSTMASTER: Send address changes to *Endocrinology and Metabolism Clinics of North America*, Elsevier Journals Customer Service, 6277 Sea Harbor Drive, Orlando, FL 32887-4800. **Customer Service: (+1) 800-654-2452 (US). From outside of the US, call (+1) 407-563-6020; e-mail: JournalsCustomerService-usa@ elsevier.com.**

Reprints. For copies of 100 or more, of articles in this publication, please contact the Commercial Rights Department, Elsevier Inc., 360 Park Avenue South, New York, NY 10010-1710; phone: (+1) 212-633-3813; fax: (+1) 212-462-1935; e-mail: reprints@elsevier.com.

Endocrinology and Metabolism Clinics of North America is covered in *Index Medicus, EMBASE/Excerpta Medica, Current Contents/Clinical Medicine, Current Contents/Life Sciences, Science Citation Index, ISI/BIOMED, BIOSIS, and Chemical Abstracts.*

Printed in the United States of America.

CONSULTING EDITOR

DEREK LEROITH, MD, PhD, Chief, Division of Endocrinology, Metabolism, and Bone Diseases, Mount Sinai School of Medicine, New York, New York

GUEST EDITOR

ARIEL L. BARKAN, MD, Professor of Internal Medicine and Neurosurgery, Department of Neurosurgery; and Division of Metabolism, Endocrinology, and Diabetes, University of Michigan Medical Center, Ann Arbor, Michigan

CONTRIBUTORS

ARIEL L. BARKAN, MD, Professor of Internal Medicine and Neurosurgery, Department of Neurosurgery; and Division of Metabolism, Endocrinology, and Diabetes, University of Michigan Medical Center, Ann Arbor, Michigan

PAOLO BECK-PECCOZ, MD, Department of Medical Sciences, University of Milan, Fondazione Ospedale Maggiore Policlinico IRRCS, Milan, Italy

ANAT BEN-SHLOMO, MD, Assistant Professor of Medicine, Cedars-Sinai Medical Center; and David Geffen School of Medicine at UCLA, Los Angeles, California

MICHAEL BRADA, BSc, FRCP, FRCR, Professor of Clinical Oncology, Academic Unit of Radiotherapy and Oncology, The Institute of Cancer Research, Sutton, Surrey; and Neuro-Oncology Unit, The Royal Marsden NHS Foundation Trust, London and Sutton, United Kingdom

MARCELLO DELANO BRONSTEIN, MD, Professor of Endocrinology and Chief, Neuroendocrine Unit, Division of Endocrinology and Metabolism, Hospital das Clinicas, University of Sao Paulo Medical School, Sao Paulo, Brazil

FELIPE F. CASANUEVA, MD, PhD, Professor, Department of Medicine, Laboratory of Molecular Endocrinology, Santiago Universitario de Santiago de Compostela; and Centro de Investigacion Biomedica en Rede de Fisiopatologia Obesidad y Nutricion, Instituto Salud Carlos III, Santiago de Compostela, Spain

WILLIAM F. CHANDLER, MD, Professor of Internal Medicine and Neurosurgery, Department of Neurosurgery; and Division of Metabolism, Endocrinology, and Diabetes, University of Michigan Medical Center, Ann Arbor, Michigan

ANNAMARIA COLAO, MD, PhD, Associate Professor, Department of Molecular and Clinical Endocrinology and Oncology, Federico II University, Naples, Italy

LAWRENCE A. FROHMAN, MD, Professor Emeritus of Medicine, Section of Endocrinology, Diabetes, and Metabolism, College of Medicine, University of Illinois at Chicago, Chicago, Illinois

ANDREA GIUSTINA, MD, Full Professor of Internal Medicine, Department of Medical and Surgical Sciences, University of Brescia, Brescia; and Head, Endocrine Service, Montichiari Hospital, Montichiari, Italy

ANDREA GLEZER, MD, Senior Clinical Fellow, Neuroendocrine Unit, Division of Endocrinology and Metabolism, Hospital das Clinicas, University of Sao Paulo Medical School, Sao Paulo, Brazil

PETRA JANKOWSKA, MRCP, FRCR, Specialist Registrar, Neuro-Oncology Unit, The Royal Marsden NHS Foundation Trust, London and Sutton, United Kingdom

NIKI KARAVITAKI, MBBS, MSc, PhD, Locum Consultant in Endocrinology, Department of Endocrinology, Oxford Centre for Diabetes, Endocrinology, and Metabolism, Headington, Oxford, United Kingdom

MONICA DE LEO, MD, In-Trainee Fellow, Department of Molecular and Clinical Endocrinology and Oncology, Federico II University, Naples, Italy

ANDY LEVY, PhD, FRCP, Professor of Endocrinology and Honorary Consultant Physician, Bristol University and United Bristol Healthcare Trust, Wellcome Labs for Integrative Neuroscience and Endocrinology, University of Bristol, Bristol, United Kindgom

JENNIFER A. LOH, MD, Fellow, Georgetown University; and Washington Hospital Center, Washington, DC

GAETANO LOMBARDI, MD, Full Professor, Department of Molecular and Clinical Endocrinology and Oncology, Federico II University, Naples, Italy

TATIANA MANCINI, MD, Medical Assistant, Internal Medicine, San Marino Hospital, Republic of San Marino

MARIA CRISTINA DE MARTINO, MD, In-Trainee Fellow, Department of Molecular and Clinical Endocrinology and Oncology, Federico II University, Naples, Italy

SHLOMO MELMED, MBChB, FRCP, Senior Vice-President, Academic Affairs, Cedars-Sinai Medical Center; and David Geffen School of Medicine at UCLA, Los Angeles, California

MARK E. MOLITCH, MD, Professor of Medicine, Division of Endocrinology, Metabolism, and Molecular Medicine, Northwestern University Feinberg School of Medicine, Chicago, Illinois

DIANE BELCHIOR PARAIBA, MD, Fellow, Neuroendocrine Unit, Division of Endocrinology and Metabolism, Hospital das Clinicas, University of Sao Paulo Medical School, Sao Paulo, Brazil

LUCA PERSANI, MD, PhD, Department of Medical Sciences, University of Milan, Instituto Auxologico Italiano, Milan, Italy

ROSARIO PIVONELLO, MD, PhD, Fellow, Department of Molecular and Clinical Endocrinology and Oncology, Federico II University, Naples, Italy

SUSAN SAM, MD, Assistant Professor of Medicine, Section of Endocrinology, Diabetes, and Metabolism, College of Medicine, University of Illinois at Chicago, Chicago, Illinois

PAUL M. STEWART, FRCP, FMedSci, Professor of Medicine, University of Birmingham, University Hospital Birmingham NHS Foundation Trust, Edgbaston, Birmingham, United Kingdom

ANDREW A. TOOGOOD, MD, FRCP, Consultant Endocrinologist and Honorary Senior Lecturer, University Hospital Birmingham NHS Foundation Trust, Edgbaston, Birmingham, United Kingdom

JOSEPH G. VERBALIS, MD, Professor of Medicine and Physiology Chief, Endocrinology and Metabolism; and Program Director, General Clinical Research Center, Georgetown University Medical Center, Washington, DC

JOHN A.H. WASS, MA, MD, FRCP, Professor of Endocrinology, University of Oxford, Department of Endocrinology, Oxford Centre for Diabetes, Endocrinology, and Metabolism, Headington, Oxford, United Kingdom

CONTENTS

The anterior pituitary is a complex heterogeneous gland that exerts a central role in the integration of several regulatory systems. Its six key hormones affect peripheral glands or target tissues and are essential for reproduction, growth and development, metabolism, adaptation to external environmental changes, and stress. Each of the pituitary hormones is regulated by the central nervous system through neuroendocrine pathways involving the hypothalamus, by feedback effects from peripheral target gland hormones, and by intrapituitary mechanisms. The hormones are secreted in a pulsatile manner, which is distinct for each hormone and reflects the influence of its individual neuroendocrine control mechanisms.

A significant proportion of pituitary macroadenomas, and by definition all microadenomas, regain trophic stability after an initial period of deregulated growth. Classical proto-oncogene activation and tumor suppressor mutation are rarely responsible, and no histologic or molecular markers reliably predict behavior. GNAS1 activation and the mutations associated with multiple endocrine neoplasia type 1 and Carney complex, aryl hydrocarbon receptor interacting protein gene mutations, and a narrowing region of chromosome 11q13 in familial isolated acromegaly together account for such a small proportion of pituitary adenomas that the pituitary adenoma pathogenic epiphany is surely yet to come.

and those who have nonsuppressed circulating thyrotropin concentrations. In the latter, it is mandatory to perform a differential diagnosis, as the management of the two disorders is completely different, and failure to recognize the presence of a thyrotropinoma may result in dramatic consequences. Adenomectomy is the firstline treatment of thyrotropinomas, followed by irradiation in the case of surgical failure. Medical treatment with somatostatin analogs is effective in reducing thyrotropin secretion in more than 90% of cases.

Cushing's syndrome is a rare endocrine disease characterized by cortisol hypersecretion, induced mainly by a pituitary tumor (Cushing's disease) or, rarely, by an adrenal or an ectopic neuroendocine tumor. Cushing's syndrome is associated with severe morbidities and an increased mortality. The major systemic complications and the main cause of death are represented by cardiovascular disease. The prognosis of the disease is mainly affected by the difficulties in the diagnosis and treatment of the disease, which remain a considerable challenge.

Clinically nonfunctioning adenomas (CNFAs) range from being completely asymptomatic, and therefore detected at autopsy or as incidental findings on head MRI or CT scans performed for other reasons, to causing significant hypothalamic/pituitary dysfunction and visual field compromise because of their large size. Patients with incidental adenomas should be screened for hypersecretion and hyposecretion. In the absence of hypersecretion, hypopituitarism, or visual field defects, patients may be followed by periodic screening by MRI for enlargement. Symptomatic patients with CNFAs are generally treated by transsphenoidal resection. Postoperative MRI scans are done at 3 to 4 months after surgery to assess for completeness of resection and then repeated yearly for 3 to 5 years and subsequently less frequently to assess for regrowth. The regrowth rate may be substantially reduced with the use of dopamine agonists and radiotherapy.

Craniopharyngiomas are epithelial tumors arising along the path of the craniopharyngeal duct and presenting with a variety of manifestations. Their optimal management remains a subject of debate. Currently, surgical excision followed by external beam irradiation is the main treatment option. Craniopharyngiomas are associated with significant long-term morbidity and mortality rates.

Sellar masses are associated most commonly with pituitary adenomas. Many other neoplastic, inflammatory, infectious, and vascular lesions, however, may affect the sellar region and mimic pituitary tumors. These lesions must be considered in a differential diagnosis. This article describes the characteristics of rare sellar masses that provide clues to their differential diagnosis.

Disorders of water and sodium homeostasis are very common problems encountered in clinical medicine. Disorders of water metabolism are divided into hyperosmolar and hypoosmolar states, with hyperosmolar disorders characterized by a deficit of body water in relation to body solute and hypoosmolar disorders characterized by an excess of body water in relation to total body solute. This article briefly reviews the physiology of hyperosmolar and hypoosmolar syndromes, then focuses on a discussion of the pathophysiology, evaluation, and treatment of specific pre- and postoperative disorders of water metabolism in patients with pituitary lesions.

Hypopituitarism is characterized by loss of function of the anterior pituitary gland. It is a rare condition that can present at any age and is caused by pathology of the hypothalamic-pituitary axis or one of many gene mutations. The symptoms and signs of hypopituitarism may evolve over several years and be nonspecific or related to the effects of the underlying disease process or to hormone deficiencies. Investigation of patients requires a combination of basal hormone levels and dynamic function tests; management requires regular monitoring. The goal of physicians managing patients who have hypopituitarism is to improve their health and long-term outcome.

FORTHCOMING ISSUES

RECENT ISSUES

THE CLINICS ARE NOW AVAILABLE ONLINE!

Access your subscription at:
http://www.theclinics.com

**ELSEVIER
SAUNDERS**

Endocrinol Metab Clin N Am
37 (2008) xiii–xvi

**ENDOCRINOLOGY
AND METABOLISM
CLINICS
OF NORTH AMERICA**

Foreword

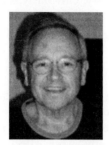

Derek LeRoith, MD, PhD
Consulting Editor

Pituitary tumors cause a number of varied endocrine disorders, sometimes developing rapidly, such as hyperprolactinemic amenorrhea, and sometimes developing gradually over years, such as acromegaly and Cushing's disease. Clinical features, diagnostic testing, and therapy are of importance to the clinical endocrinologist, and Dr. Ariel Barkan has developed an outstanding issue on this topic that is designed to update the endocrinologist on different aspects of these interesting clinical problems.

The normal physiology of hypothalamic pituitary hormonal regulation is presented by Drs. Sam and Frohman. The well-studied regulatory control of pituitary hormone production and release involves hypothalamic-produced releasing (or suppressing) hormones/factors, and peripheral feedback control mechanisms, both negative and positive, some of which are involved in short-loop, and others in long-loop, feedback regulation. More recently, there is intensive examination of the role of intrapituitary regulation of pituitary hormone release. The total effect of all these regulatory controls is the eventual circadian rhythmicity and pulsatile release that lead to normal growth and development, normal reproduction, and total body homeostasis.

The etiology of pituitary tumors is an area of basic research that has revealed interesting results. Unlike tumors that develop secondary to classic oncogenic transformation, pituitary tumors rarely do so. However, as described by Dr. Levy in his scholarly article, they are associated with genetic causes, such as gain of function mutations in GNAS1, for example.

doi:10.1016/j.ecl.2007.11.002
endo.theclinics.com

Obviously, further research will reveal the underlying genetic causes that may lead to the development of targeted therapeutics.

Pituitary tumors often require surgical removal both to reduce the level of excessive hormone secretion and to avoid or correct local effects, such as encroachment on the visual system, and thereby to prevent visual loss. Transsphenoidal surgery is the most common method, though transcranial surgery is occasionally necessary. Obviously, surgery is totally dependent on excellent pituitary imaging. Drs. Chandler and Barkan provide a concise guide to the MRI diagnosis of the most frequent pituitary lesions and discuss indications for various functioning and nonfunctioning pituitary tumors, the limitations, side effects and need for re-resection that is not uncommon.

The article by Drs. Brada and Jankowska describes the use of radiation therapy for pituitary tumors, a technique usually reserved for those tumors that are not completely "cured" by surgery or medical therapy. Conventional radiation therapy, while effective, is associated with hypopituitarism in the long term. Radiosurgery and stereotactic conformal radiotherapy is becoming more available as stereotactic "radiosurgery" and fractionated stereotactic conformal radiotherapy. The results of these techniques show distinct effectiveness, though long-term side effects are too early to assess.

Dr. Molitch describes nonfunctioning pituitary tumors and how they are detected as incidentalomas. By definition, they fail to show excess hormonal production and secretion, though they may cause hormonal deficiency, either due to a mass effect within the pituitary or on the hypothalamus. If small and not associated with symptoms or hormonal imbalance, they can be followed with periodic MRIs to assess growth. Usually, when necessary, they are treated by transsphenoidal surgery and dopamine agonists and rarely with radiotherapy to prevent regrowth after surgery.

As described by Drs. Mancini, Casanueva, and Giustina, hyperprolactinemia is a common disorder in clinical endocrine practice and is commonly associated with female and male hypogonadism. After drug-induced and secondary causes of hyperprolactinemia have been excluded, prolactinoma is the most common cause. Both serum prolactin measurements and an MRI are needed for the diagnosis. Treatment is often quite successful with the use of dopamine agonists, and transsphenoidal surgery (or radiation therapy) is usually reserved for the cases not responding to medical therapy or with large adenomas encroaching on critical structures. In their article, the authors also discuss the effect of pregnancy on prolactinomas and the treatment of prolactinomas during pregnancy, an important issue since many prolactinomas appear in women during their fertile years.

Though acromegaly may be caused by an extra-pituitary tumor producing excessive amounts of growth hormone releasing hormone (GHRH), the most common cause is a benign pituitary adenoma. Drs. Ben-Shlomo and Melmed describe the well-known clinical features and the long-term complications of inadequately treated acromegaly. Transsphenoidal surgery is the treatment of choice for micro-adenomas and the more common macroadenomas; with the latter, there is generally incomplete resection, and medical suppression of the excessive growth hormone and IGF-1 concentrations is commonly used (both somatostatin analogues and pegvisomant). Radiation is reserved for the more unusual cases, because, while it can definitively stop tumor growth, it is usually associated with hypopituitism and even long-term neurological complications.

Cushing's syndrome, while relatively rare, is commonly a challenge both for diagnosis and for therapy. The most common cause is iatrogenic, due to prolonged steroid therapy for chronic disorders. Pituitary tumors are more common than adrenal adenomas in causing Cushing's syndrome, and ectopic neuroendocrine tumors are relatively rare.

Drs. Pivonello, De Martino, De Leo, Lombardi and Colao describe, in depth, the difficulties in diagnosis that often lead to problems with therapy, how therapy is often not entirely successful, and the factors often resulting in poor prognoses.

A rare cause of hyperfunctioning pituitary tumors is thyrotropinomas. As described in the article by Drs. Beck-Peccoz and Persani, thyrotropinomas may be easily distinguished from other causes of hyperthyroidism such as Graves' disease and a toxic nodule, as the latter have suppressed thyroid stimulating hormone levels. Pituitary resistance to thyroid hormone needs to be excluded, since its treatment is thyroid ablation, whereas thyrotropinomas are surgically removed with or without radiation therapy. Incidentally, somatstostatin can suppress TSH secretion when necessary.

Drs. Karavitaki and Wass discuss the rare condition of craniopharyngioma. These tumors may be discovered in children or in adults, and are often treated with surgery and radiation therapy. Long-term morbidity results from endocrine hypofunction and neurologic (visual) morbidities, and cognitive loss stems either from the lesion or as a result of treatment.

Most pituitary tumors are either hormone producing (functional) or nonfunctional adenomas. There are, however, rare sellar masses that mimic pituitary adenomas, and these should always be considered in the differential diagnosis. They include a large and varied range of neoplastic, inflammatory, infectious, developmental, and vascular lesions. The list, as outlined in the article by Drs. Glezer, Belchior, and Bronstein, is quite long; however, the authors summarize some important features of the more common abnormalities.

Hypopituitarism may present as an isolated hormonal deficiency or as pan-hypopituitarism. The etiology ranges from primary deficiencies to secondary causes such as pituitary or suprasellar tumors, infiltrative lesions or destructive lesions seen following brain injury or radiation therapy. Drs. Toogood and Stewart describe the various hormonal deficiencies, the classic tests required to detect each deficiency, and replacement therapies. Their article offers both an academic and practical point of view.

Drs. Loh and Verbalis, in their article, discuss disorders of sodium and water metabolism, as related to pituitary diseases. Although hyponatremia is generally a more common disorder than hypernatremia, in the case of pituitary lesions, diabetes insipidus, and resultant hypernatremia are more common that the syndrome of inappropriate antidiuretic hormone (SIADH) secretion with concomitant hyponatremia. Once again, their article reveals both important information on the pathophysiology, possible complications, diagnostic testing, and therapeutic approaches.

Given the outstanding contributions by the international experts in the field, I believe the readers of this issue certainly owe all the authors and the issue editor, as I do, for the excellent, while predictable outcome!

Derek LeRoith, MD, PhD
Division of Endocrinology, Metabolism, and Bone Diseases
Mount Sinai School of Medicine
One Gustave L. Levy Place
Box 1055, Altran 4-36
New York, NY 10029, USA

E-mail address: derek.leroith@mssm.edu

ELSEVIER
SAUNDERS

Endocrinol Metab Clin N Am
37 (2008) xvii–xviii

ENDOCRINOLOGY
AND METABOLISM
CLINICS
OF NORTH AMERICA

Preface

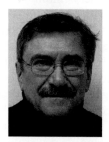

Ariel L. Barkan, MD
Guest Editor

Endocrine diseases of the hypothalamic-pituitary area have always been regarded as intellectually challenging, physiologically fascinating but... rather esoteric. Most general endocrinologists practice for years without encountering a single case of acromegaly. A proficiency in interpreting thyroid ultrasounds is expected from any endocrine fellow, but a large proportion of them will admit to having problems locating the pituitary on the MRI. Medical students and residents accept with resignation their inability to understand the logic behind the differential diagnosis of Cushing's syndrome.

Pituitary diseases are believed to be so rare that they barely register on the radar screen of public health authorities, funding agencies, hospital administrators, and training program directors. After all, even though about 20% of the general population has blips on the pituitary MRI scans and some 15% of autopsies find small and undiagnosed pituitary tumors, how many cases of clinically relevant pituitary diseases are there?

Well, as a matter of fact, quite a lot.

Dr. Albert Beckers and his colleagues found an approximate 1: 1000 prevalence of clinically important pituitary tumors in several well-defined communities in Europe, comprising a total of almost three quarters of a million individuals. Half of these tumors were prolactinomas, 25% were nonfunctioning, 12% were growth hormone–producing, and Cushing's disease and craniopharyngioma contributed 7% each (89th Meeting of the Endocrine Society, OR13-1: 2007). This is 3.5 to 5 times higher than the previously reported numbers. Similarly, the incidence of hypopituitarism increases steadily with the rising numbers of long-term survivors of cancer,

0889-8529/08/$ - see front matter © 2008 Elsevier Inc. All rights reserved.
doi:10.1016/j.ecl.2007.11.001
endo.theclinics.com

massive head trauma, or subarachnoid hemorrhage. Thus, pituitary diseases can no longer be viewed as exotic illnesses, but rather as medical problems of significant impact.

Recent years have witnessed major refinements in our ability to visualize pituitary lesions using MRI studies, and to document subtle hormonal abnormalities with the use of sensitive hormonal assays. Similarly, there have been major therapeutic advances: minimally-invasive transnasal surgery, computer-driven radiation techniques, and several new medications.

The changed landscape of pituitary endocrinology was the impetus behind assembling the leading experts in the field to summarize the contemporary state-of-the-art knowledge in this fascinating area.

This issue was designed not so much for the narrowly defined "pituitary specialists," but mainly for general clinical endocrinologists, endocrine fellows, and, hopefully, for medical students and residents. If this issue helps in solving clinical dilemmas that often arise in clinical practice and if even a single medical resident, having read it, says "That is what I want to do when I grow up!", the authors would feel that their efforts were well spent.

I would like to express my deepest gratitude to all the authors who participated in thisproject. Their dedication and generosity with their knowledge and time were outstanding.

Finally, I would like to thank W.B. Saunders for initiating this project and especially Ms. Rachel Glover, who guided it from the beginning to the end.

And, of course, Elizabeth, as ever...

Ariel L. Barkan, MD
University of Michigan Medical Center
Ann Arbor, MI, USA

E-mail address: abarkan@med.umich.edu

ELSEVIER
SAUNDERS

Endocrinol Metab Clin N Am
37 (2008) 1–22

ENDOCRINOLOGY
AND METABOLISM
CLINICS
OF NORTH AMERICA

Normal Physiology of Hypothalamic Pituitary Regulation

Susan Sam, MD[a], Lawrence A. Frohman, MD[b],*

[a]Section of Endocrinology, Diabetes, and Metabolism (M/C 640), College of Medicine,
University of Illinois at Chicago, 1819 West Polk Street, 625 CMW, Chicago, IL 60612, USA
[b]Section of Endocrinology, Diabetes, and Metabolism (M/C 275), College of Medicine,
University of Illinois at Chicago, 1747 West Roosevelt Road, Room 517,
Chicago, IL 60608, USA

The anterior pituitary is a heterogeneous gland with multiple cell types that secrete hormones with unique functions. Each of its secreted hormones participates in complex regulatory systems involving peripheral glands or target tissues, is controlled by separate and distinct hypothalamic regulatory mechanisms and by feedback systems, and is modulated by intrapituitary influences that are still only partially understood. The pituitary hormones are essential for reproduction, growth, metabolic homeostasis, and responses to stress, and they are critical for adapting to changes in the external environment. This article reviews the regulation of secretion of the individual anterior pituitary hormones and their neuroendocrine, intrapituitary (autocrine/ paracrine), and peripheral (endocrine and metabolic) control mechanisms.

Growth hormone

Growth hormone (GH) is a single-chain 191–amino acid polypeptide with a molecular size of 22 kilodaltons (kDa). It is synthesized in and released from somatotrope cells, which constitute the most numerous cell type in the anterior pituitary. GH exerts a broad spectrum of effects, resulting in growth promotion and the regulation of carbohydrate, protein, lipid, and mineral metabolism. These are mediated by direct effects on peripheral tissues and indirect effects on the liver and other tissues through the generation of insulin-like growth factor-1 (IGF-1). Nearly 80% of circulating IGF-1 is of hepatic origin. The synthesis and secretion of GH are regulated primarily

* Corresponding author.
E-mail address: frohman@uic.edu (L.A. Frohman).

0889-8529/08/$ - see front matter © 2008 Elsevier Inc. All rights reserved.
doi:10.1016/j.ecl.2007.10.007
endo.theclinics.com

through the actions of hypothalamic neuropeptides that integrate hormonal, metabolic, and neurogenic signals. In addition to its most abundant chemical form, alternative mRNA processing leads to a shorter 20-kDa molecule, referred to as "variant GH," which accounts for up to 10% to 20% of pituitary GH. It is cosecreted with 22-kDa GH and has similar growth-promoting, although reduced anti–insulin-like, activity [1]. The half-life of GH in serum is 20 to 25 minutes [2]; the secretion rate in young adult men is approximately 600 µg/d, and it is approximately 900 µg/d in young adult women [3].

Neuroendocrine control

The regulation of GH secretion occurs through the integrated action of numerous peptides and nonpeptide hormones. The neuroendocrine control is mediated primarily through the hypophysiotropic hormones growth hormone–releasing hormone (GHRH) and somatostatin (somatotrope release-inhibiting factor [SRIF]).

GHRH is a 44–amino acid peptide synthesized in and secreted from neurons in the arcuate nucleus of the hypothalamus and serves as the primary stimulatory regulator of GH [4]. It binds to a stimulatory G protein–coupled somatotrope receptor, resulting in activation of adenylyl cyclase, causing an increase in intracellular cyclic adenosine monophosphate (cAMP) levels and a mobilization of intracellular Ca^{2+}, which triggers the release of GH. In addition, GHRH stimulates the synthesis of GH and is required for somatotrope proliferation during development. When present in excess, it can result in somatotrope hyperplasia and increased GH secretion. The regulation of GHRH secretion is mediated by neuropeptides and monoaminergic neurotransmitters and by feedback from peripheral sources. A dual function of many of these neuropeptides in feeding behavior and metabolic regulation underscores the importance of nutrient control in GH secretion.

Somatostatin is a 14–amino acid peptide and has a widespread distribution within the central nervous system. SRIF-containing neurons affecting GH secretion are located primarily in the periventricular hypothalamic nucleus and, after release into the portal vascular system, bind to somatotrope receptors. There are five distinct SRIF receptors, of which types 2 and 5 exert the most potent effects on GH secretion. Binding of SRIF to its receptors results in activation of inhibitory G-proteins, which leads to lowering of cAMP levels and inhibition of GH secretion. Although SRIF does not suppress basal GH synthesis, it inhibits the stimulatory effects of GHRH. SRIF secretion is similarly regulated by neuropeptide and monoamine transmitters, in addition to peripheral feedback signals.

Ghrelin, a 28–amino acid octanoylated peptide, located primarily in the stomach but also in the hypothalamus, binds to a specific GH secretagogue (GHS) receptor on the somatotrope and stimulates GH secretion [5,6]. GHS receptors are also present in the hypothalamus, and direct effects on GHRH release have been observed in animal studies. Although peripheral levels of ghrelin are linked to nutritional status, a physiologic role for this peptide on GH secretion remains controversial.

Intrapituitary regulation

In addition to the important role of hypothalamic hormones in the generation of pulsatile GH secretion, it has recently been shown that the pituitary contains a large-scale network organization of somatotropes that are connected to one another by adherens junctions (anchoring connections of the cytoskeleton of adjacent cells). This network has been proposed as being responsible for integrated amplification during the pulses of GH secretion [7].

Pulsatility of growth hormone secretion

GH secretion occurs in a pulsatile manner in humans and in all other species examined, with from 8 to 12 pulses occurring in a 24-hour period [8]. In men, approximately 70% of GH secretion occurs during the early hours of the night, in association with deep (electroencephalographic [EEG] stage III–IV, or slow wave) sleep [9], whereas daytime pulses are of lesser magnitude and interspersed with troughs that are at or beneath the level of sensitivity of most GH assays. In women, the relative proportion of daytime GH secretion is greater and the interpeak troughs are slightly higher than in men [10]. Similar and more pronounced gender differences are seen in the rat. GH pulsatility is also affected by nutrient status, with obesity impairing and fasting enhancing pulsatile GH secretion [11]. Experimental data from animals [12] and humans [13] support the role of GHRH as the principal regulator of GH pulsatility.

Age

GH secretion is maximal during puberty and through the third decade, after which it declines progressively with age. A similar decline in slow-wave sleep occurs during this same period, suggesting at least partial entrainment of GH with sleep. Sleep-associated GH secretion can be inhibited by cholinergic muscarinic receptor blockade [14].

Feedback regulation

GH secretion is under a complex multilevel feedback regulatory control. In the hypothalamus, GH feeds back to stimulate SRIF release and inhibit GHRH release, thereby inhibiting its own secretion from the pituitary.

IGF-1 has similar actions in the hypothalamus and also feeds back at the level of the pituitary to inhibit basal and GHRH-stimulated GH secretion. SRIF inhibits GHRH release, and GHRH stimulates SRIF release within the hypothalamus. Together, these hormones create a dynamic control system that also modulates the GH responses to all other stimuli. In addition, feedback effects on the pituitary receptors for GHRH, SRIF, and ghrelin add another level of control, although they likely contribute to a greater extent to long-term rather than to short-term regulation. Studies in humans using a GHRH antagonist indicate that gender differences exist in GH feedback regulation [10].

Nutrient regulation

The profound metabolic effects of GH are associated with reciprocal effects of nutrients on GH secretion. Hyperglycemia in man leads to a marked suppression of GH secretion for 1 to 3 hours, followed by a rebound increase in GH [15]. In contrast, hypoglycemia is a profound stimulus for GH secretion [16]. Studies in mice suggest that these changes are mediated by effects on GHRH and SRIF [17]. GH enhances amino acid uptake and protein synthesis, whereas protein intake and especially certain amino acids, notably arginine, stimulate GH secretion [18]. The additive effect of arginine and GHRH and the responses to cholinergic agonists imply that this response is mediated by an inhibition of SRIF release [19]. GH exerts profound lipolytic effects and causes marked increases in free (nonesterified) fatty acids. Acute elevations in free fatty acids, in turn, cause suppression of GH secretion in response to GHRH [20], suggesting an effect mediated by enhanced SRIF release. This observation is consistent with the reduced GH secretion seen in obesity in which free fatty acids are elevated but not with food deprivation, in which free fatty acid levels are also elevated. This seeming paradox may be explained by the decreases in IGF-1 during starvation.

Gonadal hormones

The activation of gonadal steroids at puberty and their decline during aging parallel the changes in GH secretion at these periods, although a causal relation between the two has not been clearly demonstrated. Although some studies report conflicting results, most animal studies suggest that the effects of gonadal steroids occur primarily at the level of the pituitary and on GH synthesis. In humans, evidence points to a stimulatory role of estrogens but not androgens, except those that are aromatizable to estrogens [21]. These effects are seen initially at puberty and can be demonstrated throughout adult life. Estrogens and androgens also have opposite effects on hepatic IGF-1 production, with estrogens inhibiting and androgens stimulating

IGF-1 synthesis. In humans, these effects tend to complicate the interpretation of gonadal steroids on GH secretion.

Glucocorticoid and thyroid hormones

Acute administration of glucocorticoids stimulates GH secretion [22]. However, chronic glucocorticoid therapy and endogenous hypercortisolism decrease the GH response to stimulation. Although glucocorticoids have direct stimulatory effects on the somatotrope, they also have effects on the hypothalamic hormones affecting GH secretion and on the generation of IGF-1, which makes interpretation of their overall effects complex. Similarly, GH responses are reduced in both hypothyroidism and hyperthyroidism. Thyroid hormone is required for GH gene expression, but its effects on GH secretion also involve actions in the hypothalamus.

Prolactin

Prolactin is synthesized in lactotrope cells in the anterior pituitary that account for 10% to 20% of pituitary cells [23,24]. However, this percentage increases dramatically to approximately 40% in response to elevated estrogen levels, particularly during pregnancy [23–25]. Lactotropes are derived from somatomammotropes (common precursor cell line to lactotropes and somatotropes) and are the last pituitary cell line to differentiate during embryonic development [24,25]. Pituitary development and anterior pituitary cell differentiation involve the sequential expression of several transcription factors, among which Pit-1 and PROP-1 (prophet of Pit-1) are essential for differentiation of lactotropes and transcription of prolactin [26]. Mutations in these genes are a cause of combined pituitary hormone deficiency that involves GH, prolactin, and thyroid-stimulating hormone (TSH) but may also involve gonadotropins [27].

Prolactin is a single-chain protein of 198 amino acids with a molecular size of 23 kDa that shares extensive structural similarity to GH. The main physiologic function of prolactin in mammals is stimulation of lactation and modulation of maternal behavior. The physiologic effects of prolactin are mediated by the prolactin receptor, a single membrane-bound protein that belongs to the type 1 cytokine receptor family [28]. Activation of the prolactin receptor involves ligand-induced dimerization of the receptor and activation of Janus kinase 2 (JAK2), which results in tyrosine phosphorylation of the receptor and other proteins, such as the signal transducer and activator of transcription proteins (STAT 1–5) and Src-related protein kinases (SH2-PK) [24,25,28]. Prolactin receptors are present in many tissues, but the highest densities are in the liver, ovary, and mammary glands [29].

Hypothalamic regulation

In contrast to other anterior pituitary hormones, prolactin regulation is unique in that the predominant hypothalamic influence on its secretion is inhibitory rather than stimulatory. This regulation is provided primarily by tonic inhibition by hypothalamic dopamine. Hence, disruption of the hypothalamic-pituitary stalk increases prolactin secretion. The brain contains several dopaminergic systems, of which the hypothalamic tuberoinfundibular dopaminergic (TIDA) system is the main regulator of prolactin secretion [25]. Dopamine reaches the lactotropes through the hypothalamic-pituitary portal system and inhibits prolactin release, prolactin gene expression, and lactotrope proliferation. Inhibition of prolactin release occurs within seconds of exposure to dopamine on binding to type 2 (D2) dopamine receptors, followed by hyperpolarization of the cell membrane and inactivation of voltage-gated calcium channels [24,25]. Inhibition of prolactin gene expression occurs within minutes or hours. Dopamine receptors are members of the G protein–coupled receptor family, and the D2 receptor interacts with G_i proteins and inhibits adenylyl cyclase and inositol phosphate metabolism [29–31]. The inhibition of lactotrope proliferation occurs within days and is mediated by blockade of cAMP actions that are mitogenic in lactotropes [24,25].

Prolactin autoregulation

Prolactin regulates its own release through a short-loop feedback mechanism by binding to prolactin receptors on the hypothalamic dopaminergic system [24]. This feedback mechanism is mediated by modulating the activity of tyrosine hydroxylase (TH), the rate-limiting enzyme for synthesis of dopamine, in TIDA neurons [24,25]. An increase in circulating prolactin levels increases the activity of this enzyme in TIDA neurons, thereby increasing dopamine synthesis. Conversely, a reduction in circulating prolactin levels decreases TH activity in TIDA neurons and decreases dopamine synthesis and release [24,25]. The mechanisms regulating these events are not fully understood. This regulation seems to be lost in certain physiologic and pathologic conditions, such as pregnancy, lactation, and prolactinomas that are associated with elevated prolactin levels [25].

Prolactin-releasing factors

Several known stimulators of prolactin secretion include hypothalamic peptides, such as thyrotropin-releasing hormone (TRH), oxytocin, growth factors, and estrogen [23,24]. Even though TRH is a potent stimulator of prolactin release in vitro [32], its significance in vivo has been questioned, because primary hypothyroidism does not consistently lead to hyperprolactinemia [23,24]. Both oxytocin and prolactin secretion are increased during lactation [33] and in response to nipple stimulation [34]. Estrogen stimulates *PRL* gene transcription and secretion [23–25,35] and affects prolactin homeostasis in the hypothalamus and pituitary [25], leading to higher PRL levels in women of reproductive age as compared with postmenopausal women and men [36]. Prolactin levels in humans are also sleep dependent and rise with the onset of sleep [37].

Thyroid-stimulating hormone

TSH is a 28-kDa heterodimeric glycoprotein hormone consisting of two noncovalently linked subunits. TSH is secreted from thyrotrope cells, which constitute 5% of anterior pituitary cells. The α-subunit is common to TSH, follicle-stimulating hormone (FSH), and luteinizing hormone (LH) (and also chorionic gonadotropin) and contains 92 amino acids. The β-subunit, which contains 110 amino acids, is unique to the thyrotrope and confers specificity of biologic action. Both subunits are glycosylated on asparagine residues, and appropriate glycosylation is necessary for correct molecular folding and optimal biologic activity [38]. Glycosylation not only enhances TSH biologic activity on the thyroid but increases the metabolic clearance rate of the hormone. Approximately 40 to 150 mU of TSH is secreted daily, and the hormone's half-life in circulation is approximately 30 minutes [39].

Neuroendocrine regulation

The primary neuroendocrine regulation of TSH is mediated through TRH. TRH is a tripeptide present in many regions of the nervous system and in nonneural tissue. However, the TRH-containing neurons that control TSH secretion are located exclusively in the periventricular and medial parvocellular subdivisions of the hypothalamic paraventricular nucleus. TRH secretion is regulated by numerous neuropeptides, including leptin, proopiomelanocortin (POMC), neuropeptide Y (NPY), Agouti-related peptide (AGRP), and cocaine- and amphetamine-related transcript (CART), which integrate the influence of energy metabolism on thyroid hormone secretion [40,41]. The physiologic importance of TRH is reflected by the absence of an increase in serum TSH despite subnormal thyroxine (T_4) levels in patients who have hypothalamic disorders. In addition to its feedback effects on the pituitary, thyroid hormone also exerts inhibitory effects on TRH biosynthesis and secretion into the hypophyseal-portal circulation [42,43].

Somatostatin inhibits TSH as well as GH secretion, although it is less potent on the thyrotrope than on the somatotrope [44]. Even though SRIF analogues are useful in treating TSH-secreting tumors, their long-term use in acromegaly does not lead to hypothyroidism. Dopamine also suppresses TSH secretion by its inhibitory effects on adenylyl cyclase [45]. However, long-term use of dopamine agonists does not result in hypothyroidism.

Intrapituitary regulation

TSH synthesis and secretion are regulated primarily by the interplay of TRH and thyroid hormone. TRH stimulates and thyroid hormone suppresses the transcription of both α- and β-subunits. TRH, in addition, enhances posttranslational processing of TSH, primarily by increasing glycosylation. TRH action is initiated by its binding to a specific thyrotrope membrane receptor that is coupled to a G protein, with cyclic guanosine nucleotide (cGMP) serving as a second messenger. The G protein also activates phospholipase C, increasing inositol triphosphate (IP$_3$) leading to mobilization of Ca^{2+} and release of TSH from secretory granules. Thyroid hormone inhibits the stimulatory effect of TRH on TSH release. This acute inhibitory effect requires conversion of T$_4$ to triiodothyronine (T$_3$), which is produced by type II deiodinase (D2) within the pituitary.

Recent studies have implicated another pituitary cell type, the folliculo-stellate (FS) cell, as the exclusive site of D2 in the pituitary, and it has been proposed that this cell plays a critical intermediary role in the effects of thyroid hormone on the thyrotrope [46]. FS cells are organized into a three-dimensional network within which the hormone-secreting cells reside. This network forms a functional intrapituitary circuit that can transport small signaling molecules (eg, Ca^{2+} and T$_3$) throughout the anterior pituitary to various cell types [47].

Evidence also exists from animal studies for a paracrine/autocrine regulation of the thyrotrope by locally produced pituitary peptides [48]. The most consistent data relate to neuromedin B, a bombesin-like peptide, which seems to exert an inhibitory effect. The relevance of these regulatory peptides in humans is presently unclear.

Pulsatility

TSH secretion occurs in a pulsatile manner. The ultradian pattern consists of secretory pulses that occur every 2 to 3 hours with constant low levels of secretion between pulses. There is also a diurnal pattern of TSH secretion with a nocturnal surge that occurs before the onset of sleep [49]. Sleep onset seems to have an inhibitory effect, because the surge is enhanced if sleep is delayed, whereas early sleep onset and prolonged sleep result in a diminished surge and shorter duration of TSH secretion. The pulsatility is independent of circulating thyroid and glucocorticoid hormone levels, and thus is most likely neurally driven.

Aging

As individuals age, the daily secretion of TSH is reduced and the circulating levels decrease [50]. Although free T$_4$ levels in serum remain unchanged, the

T_3/T_4 ratio decreases in the eighth and ninth decades. It is uncertain whether these changes have clinical consequences other than the need for a reduction in T_4 dose (by approximately 20%) in patients receiving exogenous hormone.

Feedback control

The feedback regulation of TSH secretion occurs principally as the result of changes in peripheral thyroid hormone levels. Feedback occurs primarily in the pituitary, mediated by mechanisms described previously. The effects can be seen within a few hours of elevations of thyroid hormone levels and occur initially by reducing the TSH secretory response to TRH and later by effects on TSH synthesis. Thyroid hormone feedback also occurs on TRH-producing neurons, but these effects are believed to be of lesser magnitude than those on the thyrotrope. Suppression of the hypothalamic component of the axis can be observed after long periods of thyroid hormone administration, but the severity of hypothyroidism and the duration of the recovery of function are much less pronounced than is seen with the hypothalamic-pituitary-adrenal axis.

In addition to this classic feedback loop, evidence exists for both short-loop feedback (inhibitory effects of TSH on hypothalamic TRH) and ultrashort-loop feedback (inhibitory effects of TSH within the pituitary) mechanisms [51]. The latter is believed to involve the FS cells, which express the TSH receptor. The physiologic role of this loop may be in the fine-tuning of the secretory patterns of TSH and the generation of pulsatile hormone secretion.

Nutritional effects

TSH, T_3, and T_4 concentrations are decreased by both short-term and long-term fasting in people, as are reductions in pulsatile and circadian TSH secretion [52]. In animal studies, decreased TRH release into portal blood and reduced pro-TRH mRNA have been observed [53,54]. The mediation of these changes has been attributed to the decrease in leptin production that occurs during food deprivation. Leptin directly stimulates TRH mRNA and also indirectly affects TRH through its interactions with other hypothalamic neuropeptides that regulate nutrient homeostasis [55].

Exercise and stress

Acute physical activity induces an increase in TSH levels within minutes of its onset. The changes are most pronounced at night, when TSH secretion is normally increased [56]. The mediation of this response is not fully understood but appears to be independent of glucocorticoid activation, which would be expected to suppress TSH secretion [57]. Stress is associated with decreased activation of the hypothalamic-pituitary-thyroid axis. This inhibition is in part mediated by indirect negative feedback effects on the hippocampus that counterbalance the direct stimulatory effect of glucocorticoids on TRH production in TRH-containing neurons.

Corticotropin

The synthesis and secretion of glucocorticoids from the adrenal cortex are under the regulation of the hypothalamic-pituitary axis. Glucocorticoids are essential for maintenance of vascular tone, endothelial integrity, cardiac contractility, and response to stress. The hypothalamic-pituitary-adrenal (HPA) axis is tightly regulated to ensure adequate glucocorticoid secretion in response to stress and to avoid excess glucocorticoid release.

The corticotrope

Corticotrope cells comprise 20% of anterior pituitary cells and are the first anterior pituitary cell type to differentiate during embryonic development [23]. Transcription factor Tbx19/T-pit is essential for differentiation of pituitary corticotropes during embryonic development, and mutations in this gene are associated with isolated corticotropin (ACTH) deficiency in humans [58]. The corticotropes are located in the central median portion of the pituitary and produce ACTH by enzymatic cleavage of the precursor hormone, POMC [23,59]. The *POMC* gene coding for this precursor hormone is highly expressed in the corticotropes and is transcribed by the pituitary promoter P1 to an approximately 1200-nucleotide POMC mRNA transcript. The primary translation product of POMC is cleaved by prohormone convertase 1 in the pituitary gland, resulting in an N-terminal peptide, $ACTH_{(1-39)}$, and β-lipotropin [60]. In addition to stimulating adrenocortical steroidogenesis and secretion, ACTH is essential for maintenance of adrenal gland size and structure [23,61]. The adrenal cortex undergoes atrophy and loses its secretory capacity in the absence of ACTH [61,62].

Hypothalamic regulation of corticotropin

Pituitary ACTH release is stimulated primarily by corticotropin-releasing hormone (CRH) that is synthesized by CRH neurons located in the paraventricular hypothalamus [63,64]. These neurons project to the median eminence and release CRH into the hypophysial portal system. CRH stimulates ACTH secretion initially by the release of preformed peptide from pituitary cells but concurrently stimulates ACTH synthesis by increasing *POMC* gene expression in corticotropes [65]. These actions are mediated by CRH type 1 receptor, a G protein–coupled receptor predominantly expressed on corticotropes, which signals through cAMP [23,61,66,67]. In addition to CRH, vasopressin and oxytocin directly stimulate ACTH release, although these effects are weak. However, these hormones can act in synergy with CRH to potentiate ACTH release [61,68,69]. Furthermore, many CRH neurons express vasopressin and upregulate its expression in response to stimulation [61,70]. Additional factors regulating *POMC* gene expression include neurotransmitters, such as dopamine, serotonin, and catecholamines [59], and cytokines, such as leukemia inhibitory factor, a proinflammatory cytokine that is expressed in the pituitary and acts synergistically with CRH to stimulate the release of ACTH [71].

Glucocorticoid feedback action

Glucocorticoids suppress *POMC* expression in pituitary corticotropes [61,72] and inhibit secretion of CRH and vasopressin, leading to inhibition of ACTH secretion [73]. This feedback inhibition is classified according to time of the phenomena: fast (within 30 minutes of glucocorticoid administration), delayed (minutes to hours), and slow (hours to days) [23,61,67,72,73]. The first two occur under physiologic conditions, such as after moderate stress, and involve inhibition of stimulated ACTH secretion. Slow feedback affects basal and stimulated ACTH secretion and occurs after chronic exposure to glucocorticoids, such as in Cushing's syndrome or with sustained high-dose exogenous glucocorticoid administration [61,72].

Glucocorticoids exert their actions by binding to two receptors: glucocorticoid receptor (GR) and mineralocorticoid receptor (MR) [67]. GR is expressed widely in many peripheral tissues and the brain, including the pituitary and hypothalamus, whereas the expression of MR is generally restricted to peripheral mineralocorticoid target tissues, such as the kidney and limited areas in the brain [61,74,75]. Glucocorticoids bind to MR with greater affinity than to GR [61], but are unable to activate peripheral MR due to enzymatic inactivation [76]. The negative feedback actions of the glucocorticoids on the HPA axis involve binding to GR in the pituitary and hypothalamus and to MR in other areas of the brain, such as the hippocampus [61,74]. Although glucocorticoid feedback on basal HPA activity is mediated by MR and GR [77,78], suppression of stimulated ACTH secretion only occurs through binding to GR in pituitary corticotropes and hypothalamic CRH neurons [61,67].

Circadian rhythmicity

Levels of ACTH and glucocorticoids follow a circadian rhythm, and in humans, the levels peak in the early morning and gradually decline during the day to reach a nadir at midnight [59]. This circadian rhythm is generated in the suprachiasmatic nucleus, which sends neuronal afferents into the paraventricular nucleus of the hypothalamus and regulates CRH expression. The amplitude rather than the frequency of ACTH pulses regulates glucocorticoid levels; thus, the amplitude of ACTH pulses is much higher during the peaks of cortisol secretion. Furthermore, glucocorticoid feedback action is essential for the control of this circadian rhythm [59,61] and this feedback regulation is mediated by GR and MR actions [61,78,79].

Luteinizing hormone and follicle-stimulating hormone

The regulation of gonadal function in men and women is under the control of the hypothalamus and the pituitary gland by means of negative and positive feedback mechanisms. This regulation is complex, and the details have only begun to be understood in recent years. Endocrine, paracrine, and autocrine mechanisms are involved, and the regulators include hypothalamic and pituitary hormones, neurotransmitters, and endogenous opioids in addition to steroidal and nonsteroidal hormones from the gonads.

The hypothalamus and gonadotropin-releasing hormone

Gonadotropin-releasing hormone (GnRH)–producing neurons originate from the olfactory area and migrate during embryogenesis to their primary location within the arcuate nucleus of the hypothalamus [23]. In mammals, two forms of GnRH have been identified [80,81]. GnRH I, a 10–amino acid peptide, is synthesized in GnRH neurons and is released into the hypophyseal portal system to stimulate the synthesis and secretion of LH and FSH from anterior pituitary gonadotropes [82,83]. A second GnRH, GnRH II, differs from GnRH I by three amino acids and is found in the midbrain region and may be important in sexual behavior, although its exact physiologic function is not yet determined [84]. In this review, the term *GnRH* refers to GnRH I.

GnRH is released in a pulsatile manner, which is essential for maintenance of normal gonadotropin synthesis and secretion. The importance of the pulsatile secretion of GnRH was initially observed in monkeys with hypothalamic lesions in which normal gonadotropin secretion was restored by pulsatile but not continuous GnRH administration [85]. GnRH neurons secrete in a coordinated pulsatile manner and may have an intrinsic pulse-generating capacity [23]. The term *GnRH pulse generator* has often been used to represent this coordinated pulsatile release. The frequency of the GnRH pulses is a critical factor that determines LH and FSH synthesis and secretion. The endogenous frequency of the GnRH pulse generator in primates is approximately one pulse per hour. This pulse frequency selectively enhances pituitary LH release, whereas FSH release is favored by slower GnRH pulse frequency, one pulse every 3 to 4 hours [86]. Furthermore, the pattern of GnRH pulse frequency is crucial in differential gonadotropin β-subunit gene transcription [87,88]. In rats [89], fast-frequency GnRH pulses increase α-subunit mRNA levels and the LHβ primary transcript. However, a sustained increase in FSHβ transcription requires slower GnRH pulses [89]. The mechanisms for differential activation of gonadotropin subunit gene transcription by changes in GnRH pulse frequency have not yet been clearly identified and may involve several signaling pathways [90].

Central regulators of gonadotropin-releasing hormone

Many neurotransmitters and peptides from various brain regions convey information to GnRH neurons. These systems include neurons that contain norepinephrine, epinephrine, dopamine, serotonin, γ-aminobutyric acid (GABA), glutamate, endogenous opiate peptides, NPY, and galanin. In general, catecholamines stimulate GnRH release, whereas endogenous opioid peptides and prolactin inhibit GnRH secretion [91]. Sex steroids are important regulators of GnRH and gonadotropins, as is discussed elsewhere in this article. Recently, a new family of peptides, kisspeptins, have been identified that markedly stimulate GnRH-induced gonadotropin secretion in rodents and humans on central or peripheral administration [92]. These peptides are endogenous ligands for the G protein–coupled receptor GPR54, and mutations in the gene coding for this receptor result in hypogonadotropic hypogonadism in men [93,94]. Kisspeptin-GPR54 signaling may have a crucial role in the regulation of puberty by contributing to the pubertal re-emergence of pulsatile GnRH release [95]. Recent data also indicate that this signaling pathway may mediate the positive and negative feedback regulation of GnRH by sex steroids [92].

Gonadotropin-releasing hormone action

GnRH action on gonadotropes is initiated by binding to its cell membrane receptor. The GnRH receptor (GnRH-R) is a seven-transmembrane protein, and, on binding to its ligand, activates multiple signal transduction pathways that stimulate the synthesis and release of gonadotropins [84]. GnRH is the main regulator of GnRH-R concentrations, which increase when endogenous GnRH levels are increased [96,97]. The ability of GnRH to induce its own receptor is termed *upregulation* and only occurs with certain physiologic frequencies of pulsatile GnRH that differ among species [91]. In contrast, continuous GnRH exposure leads to GnRH-R downregulation, termed *desensitization* [91].

The pituitary gonadotropes

Gonadotropes constitute 7% to 15% of the cells in the anterior pituitary and are located in the lateral portion of the gland [91]. LH and FSH are glycoproteins with a common α-subunit and distinct β-subunits that confer specificity to each hormone. Most gonadotropes are capable of synthesizing and secreting LH and FSH. Both gonadotropins are synthesized and released in a pulsatile manner in response to pulsatile GnRH [98]. As previously discussed, the pattern of GnRH pulse frequency determines the differential synthesis of gonadotropin β-subunits, with slower GnRH pulses favoring FSH synthesis and release and faster pulses favoring LH synthesis and release [86–89]. Additionally, GnRH enhances pituitary responsiveness to subsequent pulses of GnRH, leading to increased LH secretion, a phenomenon referred to as a self-priming effect, which is further enhanced by estradiol [91] and is essential for the midcycle LH surge during the female menstrual cycle.

Intrapituitary regulation of gonadotropins

In addition to GnRH and sex steroids, inhibins, activins, and follistatin are important regulators of gonadotropin synthesis and secretion [99]. All three latter compounds were initially isolated from the gonads but are widely expressed in other tissues, including pituitary gonadotropes [99–101]. Inhibins and activins are members of the transforming growth factor-β (TGFβ) superfamily [101–103]. Inhibins are dimers of an α-subunit and a $β_A$ (inhibin A) or $β_B$ subunit (inhibin B), whereas activins are homodimers of $β_A$ or $β_B$ subunits, activin A ($β_A$, $β_A$) and activin B ($β_B$, $β_B$) [104]. Follistatin is an activin-binding protein that neutralizes, and thus modulates, all action of activins [105]. Although inhibins are considered to act in an endocrine manner to regulate FSH release, the actions of activins and follistatin seem to be of an autocrine/paracrine nature [99,102].

Activin and follistatin synthesized locally by the pituitary are important physiologic regulators of FSH production [99,102]. Activin is a potent stimulator of FSH secretion in vivo and in vitro [106,107] and has been shown to increase FSHβ mRNA expression in pituitary cell cultures [108,109]. Monoclonal antibodies against activin inhibit FSH release from pituitary cells [110]. Furthermore, transgenic mice with defects in activin receptor type IIA have reduced levels of FSH [111]. Inhibin/activin subunits, activin receptors, activin B, and follistatin are all synthesized in the pituitary [99,102], supporting an autocrine/paracrine mode of regulation. Follistatin is an activin-binding protein [112] that interferes with activin binding to its receptors (activin type-I and activin type-II), thereby inhibiting activin's actions [113]. Follistatin mRNA levels are directly regulated by GnRH pulse frequency. Fast GnRH pulses increase follistatin mRNA levels and result in activin inhibition and reduced FSH production, whereas slower frequency GnRH pulses have the opposite effect [89,114]. In addition to follistatin, inhibins antagonize activin's stimulation of FSH synthesis and release by interfering with activin binding to its receptors [102].

Sex steroid feedback

Sex steroids are important regulators of GnRH and gonadotropin release through classic feedback mechanisms in the hypothalamus and the pituitary. In the hypothalamus, estradiol, progesterone, and testosterone all slow the frequency of GnRH release by negative feedback action [23]. Even though GnRH neurons express steroid hormone receptors, such as estrogen receptor β [115], the feedback actions of sex steroids on GnRH are widely believed to be mediated by other neuronal pathways [23,116]. As an example, in primates, the progesterone-mediated negative feedback actions on GnRH secretion are mediated by hypothalamic β-endorphin–containing neurons and can be blocked by naloxone, an opiate receptor blocker [117,118]. Kisspeptins have also been implicated in sex steroid feedback regulation of GnRH secretion by acting directly on GnRH neurons [119]. Kisspeptin-secreting neurons in the hypothalamus express sex steroid receptors, and sex steroids can alter the expression of the kisspeptin gene, and hence GnRH secretion [92,119].

Sex steroids also exert negative feedback at the level of the pituitary, although this feedback is most significant for estradiol. Estradiol is unique among sex steroids in its ability to exert positive and negative feedback actions at the level of the hypothalamus and pituitary [23,91]. Estradiol's actions on gonadotropes are characterized by an initial suppression and subsequent increase in LH [91,120]. Numerous studies have confirmed these observations, and the time course of the biphasic action depends on the species and dose of estradiol. In women, GnRH administration suppresses LH levels for the first 36 hours; however, after 48 hours, the LH response is augmented and persists for several days [121,122]. The mechanisms involve enhancement of the GnRH self-priming effect [123] and increased gonadotrope sensitivity to GnRH stimulation [124]. The ability of estradiol to stimulate LH secretion by positive feedback is essential for the midcycle LH surge in women [23,91].

Inhibins and regulation of hypothalamic pituitary gonadal axis

Inhibins are an additional important regulator of FSH biosynthesis and secretion in men and women. In both genders, inhibins are synthesized and released by the gonads and act in an endocrine manner to inhibit FSH secretion [99,102]. The mechanism most likely involves interaction with an inhibin coreceptor, betaglycan (type III TGFβ receptors) [125,126]. This interaction interferes with activin binding to its receptor, and thus antagonizes activin's actions. In women, inhibin A and B are important regulators of FSH, and each is distinctly regulated. Inhibin A levels peak during the midluteal phase, and thus inhibit FSH secretion in the luteal phase of the menstrual cycle [91,99]. In contrast, inhibin B levels peak in the midfollicular phase and act synergistically with estradiol to reduce FSH levels in the late follicular phase of the cycle. In men, inhibin B is the main form of circulating inhibin [127]. It is synthesized in the testes predominantly by Sertoli cells and is regulated by spermatogenesis [99,128,129]. Inhibin B levels decrease with suppression of spermatogenesis and increase when spermatogenesis is stimulated [99].

Summary

This article has focused on the physiology of secretion of the anterior pituitary hormones. It has reviewed the individual pituitary hormones, the cells from which they are secreted, and the mechanisms of regulation of their secretion. Emphasis has been given to the integration of neural control mechanisms, intracellular pathways involved in the secretory process, feedback control by peripheral hormones, pulsatility of secretion, and the close interrelation between nutritional status and metabolic factors.

References

[1] Baumann G. Growth hormone heterogeneity: genes, isohormones, variants, and binding proteins. Endocr Rev 1991;12:424–49.

[2] Parker ML, Utiger RD, Daughaday WH. Studies on human growth hormone. II. The physiological disposition and metabolic fate of human growth hormone in man. J Clin Invest 1962;41:262–8.

[3] Thompson RG, Rodriguez A, Kowarski A, et al. Growth hormone: metabolic clearance rates, integrated concentrations, and production rates in normal adults and the effect of prednisone. J Clin Invest 1972;51:3193–9.

[4] Frohman LA, Kineman RD. Growth hormone-releasing hormone: discovery, regulation, and actions. In: Kostyo J, editor. Handbook of physiology: hormonal control of growth. New York: Oxford University Press; 1998. p. 189–221.

[5] Kojima M, Hosoda H, Date Y, et al. Ghrelin is a growth hormone-releasing acylated peptide from stomach. Nature 1999;402:656–60.

[6] Smith RG, Jiang H, Sun Y. Developments in ghrelin biology and potential clinical relevance. Trends Endocrinol Metab 2005;16:436–42.

[7] Bonnefont X, Lacampagne A, Sanchez-Hormigo A, et al. Revealing the large-scale network organization of growth hormone-secreting cells. Proc Natl Acad Sci U S A 2005;102: 16880–5.

[8] Stolar MW, Baumann G. Secretory patterns of growth hormone during basal periods in man. Metabolism 1986;35:883–8.

[9] Van Cauter E, Plat L, Copinschi G. Interrelations between sleep and the somatotropic axis. Sleep 1998;21:553–66.

[10] Jaffe CA, Ocampo-Lim B, Guo W, et al. Regulatory mechanisms of growth hormone secretion are sexually dimorphic. J Clin Invest 1998;102:153–64.

[11] Riedel M, Hoeft B, Blum WF, et al. Pulsatile growth hormone secretion in normal-weight and obese men: differential metabolic regulation during energy restriction. Metabolism 1995;44:605–10.

[12] Frohman LA, Downs TR, Clarke IJ, et al. Measurement of growth hormone-releasing hormone and somatostatin in hypothalamic-portal plasma of unanesthetized sheep: spontaneous secretion and response to insulin-induced hypoglycemia. J Clin Invest 1990;86: 17–24.

[13] Goldenberg N, Barkan A. Factors regulating growth hormone secretion in humans. Endocrinol Metab Clin North Am 2007;36:37–55.

[14] Peters JR, Evans PJ, Page MD, et al. Cholinergic muscarinic receptor blockage with pirenzepine abolishes slow wave sleep-related growth hormone release in normal adult males. Clin Endocrinol (Oxf) 1986;25:213–7.

[15] Yalow RS, Goldsmith SJ, Berson SA. Influence of physiologic fluctuations in plasma growth hormone on glucose tolerance. Diabetes 1969;18:402–8.

[16] Roth J, Glick SM, Yalow RS, et al. Hypoglycemia: a potent stimulus to secretion of growth hormone. Science 1963;140:987–8.

[17] Sato M, Frohman LA. Differential sensitivity of growth hormone-releasing hormone and somatostatin release from perifused mouse hypothalamic fragments in response to glucose deficiency. Neuroendocrinology 1993;57:1097–105.

[18] Knopf RF, Conn JW, Fajans SS, et al. Plasma growth hormone response to intravenous administration of amino acids. J Clin Endocrinol Metab 1965;25:1140–4.

[19] Kelijman M, Frohman LA. The role of the cholinergic pathway in growth hormone feedback. J Clin Endocrinol Metab 1991;72:1081–7.

[20] Imaki T, Shibasaki T, Shizume K, et al. The effect of free fatty acids on growth hormone (GH)-releasing hormone-mediated GH secretion in man. J Clin Endocrinol Metab 1985; 60:290–3.

[21] Veldhuis JD, Metzger DL, Martha PM Jr, et al. Estrogen and testosterone, but not a non-aromatizable androgen, direct network integration of the hypothalamo-somatotrope (growth hormone)-insulin-like growth factor I axis in the human: evidence from pubertal pathophysiology and sex-steroid hormone replacement. J Clin Endocrinol Metab 1997; 82:3414–20.

[22] Casanueva FF, Burguera B, Muruais C, et al. Acute administration of corticoids: a new and peculiar stimulus of growth hormone secretion in man. J Clin Endocrinol Metab 1990;70: 234–7.

[23] Cone RD, Low MJ, Elmquist JK, et al. Neuroendocrinology. In: Larsen PR, Kronenberg HM, Melmed S, et al, editors. Williams textbook of endocrinology. 10th edition. Philadelphia: Saunders; 2003. p. 81–177.

[24] Horseman ND. Prolactin. In: DeGroot LJ, Jameson JL, editors. Endocrinology. 4th edition. Philadelphia: Saunders; 2001. p. 209–19.

[25] Ben-Jonathan N, Hnasko R. Dopamine as a prolactin (PRL) inhibitor. Endocr Rev 2001; 22:724–63.

[26] Zhu X, Lin CR, Prefontaine GG, et al. Genetic control of pituitary development and hypopituitarism. Curr Opin Genet Dev 2005;15:332–40.

[27] Cohen LE, Radovick S. Molecular basis of combined pituitary hormone deficiencies. Endocr Rev 2002;23:431–42.

[28] Bole-Feysot C, Goffin V, Edery M, et al. Prolactin (PRL) and its receptor: actions, signal transduction pathways and phenotypes observed in PRL receptor knockout mice. Endocr Rev 1998;19:225–68.

[29] Nagano M, Kelly PA. Tissue distribution and regulation of rat prolactin receptor gene expression. Quantitative analysis by polymerase chain reaction. J Biol Chem 1994;269: 13337–45.

[30] Kebabian JW, Calne DB. Multiple receptors for dopamine. Nature 1979;277:93–6.

[31] Bunzow JR, Van Tol HH, Grandy DK, et al. Cloning and expression of a rat D2 dopamine receptor cDNA. Nature 1988;336:783–7.

[32] Yan GZ, Pan WT, Bancroft C. Thyrotropin-releasing hormone action on the prolactin promoter is mediated by the POU protein pit-1. Mol Endocrinol 1991;5:535–41.

[33] Hennart P, Delogne-Desnoeck J, Vis H, et al. Serum levels of prolactin and milk production in women during a lactation period of thirty months. Clin Endocrinol (Oxf) 1981;14: 349–53.

[34] McNeilly AS, Robinson IC, Houston MJ, et al. Release of oxytocin and prolactin in response to suckling. Br Med J 1983;286:257–9.

[35] Seyfred MA, Gorski J. An interaction between the 5' flanking distal and proximal regulatory domains of the rat prolactin gene is required for transcriptional activation by estrogens. Mol Endocrinol 1990;4:1226–34.

[36] Katznelson L, Riskind PN, Saxe VC, et al. Prolactin pulsatile characteristics in postmenopausal women. J Clin Endocrinol Metab 1998;83:761–4.

[37] Sassin JF, Frantz AG, Kapen S, et al. The nocturnal rise of human prolactin is dependent on sleep. J Clin Endocrinol Metab 1973;37:436–40.

[38] Magner JA. Thyroid-stimulating hormone: biosynthesis, cell biology, and bioactivity. Endocr Rev 1990;11:354–85.

[39] Melmed S, Kleinberg D. Anterior pituitary. In: Larsen PR, Kronenberg HM, Melmed S, et al, editors. Williams textbook of endocrinology. 10th edition. Philadelphia: Saunders; 2003. p. 177–280.

[40] Lechan RM, Fekete C. The TRH neuron: a hypothalamic integrator of energy metabolism. Prog Brain Res 2006;153:209–35.

[41] Popovic V, Duntas LH. Leptin, TRH and ghrelin: influence on energy homeostasis at rest and during exercise. Horm Metab Res 2005;37:533–7.

[42] Dyess EM, Segerson TP, Liposits Z, et al. Triiodothyronine exerts direct cell-specific regulation of thyrotropin-releasing hormone gene expression in the hypothalamic paraventricular nucleus. Endocrinology 1988;123:2291–7.

[43] Dahl GE, Evans NP, Thrun LA, et al. A central negative feedback action of thyroid hormones on thyrotropin-releasing hormone secretion. Endocrinology 1994;135:2392–7.

[44] Williams TC, Kelijman M, Crelin WC, et al. Differential effects of somatostatin and a somatostatin analog, SMS 201-995, on the secretion of growth hormone and thyroid-stimulating hormone in man. J Clin Endocrinol Metab 1988;66:39–45.

[45] Cooper DS, Klibanski A, Ridgway EC. Dopaminergic modulation of TSH and its subunits: in vivo and in vitro studies. Clin Endocrinol (Oxf) 1983;18:265–75.

[46] Alkemade A, Friesema EC, Kuiper GG, et al. Novel neuroanatomical pathways for thyroid hormone action in the human anterior pituitary. Eur J Endocrinol 2006;154:491–500.

[47] Fauquier T, Guerineau NC, McKinney RA, et al. Folliculostellate cell network: a route for long-distance communication in the anterior pituitary. Proc Natl Acad Sci U S A 2001;98: 8891–6.

[48] Pazos-Moura CC, Ortiga-Carvalho TM, Gaspar de ME. The autocrine/paracrine regulation of thyrotropin secretion. Thyroid 2003;13:167–75.

[49] Brabant G, Prank K, Ranft U, et al. Physiological regulation of circadian and pulsatile thyrotropin secretion in normal man and woman. J Clin Endocrinol Metab 1990;70: 403–9.

[50] Mariotti S, Franceschi C, Cossarizza A, et al. The aging thyroid. Endocr Rev 1995;16: 686–715.

[51] Prummel MF, Brokken LJ, Wiersinga WM. Ultra short-loop feedback control of thyrotropin secretion. Thyroid 2004;14:825–9.

[52] Spencer CA, Lum SM, Wilber JF, et al. Dynamics of serum thyrotropin and thyroid hormone changes in fasting. J Clin Endocrinol Metab 1983;56:883–8.

[53] Rondeel JM, Heide R, De Greef WJ, et al. Effect of starvation and subsequent refeeding on thyroid function and release of hypothalamic thyrotropin-releasing hormone. Neuroendocrinology 1992;56:348–53.

[54] Blake NG, Eckland DJ, Foster OJ, et al. Inhibition of hypothalamic thyrotropin-releasing hormone messenger ribonucleic acid during food deprivation. Endocrinology 1991;129: 2714–8.

[55] Lloyd RV, Jin L, Tsumanuma I, et al. Leptin and leptin receptor in anterior pituitary function. Pituitary 2001;4:33–47.

[56] Scheen AJ, Buxton OM, Jison M, et al. Effects of exercise on neuroendocrine secretions and glucose regulation at different times of day. Am J Physiol 1998;274:E1040–9.

[57] Nicoloff JT, Fisher DA, Appleman MD Jr. The role of glucocorticoids in the regulation of thyroid function in man. J Clin Invest 1970;49:1922–9.

[58] Lamolet B, Pulichino AM, Lamonerie T, et al. A pituitary cell-restricted T box factor, Tpit, activates POMC transcription in cooperation with Pitx homeoproteins. Cell 2001;104: 849–59.

[59] White A, Ray DW. Adrenocorticotropic hormone. In: DeGroot LJ, Jameson JL, editors. Endocrinology. 4th edition. Philadelphia: Saunders; 2001. p. 221–33.

[60] Seidah NG, Benjannet S, Hamelin J, et al. The subtilisin/kexin family of precursor convertases. Emphasis on PC1, PC2/7B2, POMC and the novel enzyme SKI-1. Ann N Y Acad Sci 1999;885:57–74.

[61] Jacobson L. Hypothalamic-pituitary-adrenocortical axis regulation. Endocrinol Metab Clin North Am 2005;34:271–92.

[62] Thomas M, Keramidas M, Monchaux E, et al. Dual hormonal regulation of endocrine tissue mass and vasculature by adrenocorticotropin in the adrenal cortex. Endocrinology 2004;145:4320–9.

[63] Saffran M, Schally AV, Benfey BG. Stimulation of the release of corticotropin from the adenohypophysis by a neurohypophysial factor. Endocrinology 1955;57:439–44.

[64] Spiess J, Rivier J, Rivier C, et al. Primary structure of corticotropin-releasing factor from ovine hypothalamus. Proc Natl Acad Sci U S A 1981;78:6517–21.

[65] DeBold CR, Decherney GS, Jackson RV, et al. Effect of synthetic ovine corticotropin-releasing factor: prolonged duration of action and biphasic response of plasma adrenocorticotropin and cortisol. J Clin Endocrinol Metab 1983;57:294–8.

[66] Timpl P, Spanagel R, Sillaber I, et al. Impaired stress response and reduced anxiety in mice lacking a functional corticotropin-releasing hormone receptor 1. Nat Genet 1998;19:162–6.

[67] Munck A, Naray-Fejes-Toth A. Glucocorticoid action: physiology. In: DeGroot LJ, Jameson JL, editors. Endocrinology. 4th edition. Philadelphia: Saunders; 2001. p. 1632–46.

[68] Liu JH, Muse K, Contreras P, et al. Augmentation of ACTH-releasing activity of synthetic corticotropin releasing factor (CRF) by vasopressin in women. J Clin Endocrinol Metab 1983;57:1087–9.

[69] Link H, Dayanithi G, Fohr KJ, et al. Oxytocin at physiological concentrations evokes adrenocorticotropin (ACTH) release from corticotrophs by increasing intracellular free calcium mobilized mainly from intracellular stores. Oxytocin displays synergistic or additive effects on ACTH-releasing factor or arginine vasopressin-induced ACTH secretion, respectively. Endocrinology 1992;130:2183–91.

[70] Whitnall MH. Regulation of the hypothalamic corticotropin-releasing hormone neurosecretory system. Prog Neurobiol 1993;40:573–629.

[71] Bousquet C, Ray DW, Melmed S. A common pro-opiomelanocortin-binding element mediates leukemia inhibitory factor and corticotropin-releasing hormone transcriptional synergy. J Biol Chem 1997;272:10551–7.

[72] Dallman MF, Akana SF, Cascio CS, et al. Regulation of ACTH secretion: variations on a theme of B. Recent Prog Horm Res 1987;43:113–73.

[73] Keller-Wood ME, Dallman MF. Corticosteroid inhibition of ACTH secretion. Endocr Rev 1984;5:859–66.

[74] Krozowski ZS, Funder JW. Renal mineralocorticoid receptors and hippocampal corticosterone-binding species have identical intrinsic steroid specificity. Proc Natl Acad Sci U S A 1983;80:6056–60.

[75] Beaumont K, Fanestil DD. Characterization of rat brain aldosterone receptors reveals high affinity for corticosterone. Endocrinology 1983;113:2043–51.

[76] Rusvai E, Naray-Fejes-Toth A. A new isoform of 11 beta-hydroxysteroid dehydrogenase in aldosterone target cells. J Biol Chem 1993;268:10717–20.

[77] Bradbury MJ, Akana SF, Cascio CS, et al. Regulation of basal ACTH secretion by corticosterone is mediated by both type I (MR) and type II (GR) receptors in rat brain. J Steroid Biochem Mol Biol 1991;40:133–42.

[78] Bradbury MJ, Akana SF, Dallman MF. Roles of type I and II corticosteroid receptors in regulation of basal activity in the hypothalamo-pituitary-adrenal axis during the diurnal trough and the peak: evidence for a nonadditive effect of combined receptor occupation. Endocrinology 1994;134:1286–96.

[79] Dallman MF, Levin N, Cascio CS, et al. Pharmacological evidence that the inhibition of diurnal adrenocorticotropin secretion by corticosteroids is mediated via type I corticosterone-preferring receptors. Endocrinology 1989;124:2844–50.

[80] Neill JD. GnRH and GnRH receptor genes in the human genome. Endocrinology 2002; 143:737–43.

[81] Sherwood NM, Lovejoy DA, Coe IR. Origin of mammalian gonadotropin-releasing hormones. Endocr Rev 1993;14:241–54.

[82] Matsuo H, Baba Y, Nair RM, et al. Structure of the porcine LH- and FSH-releasing hormone. I. The proposed amino acid sequence. Biochem Biophys Res Commun 1971; 43:1334–9.

[83] Baba Y, Matsuo H, Schally AV. Structure of the porcine LH- and FSH-releasing hormone. II. Confirmation of the proposed structure by conventional sequential analyses. Biochem Biophys Res Commun 1971;44:459–63.

[84] Millar RP, Lu ZL, Pawson AJ, et al. Gonadotropin-releasing hormone receptors. Endocr Rev 2004;25:235–75.

[85] Belchetz PE, Plant TM, Nakai Y, et al. Hypophysial responses to continuous and intermittent delivery of hypothalamic gonadotropin-releasing hormone. Science 1978;202: 631–3.

[86] Filicori M, Santoro N, Merriam GR, et al. Characterization of the physiological pattern of episodic gonadotropin secretion throughout the human menstrual cycle. J Clin Endocrinol Metab 1986;62:1136–44.

[87] Haisenleder DJ, Dalkin AC, Ortolano GA, et al. A pulsatile gonadotropin-releasing hormone stimulus is required to increase transcription of the gonadotropin subunit genes: evidence for differential regulation of transcription by pulse frequency in vivo. Endocrinology 1991;128:509–17.

[88] Shupnik MA. Effects of gonadotropin-releasing hormone on rat gonadotropin gene transcription in vitro: requirement for pulsatile administration for luteinizing hormone-beta gene stimulation. Mol Endocrinol 1990;4:1444–50.

[89] Burger LL, Dalkin AC, Aylor KW, et al. GnRH pulse frequency modulation of gonadotropin subunit gene transcription in normal gonadotropes—assessment by primary transcript assay provides evidence for roles of GnRH and follistatin. Endocrinology 2002;143:3243–9.

[90] Ferris HA, Shupnik MA. Mechanisms for pulsatile regulation of the gonadotropin subunit genes by GNRH1. Biol Reprod 2006;74:993–8.

[91] Marshall JC. Regulation of gonadotropin synthesis and secretion. In: DeGroot LJ, Jameson JL, editors. Endocrinology. 4th edition. Philadelphia: Saunders; 2001. p. 248–57.

[92] Smith JT, Cunningham MJ, Rissman EF, et al. Regulation of Kiss1 gene expression in the brain of the female mouse. Endocrinology 2005;146:623–30.

[93] Seminara SB, Messager S, Chatzidaki EE, et al. The GPR54 gene as a regulator of puberty. N Engl J Med 2003;349:1614–27.

[94] de Roux N, Genin E, Carel JC, et al. Hypogonadotropic hypogonadism due to loss of function of the KiSS1-derived peptide receptor GPR54. Proc Natl Acad Sci U S A 2003;100: 10972–6.

[95] Shahab M, Mastronardi C, Seminara SB, et al. Increased hypothalamic GPR54 signaling: a potential mechanism for initiation of puberty in primates. Proc Natl Acad Sci U S A 2005; 102:2129–34.

[96] Clayton RN, Catt KJ. Gonadotropin-releasing hormone receptors: characterization, physiological regulation, and relationship to reproductive function. Endocr Rev 1981;2: 186–209.

[97] Katt JA, Duncan JA, Herbon L, et al. The frequency of gonadotropin-releasing hormone stimulation determines the number of pituitary gonadotropin-releasing hormone receptors. Endocrinology 1985;116:2113–5.

[98] Clarke IJ, Cummins JT. The temporal relationship between gonadotropin releasing hormone (GnRH) and luteinizing hormone (LH) secretion in ovariectomized ewes. Endocrinology 1982;111:1737–9.

[99] Welt C, Sidis Y, Keutmann H, et al. Activins, inhibins, and follistatins: from endocrinology to signaling. A paradigm for the new millennium. Exp Biol Med 2002;227:724–52.

[100] Ling N, Ying SY, Ueno N, et al. Pituitary FSH is released by a heterodimer of the beta-subunits from the two forms of inhibin. Nature 1986;321:779–82.

[101] Ueno N, Ling N, Ying SY, et al. Isolation and partial characterization of follistatin: a single-chain Mr 35,000 monomeric protein that inhibits the release of follicle-stimulating hormone. Proc Natl Acad Sci U S A 1987;84:8282–6.

[102] Bilezikjian LM, Blount AL, Donaldson CJ, et al. Pituitary actions of ligands of the TGF-beta family: activins and inhibins. Reproduction 2006;132:207–15.

[103] Vale W, Rivier J, Vaughan J, et al. Purification and characterization of an FSH releasing protein from porcine ovarian follicular fluid. Nature 1986;321:1121–31.

[104] Risbridger GP, Schmitt JF, Robertson DM. Activins and inhibins in endocrine and other tumors. Endocr Rev 2001;22:836–58.

[105] Nakamura T, Takio K, Eto Y, et al. Activin-binding protein from rat ovary is follistatin. Science 1990;247:836–8.

[106] Rivier C, Vale W. Effect of recombinant activin-A on gonadotropin secretion in the female rat. Endocrinology 1991;129:2463–5.

[107] Carroll RS, Kowash PM, Lofgren JA, et al. In vivo regulation of FSH synthesis by inhibin and activin. Endocrinology 1991;129:3299–304.

[108] Attardi B, Miklos J. Rapid stimulatory effect of activin-A on messenger RNA encoding the follicle-stimulating hormone beta-subunit in rat pituitary cell cultures. Mol Endocrinol 1990;4:721–6.

[109] Weiss J, Harris PE, Halvorson LM, et al. Dynamic regulation of follicle-stimulating hormone-beta messenger ribonucleic acid levels by activin and gonadotropin-releasing hormone in perifused rat pituitary cells. Endocrinology 1992;131:1403–8.

[110] Corrigan AZ, Bilezikjian LM, Carroll RS, et al. Evidence for an autocrine role of activin B within rat anterior pituitary cultures. Endocrinology 1991;128:1682–4.

[111] Matzuk MM, Kumar TR, Bradley A. Different phenotypes for mice deficient in either activins or activin receptor type II. Nature 1995;374:356–60.

[112] McConnell DS, Wang Q, Sluss PM, et al. A two-site chemiluminescent assay for activin-free follistatin reveals that most follistatin circulating in men and normal cycling women is in an activin-bound state. J Clin Endocrinol Metab 1998;83:581–8.

[113] Thompson TB, Lerch TF, Cook RW, et al. The structure of the follistatin:activin complex reveals antagonism of both type I and type II receptor binding. Dev Cell 2005;9:535–43.

[114] Dalkin AC, Haisenleder DJ, Gilrain JT, et al. Gonadotropin-releasing hormone regulation of gonadotropin subunit gene expression in female rats: actions on follicle-stimulating hormone beta messenger ribonucleic acid (mRNA) involve differential expression of pituitary activin (beta-B) and follistatin mRNAs. Endocrinology 1999;140:903–8.

[115] Hrabovszky E, Shughrue PJ, Merchenthaler I, et al. Detection of estrogen receptor-beta messenger ribonucleic acid and 125I-estrogen binding sites in luteinizing hormone-releasing hormone neurons of the rat brain. Endocrinology 2000;141:3506–9.

[116] Herbison AE. Multimodal influence of estrogen upon gonadotropin-releasing hormone neurons. Endocr Rev 1998;19:302–30.

[117] Ropert JF, Quigley ME, Yen SS. Endogenous opiates modulate pulsatile luteinizing hormone release in humans. J Clin Endocrinol Metab 1981;52:583–5.

[118] Van Vugt DA, Lam NY, Ferin M. Reduced frequency of pulsatile luteinizing hormone secretion in the luteal phase of the rhesus monkey. Involvement of endogenous opiates. Endocrinology 1984;115:1095–101.

[119] Smith JT, Clifton DK, Steiner RA. Regulation of the neuroendocrine reproductive axis by kisspeptin-GPR54 signaling. Reproduction 2006;131:3686–92.

[120] Tsai CC, Yen SS. The effect of ethinyl estradiol administration during early follicular phase of the cycle on the gonadotropin levels and ovarian function. J Clin Endocrinol Metab 1971;33:917–23.

[121] Shaw RW, Butt WR, London DR. The effect of oestrogen pretreatment on subsequent response to luteinizing hormone releasing hormone in normal women. Clin Endocrinol (Oxf) 1975;4:297–304.

[122] Jaffe RB, Keye WR Jr. Estradiol augmentation of pituitary responsiveness to gonadotropin-releasing hormone in women. J Clin Endocrinol Metab 1974;39:850–5.

[123] Bauer-Dantoin AC, Weiss J, Jameson JL. Roles of estrogen, progesterone, and gonadotropin-releasing hormone (GnRH) in the control of pituitary GnRH receptor gene expression at the time of the preovulatory gonadotropin surges. Endocrinology 1995;136:1014–9.

[124] Smith PF, Frawley LS, Neill JD. Detection of LH release from individual pituitary cells by the reverse hemolytic plaque assay: estrogen increases the fraction of gonadotropes responding to GnRH. Endocrinology 1984;115:2484–6.

[125] Bilezikjian LM, Blount AL, Vale WW. The cellular actions of vasopressin on corticotrophs of the anterior pituitary: resistance to glucocorticoid action. Mol Endocrinol 1987;1:451–8.

[126] Lewis KA, Gray PC, Blount AL, et al. Betaglycan binds inhibin and can mediate functional antagonism of activin signalling. Nature 2000;404:411–4.

[127] Illingworth PJ, Groome NP, Byrd W, et al. Inhibin-B: a likely candidate for the physiologically important form of inhibin in men. J Clin Endocrinol Metab 1996;81:1321–5.

[128] Handelsman DJ, Spaliviero JA, Phippard AF. Highly vectorial secretion of inhibin by primate Sertoli cells in vitro. J Clin Endocrinol Metab 1990;71:1235–8.

[129] Meachem SJ, Nieschlag E, Simoni M. Inhibin B in male reproduction: pathophysiology and clinical relevance. Eur J Endocrinol 2001;145:561–71.

ELSEVIER
SAUNDERS

Endocrinol Metab Clin N Am
37 (2008) 23–50

ENDOCRINOLOGY
AND METABOLISM
CLINICS
OF NORTH AMERICA

Molecular and Trophic Mechanisms of Tumorigenesis

Andy Levy, PhD, FRCP

*Henry Wellcome Labs for Integrative Neuroscience & Endocrinology, University of Bristol,
Dorothy Hodgkin Building, Whitson Street, Bristol BS1 3NY, UK*

The aim of this article is to summarize recent advances and examine some of the conceptual background of pituitary tumor pathogenesis and propagation, rather than provide an exhaustive catalog of the qualitative and quantitative molecular differences between pituitary tumors and the normal pituitary. The latter has largely been achieved by several recent articles [1–3].

Human pituitary adenomas are the third most common intracranial neoplasm in surgery. They account for around 10% to 25% of intracranial neoplasms, and the management of intracranial neoplasms for about 10% of all neurosurgical procedures performed at the present time [3]. Estimates based on optimal MRI screening in 1994 suggested that about 10% of the general population harbor pituitary imaging abnormalities consistent with the presence of microadenomas [4]. A meta-analysis 10 years later estimated the prevalence of imaging abnormalities consistent with the presence of pituitary adenomas to be just over 22%, with an 11% to 14% prevalence of pituitary adenomas confirmed at autopsy examination [5,6], but there have been no opportunities to explore concordance between the two detection methods. Pituitary adenoma incidence, prevalence, and burden on surgical services are necessarily estimates, given different patterns of presentation, the high proportion of occult disease, and variable reference points based on radiologic, functional, histologic, and health service demographic data. Nevertheless, the overall incidence of clinically overt pituitary adenomas is likely to be around 15 to 20 per million per year, one quarter to one third of which require surgical intervention.

Approximately 50% of newly diagnosed pituitary adenomas are prolactinomas. Endocrinologically inactive adenomas (including most gonadotroph adenomas) represent about 30%, somatotroph adenomas 15% to 20%, corticotroph adenomas 5% to 10%, and thyrotroph adenomas less

---

E-mail address: a.levy@bris.ac.uk

0889-8529/08/$ - see front matter © 2008 Elsevier Inc. All rights reserved.
doi:10.1016/j.ecl.2007.10.009

endo.theclinics.com

than 1% [7]. Limited dural invasion is often seen, but pituitary carcinomas, such as metastatic anterior pituitary disease, constitutes less than 0.2% of pituitary adenomas and for a slightly higher proportion of pituitary tumors that come to surgery [8]. Interestingly, and perhaps unexpectedly given the tacit expectation of an inverse relationship between differentiation and growth rate in tumors in many organ systems, a considerably higher proportion of pituitary carcinomas are endocrinologically active compared with pituitary adenomas (42% corticotropin or ACTH, 33% prolactin, 6% growth hormone, 5% luteinizing and follicle stimulating hormone, and 1% thyrotropin) with just 12% nonhormone-secreting.

Extrapolating from the prevalence of acromegaly, which has minimal effects on longevity and is the most diagnostically secure of all pituitary adenomas, the overall prevalence of clinically overt pituitary adenomas (secreting microadenomas and secreting and space-occupying macroadenomas) is likely to be around 200 to 250 per million. Thus, more than 99.9% of pituitary adenomas remain occult microadenomas, and of the 0.025% that manifest clinically, around half are detected at the microadenoma stage (less than 1-cm in diameter with no evidence of distortion of the sella turcica) [9] and expand no further. Even though macroadenomas, particularly macroprolactinomas, must have grown through dimensions consistent with the diagnosis of microadenoma, significant enlargement of microadenomas, and microprolactinomas in particular, occurs in less than 5% [5]. These data suggest that for prolactinomas, the processes of continued growth and hormone secretion are to some extent mutually exclusive, such that early hormone secretion of sufficient magnitude to come to clinical attention is in at least 95% of cases associated with no further growth. Conversely, in macroprolactinomas, hormone secretion is unlikely to reach clinical significance until they have exceeded 1-cm in diameter.

Based in these data—assuming for argument's sake that the cellular propensity to secrete hormone autonomously remains unchanged as tumor mass increases—it would appear that unlike the case in pituitary carcinomas, a degree of pituitary adenoma cell differentiation sufficient to synthesize and secrete hormones at high level (given that a 0.5-cm diameter lesion has less than 2% of the volume of a 2-cm diameter adenoma) is associated with limitation of growth. There are no grounds for assuming that the converse, that is, a direct association between low level hormone secretion and continued growth, is true. The extent to which successive waves of estrogen exposure during normal menstrual cyclicity are implicated in the confinement, broadly speaking, of microprolactinomas to females and the exclusion of macroprolactinomas from females is also unclear, although in rats there does appear to be some longer-term programming effects of estrogen exposure [10].

The vast majority of pituitary adenomas overall, and over 50% of those that come to clinical attention, therefore exhibit the neoplastically unusual developmental pattern of a strictly limited period of growth after an inducing event or events, followed by reversion once again to trophic equilibrium in an expanded steady state. A proportion of these subsequently diminish in size spontaneously [11], and some may resolve entirely [12]. The remainder, represented by 40% to 50% of clinically overt pituitary adenomas and a fraction of a percent of all pituitary adenomas [13], continue to slowly expand. It is the latter subgroup, together with hormone secreting microadenomas, that are principally responsible for the clinical problems associated with pituitary adenomas, and from which tissue for investigation of their pathogenesis is almost invariably derived.

In summary, the prevalence of clinically significant pituitary adenomas is between 2 to 2.5 per 10,000, but may be as high as 9 per 10,000 [9]. Microadenomas make up 50% to 60% of this total and these, by definition, show no further growth even in the long term. A proportion of the remainder, macroadenomas, also appear to remain trophically static, but many can be expected to slowly expand over a period of years. More aggressive growth is sometimes seen, with re-expansion after successive surgical debulking. Even then, the rate of growth seems to remain relatively predictable and, with few exceptions [14], tends to moderate with time rather than the converse. The absence of on-going expansion of the majority of pituitary adenomas and the slow growth rate of almost all the remainder, their occasional tendency to spontaneously regress or resolve irrespective of size, their sexually dimorphic behavioral phenotypes and generally unremarkable histology, the retention of regulated secretory phenotype in many cases, their trophic response to debulking and the induction of remission after removal of histologically normal pituitary tissue [15,16], are all characteristics that are somewhat at odds with what might be expected of deregulated growth following the acquisition of genetic defects in oncogenes and tumor suppressors. As this pattern of growth and behavior is difficult to reconcile to classical mechanisms of oncogenesis, it is important to consider what is known about the trophic responses of the normal pituitary gland.

Normal pituitary structure

The human pituitary weighs about 100 mg at birth and increases to about 600 mg in adulthood. The female pituitary weighs slightly more than the male [17] and this difference is more pronounced in multiparous women [18]. The functional importance of the architecture of the pituitary on complex intercellular communication within it [19], and the potential for trophic anomalies to occur or propagate once its three dimensional geometry is disrupted, are particularly difficult to directly explore.

Estimates of the relative proportions of different cell types in the human pituitary vary but generally agree that somatotrophs, and under some circumstances lactotrophs, make up the bulk of secretory cells (50% and 15%–50% respectively), with corticotrophs contributing 15% to 20%, gonadotrophs 10%, and thyrotrophs 5% [20]. As simultaneous immunochemistry for all pituitary hormones on the same or adjacent sections is fraught with technical difficulties related to sensitivity, the overall size of the population of hormonally negative cells, which are in many respects the most interesting population of all—comprising oligopotent stem cells, nascent cells that retain mitotic potential, trophically mature cells that have yet to differentiate or undergo apoptosis, and cells that had previously exhibited a secretory phenotype but at least at the time of sampling are hormonally quiescent—can only be approximated.

The anterior pituitary responds to different stimuli not only by rapidly modifying patterns of hormone secretion and synthesis, but also by altering the relative proportions and absolute numbers of different cell subtypes that it contains, presumably to facilitate subacute hormonal responses and in some way prepare for future secretory demands. Potential mechanisms to achieve this include transient fluctuations in relative rates of cell division and cell death, differentiation of previously uncommitted cells to hormone synthesizing and secreting subtypes, a direct change from one mature secretory phenotype to another, or polarization of the secretory profiles of bihormonal or polyhormonal cells. Direct evidence for these changes in normal human pituitary under physiologic conditions is for the most part unavailable.

Pituitary size increases during pregnancy by 15% to 36% and peaks several days postpartum [21]. Concomitant with this change in size is a marked increase in lactotrophs, from around 17% antenatally [20] to 50% at term [22]. If suckling does not take place, lactotroph mass returns to almost normal within 1 to 3 weeks, but remains slightly higher after pregnancy than in nulliparous animals, indicating that pregnancy-induced changes in the size of the prolactin immunopositive population are not entirely reversible [20]. Whether a direct change from somatotrophs into mammosomatotrophs or completely into lactotrophs occurs during pregnancy, and whether nongravid lactotroph numbers are restored after weaning by the reverse of the process, or entirely by "massive programmed cell death" remains unknown. The reason for the surprising absence of reliable data, for this most ordinary of physiologic states, is that precise correlation of mitotic and apoptotic activity with changes in specific cell subpopulations is precluded by the dependence of immunochemical sensitivity on hormone synthesis and secretion, both of which change dramatically at the time that trophic events might be expected to occur.

Quantitative variations in gene expression between normal pituitary and human pituitary adenoma biopsy samples require careful interpretation, as the expression profiles of highly polarized cell populations in human pituitary adenomas are necessarily different from the composite derived from the complex admixture of different cell types that constitute the normal pituitary. Equally, inexorable expansion with increased mitotic activity seen in spontaneous rat pituitary tumors is very unusual in human pituitary adenomas. Thus, although normal rat pituitary secretory and trophic responses have informed our understanding of human pituitary adenomas, concepts derived by extrapolation from one to the other should be considered with some caution.

Pituitary trophic activity

The mature male rat anterior pituitary contains a subpopulation of cells with the characteristics of oligopotent stem cells [23]—not necessarily randomly distributed [24]—that continue to undergo mitotic activity at a steady state in adulthood. With the exception of a reduction in mitotic rate, in response to pharmacologic levels of glucocorticoids [25] and subtle diurnal variation [26], the rate of division of these cells at any age appears to be largely independent of acute changes in the hormonal milieu. Basal anterior pituitary mitotic rate, attributable to this active oligopotent stem cell pool, diminishes from around 2.5% of pituitary parenchymal cells per day (generating about 85,000 cells per day) in 4- to 6-week-old animals, to 0.02% by 16 months (generating 4,000 cells per day) [27]. Using hematopoietic stem cell behavior as a precedent, it seems likely that the reduction in cell turnover with age, from a level sufficient to completely replace the parenchymal cells of the anterior pituitary every 5 weeks in youth, is the result of continuous but unbalanced reciprocal interchange between a pool of inactive oligopotent stem cells and a smaller pool of active oligopotent stem cells that becomes further depleted with time. The identity of oligopotent stem cells remains frustratingly unclear.

In the absence of any changes in environmental, physiologic, or psychologic stress, the majority of daughter cells of asymmetric oligopotent stem cell division undergo early apoptosis (Fig. 1). Data from a number of sources suggests that the proportion that escape early apoptosis (transient amplifying cells) persist as hormone receptor-expressing but hormonally null progenitor cells [28,29], a roughly similar proportion of which are in G_1 and G_2 at any one time. Under changing (ie, not persistently abnormal) endocrine circumstances, these nascent progenitor cells are susceptible to apoptosis [25,30], or are able to undergo rapid but limited further cell division, to give rise to hormonally null daughter cells that may subsequently differentiate into hormone-secreting subtypes at some future point [31,32].

Only a small proportion of the increase in hormone-secreting cell populations, corticotrophs after adrenalectomy, gonadotrophs after gonadectomy [29], and probably a very small proportion of thyrotrophs after thyroidectomy [33], are derived from division of pre-existing hormone secreting cells or early differentiation of immediately postmitotic cells [26,34]. Instead, most of the adrenalectomy-induced increase in mitotic activity, for example, occurs in nascent, null progenitor parents, less than 2 or 3 weeks old, that give rise to hormonally null daughter cells. The nascent, hormonally null progenitor cells express somatostatin (SSTR2) receptors [35] (among others), occupation of which blocks glucocorticoid withdrawal-induced cell cycle activity [36]. More than 90% of the

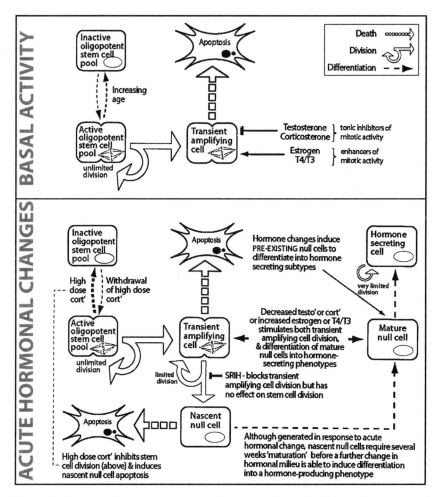

Fig. 1. Pituitary trophic responses to acute changes in glucocorticoids, sex hormones, and thyroid hormones. Under basal conditions (*top panel*), continuous oligopotent stem cell activity is balanced predominantly by early apoptotic death of nascent cells (transient amplifying cells). In response to a reduction in testosterone or corticosterone (or an increase in thyroid hormones or estrogen) (*bottom panel*), transient amplifying cells undergo several, self-limiting cycles of cell division, giving rise to nascent, null cells. The same hormonal changes simultaneously induce pre-existing null cells to differentiate into hormone secreting subtypes. Only a small proportion of new hormone secreting cells are derived from division of pre-existing hormone secreting cells. Whether the predisposition to specific secretory subtypes conferred by the genetic mutations of Carney complex and familial acromegaly affect the latter population, rather than oligopotent stem cell or transient amplifying cell populations, remains to be seen.

immunohistochemically-identified increase in corticotrophs after adrenalectomy results from differentiation of pre-existing null cells, rather than differentiation of nascent null cells (ie, transient amplifying cells) or division of pre-existing corticotrophs.

In the normal pituitary, progenitor cell turnover is under tonic inhibitory control by physiologic circulating levels of corticosterone [25,26,37] and testosterone [38–40], withdrawal of either of which produces similar, self-limiting waves of mitosis, with two peaks of increased activity at around 24 hours and 48 to 72 hours. The tonic inhibitory effects of physiologic circulating levels of corticosterone and testosterone on pituitary mitosis are exerted on the same nascent progenitor cell population, as the effects of their concurrent withdrawal (bilateral adrenalectomy plus bilateral gonadectomy) are not additive [29]. Significantly, the biphasic increase in the anterior pituitary mitotic index returns to baseline levels over the next 14 days or so, despite the continued absence of circulating glucocorticoids or testosterone [38]. Independent control of pituitary secretory and trophic responses allows a persistent physiologic stimulus to elicit a short-term adjustment to the numbers of cells within specific anterior pituitary cell sub-populations, to accompany a long-term or longer-term secretory response. In this respect, however, the temporal effects of estrogens might be slightly different and lead to a more prolonged mitotic response.

Supraphysiologic levels of corticotropin-releasing hormones (CRH) have also been shown to have trophic effects on corticotrophs, but at maximal nongravid physiologic levels, that is after bilateral adrenalectomy, the wave of increased pituitary mitosis is entirely caused by a reduction in direct glucocorticoid feedback at the level of the pituitary, rather than the concurrent increase in hypothalamo-hypophyseal portal corticotrophin-releasing factors [37]. Despite being associated with a higher incidence of corticotroph adenoma propagation [41], adrenal failure with glucocorticoid replacement insufficient to suppress ACTH to within the normal range, in the long term, has not been reported to be associated with pituitary tumor induction.

Basal turnover in the rat anterior pituitary progenitor cell compartment is also dependent on low levels of thyroid hormones and enhanced, perhaps unexpectedly, by supraphysiologic thyroid hormone supplementation in intact animals [33], implicating persistently raised thyrotropin-releasing hormone levels, rather than direct thyroid hormone withdrawal, in the induction of thyrotroph and lactotroph hyperplasia when thyroid hormones are low. Growth hormone releasing hormone (GHRH) is believed to be trophic, but increased gonadotropin-releasing hormone does not contribute to increased mitosis following gonadectomy [39].

When considering trophic activity in the pituitary, it is worth bearing in mind that both normal pituitary and pituitary adenomas in man and rats have structurally and functionally sexually dimorphic features. Microprolactinomas and corticotroph adenomas are more common in human females, and macroprolactinomas in males. In rodent models, cross-sex hormone treatment can induce cross-sex pituitary behavioral and trophic responsiveness [42]. It has been suggested that the increased abundance of multifunctional anterior pituitary cells in females, compared with males, indicates increased transdifferentiation because of hormonal fluctuations during the sexual cycle [43], and that estrogen protects lactotrophs from dopamine agonist-induced cell death [42]. Repeated fluctuations in estrogen levels, and possibly relatively high steady-state estrogen exposure, appears to be responsible for these differences. In males, lower levels of estrogen may provide less impetus to prolactin production and mitosis, but are more constant, and perhaps lead to a prolactinoma phenotype characterized by lower levels of hormone secretion per unit tumor mass, but without opportunities for waves of cell death to moderate net trophic characteristics. That is, a sexually dimorphic prolactinoma phenotype is generated in females as much by successive waves of relative estrogen withdrawal as absolute levels of circulating estrogen [10,42]. Such a mechanism would also be supported by the enhanced likelihood of spontaneous remission of microprolactinomas after pregnancy [12].

In summary, the pituitary mitotic response to changes in the hormone environment mostly occur in relatively newly formed hormonally null progenitor cells (transient amplifying cells) derived from an oligopotent active stem cell pool. Hormonally-defined cells are not entirely postmitotic, but their contribution to overall- and hormone axis-specific trophic activity in the pituitary is relatively modest. It is not clear whether pituitary cells that were believed to have undergone terminal commitment are able to de-differentiate and contribute further to trophic activity and to new differentiated cellular subtypes. Normal, male (and probably female) rat pituitary mitotic activity is thyroid hormone-dependent and stimulated by supraphysiologic thyroid hormone levels. Mitotic activity is tonically inhibited by physiologic circulating levels of testosterone and corticosterone, and stimulated by estrogen in a dose- and time-dependent manner, at least in the short term. The trophic responses elicited by persistent changes in these hormone levels (with the possible exception of estrogen exposure) are transient. Direct identification and quantification of trophic activity, with careful analysis of nascent cell characteristics, indicates that the processes of mitosis, survival decisions made by nascent cells, and differentiation of hormonally undifferentiated cells to hormone-secreting subpopulations are distinct processes that do not follow one from the other.

Human pituitary tumor phenotypes

Given the number of distinct cell populations in the normal pituitary, it is no surprise that pituitary adenomas express a wide variety of trophic and secretory phenotypes. Like other benign endocrine neoplasms, autonomy of function and growth do not necessarily go together, and adenomas with various patterns of dissociated hormone gene transcription, translation, and secretion (such as silent somatotroph, corticotroph, and thyrotroph adenomas), account for up to 20% of adenomas in some series. While symptom- or syndrome-producing secretion of more than one hormone occurs in only around 5% to 7% of pituitary adenomas, examination of biopsy samples reveals that activation of multiple hormone genes is common, despite their monomorphous appearance. This phenomenon is most frequent in adenomas secreting growth hormone and, surprisingly, can encompass all possible combinations of pituitary, and even classical, hypothalamic hormones in subpopulations of cells. Estimates of pleurihormonality range from 10% to 30% of all adenomas [44,45], from 18% to more than 50% of somatotroph adenomas, and from 20% to 100% of prolactinomas [45–47]. Multifunctionality in normal anterior pituitary cells (in rodents at least [48]) suggests that the finding of the same in pituitary adenomas does not necessarily suggest a radical departure from normal pituitary cellular phenotype, or conflict with the widely held belief that pituitary adenomas invariably arise following the acquisition of genetic defects in single cells.

Polyhormonality as a result of transdifferentiation of monohormonal cells cannot be easily distinguished from a primary differentiated state of polyhormonality in which an apparently monohormonal state is achieved through skewing of synthetic capability toward a single peptide. The observation that intracellular calcium responses to hypothalamic-releasing hormones tend to be less robust in polyhormonal than monohormonal cells [43], contributes further to a picture of a broad gamut of secretory and trophic phenotypes in the normal and neoplastic pituitary, in which not only is total hormonal synthetic activity sometimes offset against trophic activity (distinguishing micro- from macroprolactinomas), but in which total hormone synthetic activity is limited, such that when spread across several hormones, it tends to be relatively low level in each.

The familiar but relatively unusual finding of unequivocal pituitary-dependent Cushing's syndrome, without abnormalities on high definition pituitary MRI scan, and the induction of remission through removal of histologically normal tissue [16], albeit harbouring similar molecular aberrations to corticotroph adenomas [49], emphasizes the fact that high level inappropriate hormone secretion can occur entirely without unbalanced mitotic and apoptotic activity. Still, complex classifications of pituitary adenomas, based on ultrastructural and histomorphometric rather than functional characteristics, have thus far had very limited clinical impact. A more complete description of trophic behavior may have some utility, as, for example, the management of scan negative and adenoma negative pituitary-dependent Cushing's syndrome, based on the assumption that it is nothing more than an early stage of microadenomatous or macroadenomatous disease, or that macroadenomatous disease might limit to some extent the rational choice of therapeutic agent.

The intriguing propensity of corticotroph adenomas to cycle between physiologically appropriate ACTH secretion and unequivocal but still regulated ACTH hypersecretion, with a frequency of anywhere between 2 days and 4 years, has been described not only in pituitary dependent hypercortisolemia, but also in ectopic ACTH hypersecretion. Whether the phenomenon is mediated entirely through changes in secretion, or whether long period cyclicity implicates reciprocal transdifferentiation or cyclical trophic activity, remains unknown and, unfortunately, is likely to remain so, as opportunities to collect suitable evidence are extremely scarce. A report of temporary resolution of ACTH hypersecretion from an ectopic (but unknown) source during a chest infection, suggests that exogenous stimuli have a significant role in at least a proportion of these cases [50], and contributes further to evidence that pituitary adenoma microenvironment can be a potent modifier of pituitary adenoma phenotype.

In summary, given the discrepancies between the clear groupings of hormones expected by discrete induction of specific transcription factors and the more diverse combinations of hormones seen in normal and neoplastic pituitary cells, it seems that the induction of permanent enhancer autoregulation during development is not necessarily immutable. This suggests that long-term active repression required to maintain terminal cell type differentiation remains to some extent subject to extracellular signaling, and does not necessarily imply permanent commitment. If transient signaling gradients do allow for some flexibility in the identity of cell types, then not only might the varying structural anomalies associated with pituitary adenoma formation directly contribute to the particular range of pituitary hormones expressed, but the unexpected efficacy of surgical decompression, and even removal of apparently normal tissue from adjacent to corticotroph adenomas, might be more easily explained.

Clonality

The clonality of a cellular expansion is assumed to be a secure molecular marker capable of distinguishing the result of an intracellular insult or insults from a relatively exuberant, but nevertheless potentially reversible, trophic response to stromal or micro-environmental signals. Apparent clonal skewing provides, for many commentators in the field, irrefutable evidence that pituitary adenomas are induced by single cell somatic mutation, either because such mutations are believed to be sufficient in themselves to lead to subsequent propagation irrespective of the hormonal milieu, or because they predispose their daughter cells to quantitatively or qualitatively inappropriate trophic responses to physiologic hormonal stimuli. Because of this, assessment of clonal status has been embraced as a predictor of behavior and as a central guide to research on pituitary adenoma pathogenesis. The questions that follow from this are whether the observed phenotypes of pituitary adenomas fits with those expected of true monoclonal expansions, whether techniques used to establish clonality are specific, and whether clonal skewing is a sine qua non of malignancy. In short, does pituitary adenoma clonality analysis have any diagnostic, pathogenic, or prognostic utility?

At around the time of implantation during early female embryogenesis, each cell randomly but permanently inactivates genes on either the maternally- or paternally-derived X-chromosome, by cytosine methylation of promoter regions. Once methylated, the pattern of functional inactivation is believed to be stably inherited by the progeny of each cell [51]. With hematologic precursors, this wave of irreversible methylation occurs when the total number of hematopoietic stem cell precursors is around 15 [52], and it is not unreasonable to expect the number of pituitary precursors to be of this order at lyonization. Dogma has it that all female tissues consist of a mosaic of cells, in each of which genes on either the maternal or paternal X-chromosome have been inactivated. Therefore, if the relative methylation status of different alleles of an X-linked gene can be determined, and one of each allele has been inherited from each parent, quantitative differences in allele methylation in DNA extracted from a tissue sample implies that all of the cells in that sample are derived from a single cell source. This assumption should hold true if migration and dispersal of cells between assignment of clonality during embryogenesis and post-natal life leads to the formation of a mosaic at the single cell level, and if the turnover of mature cells is either switched off or balanced, that is, not confined or skewed toward cells bearing a particular methylation pattern. If these conjectures are true, and ignoring several important technical considerations, unless motile cells of similar identity and clonality spontaneously cosegregate in differentiated tissue, or a polyclonal field spontaneously undergoes differential apoptosis leaving a single clone, a monoclonal cellular expansion in a polyclonal field should indeed represent the progeny of a single cell [53].

If an expansion is polyclonal at inception, selection pressure between several subclones is very likely to lead to a reduction in the number of clones with time. Shuttling of clonal architecture between apparent monoclonality and polyclonality [54], and clonal cooperation where the survival of one clone depends on the presence of another [55], have also been described. If one of these scenarios arises during the propagation of pituitary adenomas, opportunities to examine further biopsy samples in recurrent adenomas months or years after the first analysis should reveal examples in which not only additional mutations and allelic losses are represented (as might be expected of an aneuploid tumor over time), but also examples where the original allelic losses have apparently been restored. This latter pattern was indeed exactly what was seen in more than half of 49 informative cases in which tissue became available for re-examination at repeat surgery [56]. If a technically secure finding, this strongly suggests that more than one abnormal clone may well be present at tumor inception in at least 50% of human pituitary adenomas [57,58].

As a stimulus affecting a pre-existing trophically-responsive monoclonal patch may lead to a clonal expansion derived from several or all of its constituent cells, an understanding of normal clonal architecture of the pituitary is fundamental mechanistically to allow the significance of clonal skewing to be determined. Assuming that relative migration of populations of cells within the substance of the pituitary is minimal, replenishment of pituitary cell populations by a diminishing population of stem cells is likely to lead to an expansion of average clonal patch sizes with time. A reduction in the number of active stem cells necessarily predisposes to clonal skewing; in bone marrow, where the same senescent changes have been extensively studied, clonal skewing at the human androgen receptor locus increases from about 2% in neonates to almost 40% in healthy elderly women, even when a stringent allele prevalence cut-off ratio of greater than 10 to 1 is used [59]. Cellular turnover in the pituitary is much more modest than that seen in bone marrow, but these changes remain a potentially significant cause of false-positive findings in X inactivation-based clonality assays, unless care is taken to compare findings to age-matched control tissue.

The normal clonal architecture of human and rodent pituitary has not been determined, but in several other human tissues in which it has been possible to analyze clonal structure, macroscopic monoclonality is normal. Macroscopic monoclonality has been clearly demonstrated in bladder urothelium, the 120-mm square tessellations of which are derived from about 200 founder cells [60], and in the smooth muscle and intima of the aorta as a patchwork of contiguous 4-mm patches skewed to the same allele [61]. Given the difficulty in matching sample size to patch size and orientation, macroscopic monoclonality might well be expected to be a poorly recognized feature of most normal tissues. Not surprisingly, therefore, in many monoclonal pathophysiologic states, such as uterine fibromyomata [62], the cirrhotic liver [63], parathyroid hyperplasia [64], tertiary hyperparathyroidism [65], and the nodules of primary multinodular goiters [66], analysis of clonality fails to provide a useful prediction of tissue trophic behavior, or even a secure guide to pathogenesis.

The consequences of trophic activity within the relatively small population of hormonally defined cells that retain limited mitotic potential in the pituitary is unclear, but might lead, if exposed to specific trophic stimuli, to the emergence of nonneoplastic clonal skewing, as relatively quiescent cells are displaced by the expansion of a pre-existing patch rather than expansion being derived from a single disinhibited cell [67]. With all of these considerations, the finding in female human pituitary adenomas biopsied at surgery that three out of three somatotrophinomas [68], eight out of eight endocrinologically inactive adenomas [68,69], four out of four prolactinomas [68], and 27 out of 31 corticotroph adenomas [68,70–72] are clonally skewed, may not be overly informative. Irrespective of the omission of age-matched control tissue analysis and variability of allelic ratio cutoffs and reporting bias (as an apparently monoclonal cellular expansion in a polyclonal field need not represent the progeny of a single, trophically disinhibited cell), it is not entirely surprising that clonal architecture in this context too, correlates relatively poorly with histologic characteristics, behavior, and ultimately with prognosis.

In summary, clonal skewing does not necessarily mean that pituitary adenomas are universally derived from single, trophically disinhibited cells. The restoration of allelic loss, originally identified in 50% of pituitary adenomas that come to repeat debulking surgery [56], certainly if confirmed by additional studies, indicates that polyclonality or oligoclonality rather than monoclonality may be more likely at induction, with selection pressure suppressing most of the original clones to below the level of detection or eliminating them altogether. Irrespective of clonality, the strikingly sexually dimorphic phenotype of prolactinomas suggests that the hormonal microenvironment has a very major role in adenoma propagation and behavior, if not induction, and even if monoclonality does turn out to be the norm, as the phenotype of pituitary adenomas remains highly unusual for a typical clonal malignancy, the utility of the finding is rather limited.

Aneuploidy

Persistent abnormal growth is a feature of a very small proportion of pituitary adenomas, and for most of this subgroup is relatively modest. If mutations in proto-oncogenes and tumor suppressor genes—the classical mechanisms of tumor formation—are responsible rather than just passengers in the process, then additional growth-modifying events or circumstances may need to be adduced. Aneuploidy, resulting from chromosomal rearrangement, has a much greater propensity to cause neoplasia than whole chromosome aneuploidy caused by errors in mitosis [73]. Tumor induction is not an obligatory outcome of either, and arguments about whether such changes are causes or consequences of neoplastic events remain unresolved.

Gross aneuploidy is reported in sporadic pituitary adenomas at a prevalence of around 50% [74]. A sufficient number of chromosomal regions have been implicated at the level of loss of heterozygosity, to make any particular relationship between the pattern of loss and the induction and subsequent behavior of particular pituitary adenoma subtypes difficult to substantiate. The relatively high percentage of diploid tumors among invasive adenomas indicates that aneuploidy is not a basic property of aggressive adenomas [3,75]. Histologic pleomorphism, rather than labelling index, is also a poor predictor of pituitary adenoma growth characteristics or metastatic potential [76]. Studies using comparative genomic hybridization have predictably shown high rates of gross chromosomal gains and losses in pituitary adenomas, but again, there is a lack of concordance between the sites and nature of chromosomal involvement and phenotype.

In summary, aneuploidy in human pituitary adenomas that come to surgery is very common, but the significance of multiple areas of loss of heterozygosity caused by chromosomal rearrangements, such as deletions, translocations and amplifications, remains unknown in this context.

Proliferation markers and cell cycle protein abnormalities

The association of clinically significant enlargement with a trend toward raised proliferating cell nuclear markers is of limited prognostic utility in pituitary adenomas. Despite early hopes that histologic indices of proliferation rate would help predict tumor recurrence, in a prospective study of 101 consecutive endocrinologically inactive adenomas, followed-up for an average of over 3 years, higher Ki-67 labeling indices had no such predictive value [77]. The only correlation between Ki-67 and pituitary adenoma characteristics was that tumors from young patients tend to have higher labeling indices, a finding that appears to correlate with the age-related decline in mitotic activity in the normal pituitary, but in itself is otherwise difficult to interpret. Isolated analyses of any marker of mitotic activity, irrespective of its sensitivity, specificity, and reproducibility, without concurrent analysis of apoptotic activity and age-matched control tissue, may not be sufficient to allow useful predictions about the consequences of net trophic activity to be made.

While mitosis and apoptosis are completely independent molecular mechanisms, accelerated apoptosis that accompanies the action of a pure stimulus to mitosis [78], and increased mitosis that follows a specific apoptotic stimulus [79], ensure that a single insult to one or other trophic pathway has very little effect on overall growth. This observation has led to the general concept in tumor biology that mutations that specifically increase mitosis or decrease apoptosis alone may not be sufficient, in isolation, to induce neoplasia. A net trophic response to a physiologic stimulus, resulting in tissue growth, calls for the link between mitosis and apoptosis to be temporarily loosened. Subsequent restoration of the original rates of mitosis and apoptosis without a period of reciprocal disequilibrium presumably results in persistence of an excess of histologically and functionally normal cells, typical of an occult pituitary microadenoma.

The activity of three genes has recently been described as playing a key role in the coregulation of the distinct processes of cell cycling and apoptosis. These are Lats-1 (a protein kinase tumor suppressor and regulator of cell cycle progression and apoptosis), the proapoptotic protein kinase Mst2 (a member of the GCKII family of proteins [80]), and hSav1 (also known as hWW45, the human homolog of Salvador, a scaffold protein that binds simultaneously to Mst2 and Lats-1). Operating putatively as a heterotrimer, they concurrently inhibit both cyclin E, which drives cell cycle activity, and several inhibitors of apoptosis. Mice deficient in Lats1 develop tumors in several systems as well as pituitary dysfunction [81]. Thus far, the specific roles of these genes in pituitary adenoma propagation, and potentially in the therapeutics of pituitary adenomas, have not been explored.

In summary, there appears to be a modest association between markers of proliferation, particularly Ki-67 and tumor size, in some studies (recognized in the World Health Organization classification of pituitary adenomas), but little evidence that they correlate with propensity to recurrence, or that they can be used prospectively to predict the same. At the present time, the most reliable prognostic indicators for pituitary adenomas remain adenoma size, secretory subtype (prolactinoma, for example), and the persistence or otherwise of tumor expansion identified on sequential MRI assessments. A descriptive sentence or two of the extent and direction of spread in plain English—made very much more powerful by comparison with previous scans—carries more practical information than a radioanatomic grading or histologic or ultrastructural classification. This is irrespective of its complexity, the earnestness of its creators, or their enthusiasm for immunostaining for putative proliferation markers, such as cyclins A, B, D, and E, p16, p27, p53, matrix metalloproteinase-9, DNA topoisomerase II alpha, E-cadherin, E-catenin, or for that matter, Ki-67 with Mib-1.

Familial syndromes associated with pituitary adenoma formation

Several familial conditions associated with pituitary adenoma formation have been described. These include multiple endocrine neoplasia type 1, Carney complex [82], and isolated familial acromegaly, as well as the less clearly defined and potentially overlapping "non-MEN1/non-Carney complex familial isolated pituitary adenoma" [83]. The recently described aryl hydrocarbon receptor interacting protein (AIP) inactivation [84] may also confer a modest familial predisposition to an otherwise rare condition.

Multiple endocrine neoplasia type 1

Multiple endocrine neoplasia type 1 (MEN1) is an autosomal dominant condition associated in 40% to 60% of patients with pituitary adenomas, similar overall in hormone secretory subtype distribution to those occurring sporadically, but varying between kindreds and sometimes between branches of the same extended kindred. Endocrinologists, gastroenterologists, dermatologists, and oncologists have all hoped that MEN1, which is associated with the broadest range of tumor types of any such condition, would provide clear insights into tumor pathogenesis. Menin, however, has been shown to interact with a broad range of targets, none of which is solely culpable. Germline MEN1 mutations, evident in 70% to 90% of MEN1 families, are not found in at least 10% of patients with the unequivocal MEN1 phenotype [83], suggesting that an additional tumor-promoting factor may be required. In sporadic pituitary adenomas, MEN1 gene polymorphisms occur in 30% of cases, loss of heterozygosity on 11q13 in 14%, and inactivating mutations in the coding region of the menin gene in just over 1% (see [2]).

In summary, MEN1 gene defects do not play a significant role in sporadic pituitary adenomas. The predisposition in MEN1 to pituitary adenomas of secretory phenotypes that match the frequency of those seen in sporadic disease is intriguing, and at a simple level might suggest that prevalent somatic factors implicated in sporadic adenoma induction are also implicated in second hits in MEN1.

Carney complex

Carney complex is a rare autosomal dominant condition characterized by myxomas of the heart, skin, and breast, spotty skin pigmentation (multiple skin lentigines and blue nevi), schwannomas, ovarian cysts, adrenal, testicular, and thyroid tumors, as well as pituitary adenomas in 6% to 21% of patients [82]. Unlike MEN1, only growth hormone-secreting adenomas have been described in Carney complex, although some of these also transcribe prolactin. Approximately half of all patients with Carney complex have germline inactivating mutations in the regulatory subunit type 1 of the cAMP-dependent protein kinase A gene (PRKAR1A). In Carney complex-associated somatotroph adenomas, the normal allele of the PRKAR1A gene located at 17q23 is lost [85], leading to enhanced activity of the GHRH-induced signal transduction pathway [86]. PRKAR1A mutations are infrequently associated with sporadic growth hormone-secreting adenomas [85]. Some reports suggest that the gene responsible for many, but not all of the remaining non-PRKAR1A kindreds—which appear to share an indistinguishable phenotype—maps to chromosome 2p16, but this association has yet to be fully defined.

Isolated familial acromegaly

Isolated familial acromegaly remains a diagnosis of exclusion, if a kindred with two or more cases of acromegaly or gigantism is not associated with MEN1, Carney complex, or AIP gene inactivation. Isolated familial acromegaly is only associated with growth hormone producing adenomas, and is therefore distinct from the heterogeneous and nonsomatotroph kindreds of "familial isolated pituitary adenoma." The behavior of isolated familial acromegaly suggests that it is an autosomal dominant condition with incomplete penetrance. Individuals with isolated familial acromegaly tend to develop gigantism, or acromegaly, at a relatively young age and are currently believed to harbor a candidate gene in proximity to, but nevertheless distinct from, the MEN1 gene in a 2.21Mb area of chromosome 11q13 [85,87]. Menin gene mutations, and activating mutations in the RET proto-oncogene [88,89], have not been found in tumors from patients with isolated familial acromegaly, and loss of function of the AIP gene is infrequently associated, certainly in Japan [90]. Reports of changes in menin gene expression are inconsistent.

Non-multiple endocrine neoplasia type 1 and non-Carney complex familial isolated pituitary adenomas

Familial pituitary adenomas, in the absence of MEN1 and Carney complex are rare, but a retrospective study of clinical characteristics of familial, isolated pituitary adenomas at 22 centers across Western Europe yielded 64 such kindreds, with 138 affected individuals. In 75% of cases, first degree relatives were involved, and although the proportions of tumor secretory subtypes were little different from those seen in sporadic adenomas, in 30 of the 64 kindreds, a single tumor secretory phenotype was observed. Patients with familial, isolated pituitary adenomas were younger than sporadic cases but did not show anticipation in sequential generations [83].

Aryl hydrocarbon receptor interacting protein

Vierimaa and colleagues [84] recently described three small clusters of pituitary adenomas occurring in families in Northern Finland. By combining chip-based technologies with genealogy data going back to the 18th century, they traced the predisposition to pituitary adenomas to a germline mutation in the AIP gene located on chromosome 11q13.

The aryl hydrocarbon receptor itself was first identified as the receptor for polycyclic aromatic hydrocarbons and related compounds, many of which, such as dioxins, are considered environmental contaminants. The phenotype of the aryl hydrocarbon receptor knockout mouse suggests that the receptor also has significant roles in development and physiology, and in addition to altering the expression of matrix metalloproteinases (the activity of which is critical in normal tissue remodelling), it binds to a variety of unrelated endogenous and exogenous compounds [91].

One of two AIP mutations account for 16% of all patients in Northern Finland diagnosed with pituitary adenomas secreting growth hormone. In patients from the same population presenting with gigantism or acromegaly before the age of 35 years, AIP mutations are found in 40% of apparently sporadic cases, indicating that AIP is a low-penetrance tumor suppressor in this population [84]. In other populations, the association is somewhat weaker, with 0 of 71 unselected acromegalic patients from Italy harboring AIP mutations, 2 of 113 unselected pituitary adenomas from the United States (patients aged 8 years and 20 years at diagnosis, both somatotroph adenomas, of a total of 13 in the cohort), 2 out of 27 from Germany (both less than 30 years old), 1 out of 122 from Poland, 1 of 55 from Spain, and 1 out of 36 from the Netherlands, giving a total of 9 cases out of 460 (2%), of which 2 (less than 0.5%, both acromegalics) had a family history of pituitary adenomas [92]. With the exception of the Finnish cases, all of the remainder were less than 30 years old.

In a further study from Japan, a single case of presumptive isolated familial somatotrophinoma was found to have a germline mutation of AIP, but none of 40 sporadic somatotroph adenomas were associated with a mutation [90]. Furthermore, AIP mutations were not detected in 66 patients with sporadic pituitary adenomas from the United States, 52 of whom had acromegaly or a prolactinoma [93]. A novel germline mutation in the AIP gene was detected in four of a family of 18 from Brazil, two of whom, siblings, had developed early onset acromegaly. The remaining two mutations were found in a 41-year-old family member and his 3-year-old son, neither of whom had symptomatic disease [94]. Of 107 patients (including 49 prolactinomas and 26 somatotrophinomas) from France, Belgium, and Italy, none of whom had familial disease, no germline mutations of AIP were demonstrated [95]. A further study was performed using archival material from 41 additional patients, in one of whom an AIP mutation was found and a germline mutation detected at follow-up screening [95]. In a collaborative study of 73 familial isolated pituitary adenoma kindreds in 34 centers across nine countries, 156 patients with pituitary adenomas were found to harbor 10 germline AIP mutations (an AIP mutation rate of approximately 15%). Adenomas in AIP mutation-positive patients tended to be larger, and occur at a younger age than AIP negative tumors. Most were somatotrophinomas, mammosomatotroph, or prolactinomas, and a single nonsecreting adenoma also occurred (but no corticotroph or thyrotroph adenomas) [96].

In summary, AIP mutations in sporadic pituitary adenomas occurs with a frequency of just over 1%, and are most prevalent in patients with a younger onset of disease where the condition may behave slightly more aggressively. The prevalence is considerably higher in Northern Finland and in familial isolated pituitary adenoma kindreds. The mutation has not yet, but may in future be shown to have specificity for familial adenomas of the pituitary, as opposed to tumors in other organ systems. Although somatic AIP mutations are not common in colorectal cancers (2 of 373) and have not yet been described in breast (0 of 82) or prostate cancers (0 of 44), at this prevalence, overall numbers studied thus far are insufficient to exclude other associations [97].

Oncogenes and tumor suppressors

Members of the $p21^{Cip1}$, $p57^{Kip2}$ and $p27^{Kip1}$ cyclin-kinase inhibitor family of proteins inhibit progression from G_1 into synthesis (S) phase in the cell cycle (Fig. 2) [98]. Chromosomal $p27^{Kip1}$ sequence abnormalities, loss of heterozygosity, and quantitative discrepancies in $p27^{Kip1}$ transcript prevalence have not been found consistently in pituitary adenomas, and the potential contribution of different cyclin D1 alleles, p16 amplification, and methylation patterns are equally obscure. Classic proto-oncogenes, such as N-ras, mycL1, mycN, H-ras, bcl1, H-stf1, sea, kraS2, c-erbB-2 and fos, and tumor suppressors such as retinoblastoma gene (RB)1 and p53 do not appear to have a significant role in pituitary adenoma pathogenesis.

Securin (aslo known as pituitary tumor-transforming gene or hPTTG), is responsible for inhibiting the action of a group of proteins called separins. When activated, separins terminate the activity of cohesin, which in turn allows segregation of sister chromatids to occur once all of the chromosomes are attached to the metaphase plate at the opposite poles of the mitotic spindle (Fig. 3). Securin is expressed in proliferating cells in a cell cycle-dependent manner, and when disrupted predisposes to aneuploidy through inappropriate timing of chromosomal segregation. Securin has

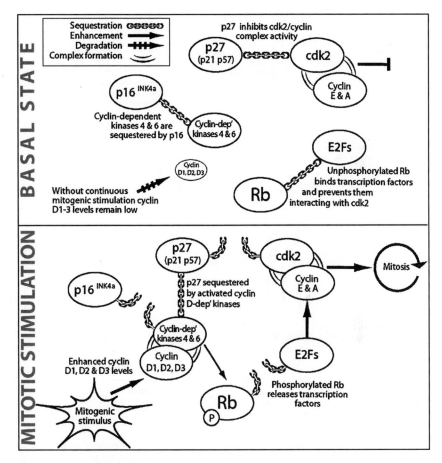

Fig. 2. Highly simplified cartoon depicting cell cycle regulatory pathways in which the disposition of controlling proteins and protein complexes are indicated under basal conditions (*top panel*) and in response to mitogenic stimuli (*bottom panel*). The interaction of D-type cyclins with cyclin-dependent kinases in response to persistent mitotic stimulation, leads to the sequestration of Cip/Kip proteins (p27^{Kip1}, p21^{Cip1} and p57^{Kip2}) that had, until that time, inhibited the actions of cyclin E/cdk2. Persistent mitogenic stimulation is therefore characterized by high levels of cyclin D-dependent kinase activity and low levels of p27Kip1, most of which is bound to cyclin D-cdks. The cyclin D-cdk4/6-Cip/Kip complex phosphorylates retinoblastoma protein (Rb) allows transcription factors, such as the E2Fs, to induce cyclin E and A. The p16^{INK4a}/cyclin D/cdk4/retinoblastoma pathway and the ARF/Mdm2/p53 pathway (not shown) are the two principal inhibitory pathways, disruption of which are implicated in many human tumors.

been reported to be present at very low levels in normal pituitary tissue, and at higher levels in many pituitary adenomas [99]. Activating mutations, promoter insertions, deletions or point mutations of hPTTG [100], or a clear correlation between hPTTG expression and mitotic index in human pituitary tumors have not been described. It remains unclear as yet whether over-expression of normal PTTG has any true transforming activity or role in human pituitary tumor propagation.

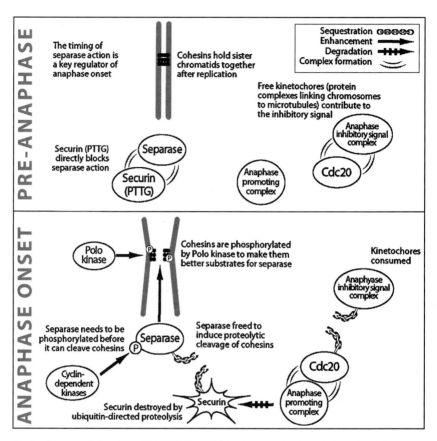

Fig. 3. Cartoon of the place of hPTTG (securin) in the control of the timing of anaphase. Pre-anaphase, hPTTG blocks separase action. The combined stimuli of phosphorylation of cohesins by Polo kinase (to make them better substrates for separase), phosphorylation of separase itself (probably by cyclin dependent kinases), and destruction of hPTTG by ubiquitin-directed proteolysis directed by the anaphase promoting/Cdc20 complex, allows the final cohesin ligatures at the centromeres to be cleaved, leading to timed separation of chromosomes and subsequent completion of anaphase.

In summary, the tacit and frequent assumption that cell cycle control is necessarily disrupted in human pituitary adenomas, and that apparent up-regulation of any gene implicated in the process (even when compared with vanishingly low levels in normal pituitary) is of causal significance, requires careful reflection, not least because an increased mitotic index in pituitary adenomas is far from universal, and the potential contribution of subtle but crucial changes in apoptotic control are largely unexplored. The panoply of subtle abnormalities in cell cycle regulatory pathways, particularly the two families of cyclin-dependent kinase inhibitors (INK: p16, p15, p18 and p19, and WAF/KIP: p21, p27 and p57), is somewhat unexpected, given the rather tenuous link between proliferation markers and clinical pituitary adenoma behavior, but presumably suggests that concurrent and essentially independent up-regulation of apoptotic activity must be occurring.

Cell signaling

The association between activation of the gsp oncogene through gain-of-function mutation of the GNAS1 gene on chromosome 20q13, and the development of somatotroph adenomas, remains the strongest potentially pathogenic mechanism yet defined for human pituitary adenomas. One of two GNAS1 single point mutations (at residue 201 (Arg substituted by Cys or His) or 227 (Gln substituted by Arg or Leu)), identified in approximately 40% of somatotrophinomas, results in increased resistance of guanosine triphosphate (GTP)-bound $G_{s\alpha}$ to hydrolysis, and a concomitant increase in adenylyl cyclase activity. The mechanism is supported but not confirmed by a transgenic mouse model, in which intrasomatotrophic cAMP levels, constitutively increased by expression of cholera toxin, develop somatotroph proliferation and pituitary hyperplasia [101], and by the finding of amplification of wild-type $G_{s\alpha}$ in somatotroph adenomas (Fig. 4) [102,103]. It is interesting and unexpected that there is no difference in the age and sex, and the duration and clinical features of acromegaly in groups with and without the GNAS1 mutation, and only trivial differences

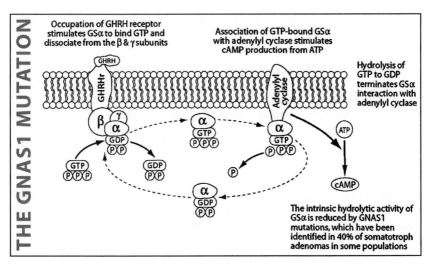

Fig. 4. The gsp oncogene (GNAS1 mutation) in GHRHr signaling. Occupation of the GHRH receptor triggers GTP binding by $G_{s\alpha}$, which dissociates from the bg subunits and interacts instead with adenylyl cyclase to stimulate production of cyclic AMP. The interaction is timed out by hydrolysis of GTP through the combined actions of GTPase activating peptides in the cytosol, the activity of adenylyl cyclase, and the intrinsic hydrolytic activity of $G_{s\alpha}$. The latter is diminished by GNAS1 mutations, which therefore increase the duration of adenylyl cyclase activity in response to GHRHr signaling.

in tumor size and circulating growth hormone levels [104], although transcript levels of cyclic AMP-response element binding protein and inducible cAMP early repressor tended to be higher in GNAS1 mutation-positive than GNAS1 mutation-negative tumors [105]. Activating mutations of GNAS1 have also been reported in a minority of endocrinologically inactive adenomas and corticotroph adenomas [106], but not in macroprolactinomas [107].

Receptor modulation

A truncated fibroblast growth factor receptor 4 (FGFR-4) has been identified in human pituitary adenomas, but its expression is not correlated with pituitary tumor type, size, or aggressiveness [108]. Abnormalities of fibroblast growth factor 2 and its receptor FGFR1 [109], and the transforming growth factor-beta receptor gene have also been described [110]. There is no evidence of constitutively active CRH receptor mutations [111] or GHRH receptor mutations [112] in sporadic pituitary adenomas or isolated familial acromegaly [113], and although GHRH is important in somatotroph lineage expansion during development, and has a role in growth hormone secretion from somatotroph adenomas [114], there is no consistent correlation between GHRH receptor expression and pituitary adenoma propagation [112,115]. Single cases of Cushing's disease, preceded by generalized glucocorticoid resistance resulting from a dominant-negative glucocorticoid receptor mutation [116], and of Nelson's syndrome, in which a glucocorticoid receptor frame shift mutation may have modified glucocorticoid sensitivity, have been reported [117].

No evidence of somatostatin receptor SSTR2 mutations have been found in pituitary adenomas, irrespective of clinical somatostatin sensitivity, but a germline SSTR5 mutation has been reported in a single somatostatin analog-resistant somatotroph adenoma [118]. Among 13 informative samples, one somatotroph and one thyrotroph adenoma showed loss of heterozygosity at the SSTR5 gene locus [119]. Expression levels of SSTR2 and SSTR5 have not been significantly correlated with growth hormone levels, tumor size [120], invasiveness, the presence or absence of GNAS1 mutation [121], or growth hormone secretory sensitivity to octreotide [122]. A proportion of prolactinomas respond slowly or incompletely to dopamine agonists, and defects in dopamine receptor expression have been adduced to explain this [123].

The increase in pituitary size and lactotroph mass during human pregnancy reverse rapidly but incompletely on weaning, or if suckling does not take place. High dose estrogen in elderly men with prostate cancer, and in male-to-female transsexuals, is not associated with an increased risk of prolactinoma formation, and differential expression of estrogen receptors does not explain the sexually dimorphic behavior of macroprolactinomas. Gender, age, menstrual status, Ki-67 proliferative indices, exposure to dopamine agonists, preoperative prolactin level, tumor size, and invasiveness have also not been related either positively or negatively to estrogen receptor status in prolactinomas [124], or endocrinologically inactive adenomas for that matter [125].

References

[1] Farrell WE, Clayton RN. Molecular pathogenesis of pituitary tumors. Front Neuroendocrinol 2000;21(3):174–98.

[2] Levy A, Lightman SL. Molecular defects in the pathogenesis of pituitary tumors. Front Neuroendocrinol 2003;24(2):94–127.

[3] Scheithauer BW, Gaffey TA, Lloyd RV, et al. Pathobiology of pituitary adenomas and carcinomas. Neurosurgery 2006;59(2):341–53.

[4] Hall WA, Luciano MG, Doppman JL, et al. Pituitary magnetic resonance imaging in normal human volunteers: occult adenomas in the general population. Ann Intern Med 1994; 120(10):817–20.

[5] Molitch ME. Pituitary incidentalomas. Endocrinol Metab Clin North Am 1997;26:725–40.

[6] Ezzat S, Asa SL, Couldwell WT, et al. The prevalence of pituitary adenomas: a systematic review. Cancer 2004;101(3):613–9.

[7] Lindholm J, Juul S, Jorgensen JOL, et al. Incidence and late prognosis of Cushing's syndrome: a population-based study. J Clin Endocrinol Metab 2001;86(1):117–23.

[8] Scheithauer RF, Young WFJ, Horvath E, et al. Silent corticotroph carcinoma of the adenohypophysis: a report of five cases. Am J Surg Pathol 2003;27(4):477–86.

[9] Daly AF, Rixhon M, Adam C, et al. High prevalence of pituitary adenomas: a cross-sectional study in the province of Liege, Belgium. J Clin Endocrinol Metab 2006;91(12): 4769–75.

[10] Console GM, Gomez Dumm CL, Brown OA, et al. Sexual dimorphism in the age changes of the pituitary lactotrophs in rats. Mech Ageing Dev 1997;95(3):157–66.

[11] Donovan LE, Corenblum B. The natural history of the pituitary incidentaloma. Arch Intern Med 1995;155(2):181–3.

[12] Jeffcoate WJ, Pound N, Sturrock NDC, et al. Long-term follow-up of patients with hyperprolactinaemia. Clin Endocrinol (Oxf) 1996;45:299–303.

[13] Nammour GM, Ybarra J, Hossain Naheedy M, et al. Incidental pituitary macroadenoma: a population-based study. Am J Med Sci 1997;314:287–91.

[14] Adler I, Barsi P, Czirjak S, et al. Rapid re-enlargement of a macroprolactinoma after initial shrinkage in a young woman treated with bromocriptine. Gynecol Endocrinol 2005;20(6): 317–21.

[15] Burke CW, Adams CB, Esiri MM, et al. Transsphenoidal surgery for Cushing's disease: does what is removed determine the endocrine outcome? Clin Endocrinol (Oxf) 1990; 33(4):525–37.

[16] Kruse A, Klinken L, Holck S, et al. Pituitary histology in Cushing's disease. Clin Endocrinol (Oxf) 1992;37(3):254–9.

[17] Denk CC, Onderoglu S, Ilgi S, et al. Height of normal pituitary gland on MRI: differences between age groups and sexes. Okajimas Folia Anat Jpn 1999;76(2–3):81–7.

[18] Chanson P, Daujat F, Young J, et al. Normal pituitary hypertrophy as a frequent cause of pituitary incidentaloma: a follow-up study. J Clin Endocrinol Metab 2001;86(7):3009–15.

[19] Schwartz J. Intercellular communication in the anterior pituitary. Endocr Rev 2000;21(5): 488–513.

[20] Asa SL, Penz G, Kovacs K, et al. Prolactin cells in the human pituitary. A quantitative immunocytochemical analysis. Arch Pathol Lab Med 1982;106(7):360–3.

[21] Dinc H, Esen F, Demirci A, et al. Pituitary dimensions and volume measurements in pregnancy and post partum. MR assessment. Acta Radiol 1998;39(1):64–9.

[22] Haggi ES, Torres AI, Maldonado CA, et al. Regression of redundant lactotrophs in rat pituitary gland after cessation of lactation. J Endocrinol 1986;111(3):367–73.

[23] Chen J, Hersmus N, Van Duppen V, et al. The adult pituitary contains a cell population displaying stem/progenitor cell and early embryonic characteristics. Endocrinology 2005; 146(9):3985–98.

[24] Lepore DA, Jokubaitis VJ, Simmons PJ, et al. A role for angiotensin-converting enzyme in the characterization, enrichment, and proliferation potential of adult muring pituitary colony-forming cells. Stem Cells 2006;24(11):2382–90.

[25] Nolan LA, Kavanagh E, Lightman SL, et al. Anterior pituitary cell population control: basal cell turnover and the effects of adrenalectomy and dexamethasone treatment. J Neuroendocrinol 1998;10:207–15.

[26] McNicol AM, Carbajo-Perez E. Aspects of anterior pituitary growth, with special reference to corticotrophs. Pituitary 1999;1(3–4):257–68.

[27] Nolan LA, Lunness HR, Lightman SL, et al. The effects of age and spontaneous adenoma formation on trophic activity in the rat pituitary gland: a comparison with trophic activity in the human pituitary and in human pituitary adenomas. J Neuroendocrinol 1999;11:393–401.

[28] Taniguchi Y, Tamatani R, Yasutaka S, et al. Proliferation of pituitary corticotrophs following adrenalectomy as revealed by immunocytochemistry combined with bromodeoxyuridine-labeling. Histochem Cell Biol 1995;103:127–30.

[29] Nolan LA, Levy A. A population of non-LH/non-ACTH-positive cells in the male rat anterior pituitary responds mitotically to both gonadectomy and adrenalectomy. J Neuroendocrinol 2006;18(9):655–61.

[30] Nolan LA, Levy A. Anterior pituitary trophic responses to dexamethasone withdrawal and repeated dexamethasone exposures. J Endocrinol 2001;169:263–70.

[31] Potten CS, Schofield R, Lajtha LG. A comparison of cell replacement in bone marrow, testis and three regions of surface epithelium. Biochim Biophys Acta 1979;560(1):281–99.

[32] Fuchs E, Segre JA. Stem cells: a new lease on life. Cell 2000;100:143–55.

[33] Nolan LA, Thomas CK, Levy A. Permissive effects of thyroid hormones on rat anterior pituitary mitotic activity. J Endocrinol 2004;180:35–43.

[34] Taniguchi Y, Yasutaka S, Kominami R, et al. Proliferation and differentiation of rat anterior pituitary cells. Anat Embryol (Berl) 2002;206(1–2):1–11.

[35] Park S, Kamegai J, Kineman RD. Role of glucocorticoids in the regulation of pituitary somatostatin receptor subtype (sst1–sst5) mRNA levels: evidence for direct and somatostatin-mediated effects. Neuroendocrinology 2003;78(3):1163–75.

[36] Nolan LA, Schmid HA, Levy A. Octreotide and the novel multi-receptor ligand somatostatin receptor agonist pasireotide (SOM230), block the adrenalectomy-induced increase in mitotic activity in male rat anterior pituitary. Endocrinology 2007;148:2821–7.

[37] Nolan LA, Thomas CK, Levy A. Pituitary mitosis and apoptotic responsiveness following adrenalectomy are independent of hypothalamic paraventricular nucleus CRH input. J Endocrinol 2004;181(3):521–9.

[38] Nolan LA, Levy A. The effects of testosterone and estrogen on gonadectomized and intact male rat anterior pituitary mitotic and apoptotic activity. J Endocrinol 2006;188(3):387–96.

[39] Sakuma S, Shirasawa N, Yoshimura F. A histometrical study of immunohistochemically identified mitotic adenohypophysial cells in immature and mature castrated rats. J Endocrinol 1984;100:323–8.

[40] Inoue K, Tanaka S, Kurosumi K. Mitotic activity of gonadotropes in the anterior pituitary of the castrated male rat. Cell Tissue Res 1985;240(2):271–6.

[41] Nagesser SK, van Seters AP, Kievit J, et al. Long-term results of total adrenalectomy for Cushing's disease. World J Surg 2000;24(1):108–13.

[42] Aoki MP, Aoki A, Maldonado CA. Sexual dimorphism of apoptosis in lactotrophs induced by bromocryptine. Histochem Cell Biol 2001;116(3):215–22.

[43] Nunez L, Villalobos C, Senovilla L, et al. Multifunctional cells of mouse anterior pituitary reveal a striking sexual dimorphism. J Physiol 2003;549(Pt 3):835–43.

[44] Scheithauer BW, Horvath E, Kovacs K, et al. Plurihormonal pituitary adenomas. Semin Diagn Pathol 1986;3:69–82.

[45] Ho DM, Hsu CY, Ting LT, et al. Plurihormonal pituitary adenomas: immunostaining of all pituitary hormones is mandatory for correct classification. Histopathology 2001;39(3): 310–9.

[46] Furuhata S, Kameya T, Otani M, et al. Prolactin presents in all pituitary tumors of acromegalic patients. Hum Pathol 1993;24(1):10–5.

[47] Ma W, Ikeda H, Yoshimoto T. Clinicopathologic study of 123 cases of prolactin-secreting pituitary adenomas with special reference to multihormone production and clonality of the adenomas. Cancer 2002;95(2):258–66.

[48] Villalobos C, Nunez L, Frawley LS, et al. Multi-responsiveness of single anterior pituitary cells to hypothalamic-releasing hormones: a cellular basis for paradoxical secretion. Proc Natl Acad Sci USA 1997;94(25):14132–7.

[49] Simpson DJ, McNicol AM, Murray DC, et al. Molecular pathology shows p16 methylation in nonadenomatous pituitaries from patients with Cushing's disease. Clin Cancer Res 2004; 10(5):1780–8.

[50] Peri A, Bemporad D, Parenti G, et al. Cushing's syndrome due to intermittent ectopic ACTH production showing a temporary remission during a pulmonary infection. Eur J Endocrinol 2001;145:605–11.

[51] Gartler SM, Riggs AD. Mammalian X-chromosome inactivation. Annu Rev Genet 1983; 17:155–90.

[52] Tonon L, Bergamaschi G, Dellavecchia C, et al. Unbalanced X-chromosome inactivation in haemopoietic cells from normal women. Br J Haematol 1998;102(4):996–1003.

[53] Levy A. Monoclonality of endocrine tumours: what does it mean? Trends Endocrinol Metab 2001;12(7):301–7.

[54] Schmidt GH, Mead R. On the clonal origin of tumours—lessons from studies of intestinal epithelium. Bioessays 1990;12(1):37–40.

[55] Woodruff MF, Ansell JD, Forbes GM, et al. Clonal interaction in tumours. Nature 1982; 299(5886):822–4.

[56] Clayton RN, Pfeifer M, Atkinson AB, et al. Different patterns of allelic loss (loss of heterozygosity) in recurrent human pituitary tumors provide evidence for multiclonal origins. Clin Cancer Res 2000;6(10):3973–82.

[57] Clayton RN, Farrell WE. Clonality of pituitary tumours: more complicated than initially envisaged? Brain Pathol 2001;11(3):313–27.

[58] Zahedi A, Booth GL, Smyth HS, et al. Distinct clonal composition of primary and metastatic adrencorticotrophic hormone-producing pituitary carcinoma. Clin Endocrinol (Oxf) 2001;55:549–56.

[59] Busque L, Mio R, Mattioli J, et al. Nonrandom X-inactivation patterns in normal females: lyonization ratios vary with age. Blood 1996;88(1):59–65.

[60] Tsai YC, Simoneau AR, Spruck CHR, et al. Mosaicism in human epithelium: macroscopic monoclonal patches cover the urothelium. J Urol 1995;153(5):1698–700.

[61] Schwartz SM, Murry CE. Proliferation and the monoclonal origins of atherosclerotic lesions. Annu Rev Med 1998;49:437–60.

[62] Tiltman AJ. Smooth muscle neoplasms of the uterus. Curr Opin Obstet Gynecol 1997;9(1): 48–51.

[63] Aihara T, Noguchi S, Sasaki Y, et al. Does monoclonality mean malignancy. Hepatology 1996;24(6):1550.

[64] Arnold A, Brown MF, Urena P, et al. Monoclonality of parathyroid tumors in chronic renal failure and in primary parathyroid hyperplasia. J Clin Invest 1995;95(5):2047–53.

[65] Tominaga Y, Kohara S, Namii Y, et al. Clonal analysis of nodular parathyroid hyperplasia in renal hyperparathyroidism. World J Surg 1996;20(7):744–50.

[66] Aeschimann S, Kopp PA, Kimura ET, et al. Morphological and functional polymorphism within clonal thyroid nodules. J Clin Endocrinol Metab 1993;77(3):846–51.

[67] Levy A. Is monoclonality in pituitary adenomas synonymous with neoplasia? Clin Endocrinol (Oxf) 2000;52:393–7.

[68] Herman V, Fagin J, Gonsky E, et al. Clonal origins of pituitary adenomas. J Clin Endocrinol Metab 1990;71:1427–33.

[69] Alexander JM, Biller BM, Bikkal H, et al. Clinically nonfunctioning pituitary tumors are monoclonal in origin. J Clin Invest 1990;86:336–40.

[70] Biller BMK, Alexander JM, Zervas NT, et al. Clonal origins of adrenocorticotropin-secreting pituitary tissue in Cushing's disease. J Clin Endocrinol Metab 1992;75(5): 1303–9.

[71] Schulte HM, OldFFfield EH, Allolio B, et al. Clonal composition of pituitary adenomas in patients with Cushing's disease: determination by X-chromosome inactivation analysis. J Clin Endocrinol Metab 1991;73:1302–8.

[72] Gicquel C, Le Bouc Y, Luton JP, et al. Monoclonality of corticotroph macroadenomas in Cushing's disease. J Clin Endocrinol Metab 1992;75(2):472–5.

[73] Sotillo R, Hernando E, Díaz-Rodríguez E, et al. Mad2 overexpression promotes aneuploidy and tumorigenesis in mice. Cancer Cell 2007;11(1):9–23.

[74] Anniko M, Tribukait B, Wersall J. DNA ploidy and cell phase in human pituitary tumors. Cancer 1984;53(8):1708–13.

[75] Gaffey TAJ, Scheithauer BW, Leech RW, et al. Pituitary adenoma: a DNA flow cytometric study of 192 clinicopathologically characterized tumors. Clin Neuropathol 2005;24(2): 56–63.

[76] Pegolo G, Buckwalter JG, Weiss MH, et al. Pituitary adenomas. Correlation of the cytologic appearance with biologic behavior. Acta Cytol 1995;39(5):887–92.

[77] Losa M, Franzin A, Mangili F, et al. Proliferation index of nonfunctioning pituitary adenomas: correlations with clinical characteristics and long-term follow-up results. Neurosurgery 2000;47(6):1313–8.

[78] Neufeld TP, de la Cruz AF, Johnston LA, et al. Coordination of growth and cell division in the Drosophila wing. Cell 1998;93(7):1183–93.

[79] Stowers RS, Schwarz TL. A genetic method for generating Drosophila eyes composed exclusively of mitotic clones of a single genotype. Genetics 1999;152(4):1631–9.

[80] O'Neill EE, Matallanas D, Kolch W. Mammalian sterile 20-like kinases in tumor suppression: an emerging pathway. Cancer Res 2005;65(13):5485–7.

[81] St John MA, Tao W, Fei X, et al. Mice deficient of Lats1 develop soft-tissue sarcomas, ovarian tumours and pituitary dysfunction. Nat Genet 1999;21:182–6.

[82] Carney JA. The Carney complex (myxomas, spotty pigmentation, endocrine overactivity, and schwannomas). Dermatol Clin 1995;13(1):19–26.

[83] Daly AF, Jaffrain-Rea ML, Ciccarelli A, et al. Clinical characterization of familial isolated pituitary adenomas. J Clin Endocrinol Metab 2006;91(9):3316–23.

[84] Vierimaa O, Georgitsi M, Lehtonen R, et al. Pituitary adenoma predisposition caused by germline mutations in the AIP gene. Science 2006;312(5777):1228–30.

[85] Lytras A, Tolis G. Growth hormone-secreting tumors: genetic aspects and data from animal models. Neuroendocrinology 2006;83:166–78.

[86] Frohman LA, Eguchi K. Familial acromegaly. Growth Horm IGF Res 2004;14(Suppl A): S90–6.

[87] Soares B, Eguchi K, Frohman LA. Tumor deletion mapping on chromosome 11q13 in eight families with isolated familial somatotropinoma and in 15 sporadic somatotropinomas. J Clin Endocrinol Metab 2005;90(12):6580–7.

[88] Komminoth P, Roth J, Muletta-Feurer S, et al. RET proto-oncogene point mutations in sporadic neuroendocrine tumors. J Clin Endocrinol Metab 1996;81(6):2041–6.

[89] Yoshimoto K, Tanaka C, Moritani M, et al. Infrequent detectable somatic mutations of the RET and glial cell line-derived neurotrophic factor (GDNF) genes in human pituitary adenomas. Endocr J 1999;46(1):199–207.

[90] Iwata T, Yamada S, Mizusawa N, et al. The aryl hydrocarbon receptor-interacting protein gene is rarely mutated in sporadic GH-secreting adenoma. Clin Endocrinol (Oxf) 2007; 66(4):499–502.

[91] Hillegass JM, Murphy KA, Villano CM, et al. The impact of aryl hydrocarbon receptor signaling on matrix metabolism: implications for development and disease. Biol Chem 2006;387(9):1159–73.

[92] Georgitsi M, Raitila A, Karhu A, et al. Molecular diagnosis of pituitary adenoma predisposition caused by aryl hydrocargon receptor-interacting protein gene mutations. Proc Natl Acad Sci USA 2007;104(10):4101–5.

[93] Yu R, Bonert V, Saporta I, et al. Aryl hydrocarbon receptor interacting protein variants in sporadic pituitary adenomas. J Clin Endocrinol Metab 2006;91:5126–9.

[94] Toledo RA, Lourenco DMJ, Liberman B, et al. Germline mutation in the Aryl Hydrocarbon Receptor Interacting Protein (AIP) Gene in Familial Somatotropinoma. J Clin Endocrinol Metab 2007;92(5):1934–7.

[95] Barlier A, Vanbellinghen JF, Daly AF, et al. Mutations in the aryl hydrocarbon receptor interacting protein gene are not highly prevalent among subjects with sporadic pituitary adenomas. J Clin Endocrinol Metab 2007;92(5):1952–5.

[96] Daly AF, Vanbellinghen JF, Khoo SK, et al. Aryl hydrocarbon receptor interacting protein gene mutations in familial isolated pituitary adenomas: analysis in 73 families. J Clin Endocrinol Metab 2007;92(5):1891–6.

[97] Georgitsi M, Karhu A, Winqvist R, et al. Mutation analysis of aryl hydrocarbon receptor interacting protein (AIP) gene in colorectal, breast, and prostate cancer. Br J Cancer 2007; 96(2):352–6.

[98] Sherr CJ, Roberts JM. Inhibitors of mammalian G1 cyclin-dependent kinases. Genes Dev 1995;9(10):1149–63.

[99] Zhang X, Horwitz GA, Heaney AP, et al. Pituitary tumor transforming gene (PTTG) expression in pituitary adenomas. J Clin Endocrinol Metab 1999;84(2):761–7.

[100] Kanakis D, Kirches E, Mawrin C, et al. Promoter mutations are no major cause of PTTG overexpression in pituitary adenomas. Clin Endocrinol (Oxf) 2003;58(2):151–5.

[101] Burton FH, Hasel KW, Bloom FE, et al. Pituitary hyperplasia and gigantism in mice caused by a cholera toxin transgene. Nature 1991;350:74–7.

[102] Bertherat J, Chanson P, Montminy M. The cyclic adenosine 3′,5′-monophosphate-responsive factor CREB is constitutively activated in human somatotroph adenomas. Mol Endocrinol 1995;9(7):777–83.

[103] Hamacher C, Brocker M, Adams EF, et al. Overexpression of stimulatory G protein alpha-subunit is a hallmark of most human somatotrophic pituitary tumours and is associated with resistance to GH-releasing hormone. Pituitary 1998;1(1):13–23.

[104] Spada A, Arosio M, Bochicchio D, et al. Clinical, biochemical, and morphological correlates in patients bearing growth hormone-secreting pituitary tumors with or without constitutively active adenylyl cyclase. J Clin Endocrinol Metab 1990;71(6): 1421–6.

[105] Peri A, Conforti B, Baglioni-Peri S, et al. Expression of cyclic adenosine 3′,5′-monophosphate (cAMP)-responsive element binding protein and inducible-cAMP early repressor genes in growth hormone-secreting pituitary adenomas with or without mutations of the Gsalpha gene. J Clin Endocrinol Metab 2001;86(5):2111–7.

[106] Williamson EA, Ince PG, Harrison D, et al. G-protein mutations in human pituitary adrenocorticotrophic hormone-secreting adenomas. Eur J Clin Invest 1995;25(2): 128–31.

[107] Tordjman K, Stern N, Ouaknine G, et al. Activating mutations of the Gs alpha-gene in nonfunctioning pituitary tumors. J Clin Endocrinol Metab 1993;77(3):765–9.

[108] Abbass SA, Asa SL, Ezzat S. Altered expression of fibroblast growth factor receptors in human pituitary adenomas. J Clin Endocrinol Metab 1997;82(4):1160–6.

[109] McCabe CJ, Khaira JS, Boelaert K, et al. Expression of pituitary tumour transforming gene (PTTG) and fibroblast growth factor-2 (FGF-2) in human pituitary adenomas: relationships to clinical tumour behaviour. Clin Endocrinol (Oxf) 2003;58(2):141–50.

[110] Fujiwara K, Ikeda H, Yoshimoto T. Abnormalities in expression of genes, mRNA, and proteins of transforming growth factor-beta receptor type I and type II in human pituitary adenomas. Clin Neuropathol 1998;17(1):19–26.

[111] Asa SL, Ezzat S. The cytogenesis and pathogenesis of pituitary adenomas. Endocr Rev 1998;19(6):798–827.

[112] Hashimoto K, Koga M, Motomura T, et al. Identification of alternatively spliced messenger ribonucleic acid encoding truncated growth hormone-releasing hormone receptor in human pituitary adenomas. J Clin Endocrinol Metab 1995;80(10):2933–9.

[113] Jorge BH, Agarwal SK, Lando VS, et al. Study of the multiple endocrine neoplasia type 1, growth hormone-releasing hormone receptor, Gs alpha, and Gi2 alpha genes in isolated familial acromegaly. J Clin Endocrinol Metab 2001;86(2):542–4.

[114] Dimaraki EV, Chandler WF, Brown MB, et al. The role of endogenous growth hormone-releasing hormone in acromegaly. J Clin Endocrinol Metab 2006;91(6):2185–90.

[115] Thapar K, Kovacs K, Stefaneanu L, et al. Overexpression of the growth-hormone-releasing hormone gene in acromegaly-associated pituitary tumors. An event associated with neoplastic progression and aggressive behavior. Am J Pathol 1997;151(3):769–84.

[116] Karl M, Lamberts SW, Koper JW, et al. Cushing's disease preceded by generalized glucocorticoid resistance: clinical consequences of a novel, dominant-negative glucocorticoid receptor mutation. Proc Assoc Am Physicians 1996;108(4):296–307.

[117] Karl M, Von Wichert G, Kempter E, et al. Nelson's syndrome associated with a somatic frame shift mutation in the glucocorticoid receptor gene. J Clin Endocrinol Metab 1996;81(1):124–9.

[118] Ballare E, Persani L, Lania AG, et al. Mutation of somatostatin receptor type 5 in an acromegalic patient resistant to somatostatin analog treatment. J Clin Endocrinol Metab 2001;86(8):3809–14.

[119] Filopanti M, Ballare E, Lania AG, et al. Loss of heterozygosity at the SS receptor type 5 locus in human GH- and TSH-secreting pituitary adenomas. J Endocrinol Invest 2004;27(10):937–42.

[120] Greenman Y, Melmed S. Heterogeneous expression of two somatostatin receptor subtypes in pituitary tumors. J Clin Endocrinol Metab 1994;78(2):398–403.

[121] Corbetta S, Ballare E, Mantovani G, et al. Somatostatin receptor subtype 2 and 5 in human GH-secreting pituitary adenomas: analysis of gene sequence and mRNA expression. Eur J Clin Invest 2001;31(3):208–14.

[122] Murabe H, Shimatsu A, Ihara C, et al. Expression of somatostatin receptor (SSTR) subtypes in pituitary adenomas: quantitative analysis of SSTR2 mRNA by reverse transcription-polymerase chain reaction. J Neuroendocrinol 1996;8(8):605–10.

[123] Caccavelli L, Feron F, Morange I, et al. Decreased expression of the two D2 dopamine receptor isoforms in bromocriptine-resistant prolactinomas. Neuroendocrinology 1994;60(3):314–22.

[124] Kaptain GJ, Simmons NE, Alden TD, et al. Estrogen receptors in prolactinomas: a clinico-pathological study. Pituitary 1999;1(2):91–8.

[125] Gittoes NJ, McCabe CJ, Sheppard MC, et al. Estrogen receptor beta mRNA expression in normal and adenomatous pituitaries. Pituitary 1999;1(2):99–104.

ELSEVIER
SAUNDERS

Endocrinol Metab Clin N Am
37 (2008) 51–66

ENDOCRINOLOGY
AND METABOLISM
CLINICS
OF NORTH AMERICA

Treatment of Pituitary Tumors: a Surgical Perspective

William F. Chandler, MD[a,b,*], Ariel L. Barkan, MD[a,b]

[a]Department of Neurosurgery, University of Michigan Medical Center, 3552 Taubman Center,
Box 5338, 1500 East Medical Center Drive, Ann Arbor, MI 48109, USA
[b]Division of Metabolism, Endocrinology, and Diabetes, University of Michigan Medical
Center, Ann Arbor, MI 48109, USA

This article is intended to provide the clinical endocrinologist with a better understanding of the surgical aspects of diseases affecting the hypothalamic-pituitary area. This understanding requires a working knowledge of radiologic diagnosis of the most prevalent pituitary diseases, indications for surgical intervention, the choice of surgical approach to the lesion, and the expected extent of resection.

Clinical neuroanatomy of the pituitary

Normal pituitary is approximately 10 to 12 mm in the largest dimension. It is located in the sella turcica and is a part of skull-base structures. The gland is separated from the suprasellar cistern by a thin diaphragm that is penetrated by the pituitary stalk. Approximately 10 to 15 mm above the diaphragm lies the optic chiasm, anterior to which are the optic nerves and posterior to which are the optic tracts. Thus, to cause diminution in visual acuity or fields defect, the tumor must expand more than 1 to 1.5 cm above the level of the diaphragm and distort the optic pathways.

The sella is bordered laterally by the cavernous sinuses. Each contains the carotid artery and cranial nerves III, IV, V_1, V_2, and VI. Impairment of cranial nerves III, IV, and VI causes ipsilateral ophthalmoplegia, double vision, ptosis, and dilatation of the pupil. In addition, damage to cranial nerve

* Corresponding author. Department of Neurosurgery, University of Michigan Medical Center, 3552 Taubman Center, Box 5338, 1500 East Medical Center Drive, Ann Arbor, MI 48109.
    E-mail address: wchndlr@med.umich.edu (W.F. Chandler).

0889-8529/08/$ - see front matter © 2008 Elsevier Inc. All rights reserved.
doi:10.1016/j.ecl.2007.10.006   *endo.theclinics.com*

V may cause diminished corneal reflex and ipsilateral pain or paresthesia in the forehead and the upper cheek.

The inferior surface of the gland is separated by a thin bony wall from the sphenoid sinus. Extension of the tumor into the sphenoid sinus is most often asymptomatic. Occasionally, cerebrospinal fluid (CSF) rhinorrhea may be a consequence of sphenoidal tumor invasion.

Goals of pituitary surgery

Pituitary lesions may be asymptomatic or may present with mass effects (impaired visual acuity, constricted visual fields, or ophthalmoplegia), with syndromes of hormone excess, or with hypopituitarism.

The goals of surgery need to be firmly established in each individual patient. The risks of pituitary surgery performed by an experienced operator are small but never absent. These risks need to be clearly communicated to the patient. When surgery is chosen as a treatment option, the following priorities must be adhered to:

1. Remove as much tumor as possible to relieve compression of the optic pathways and to eliminate as much hormonally active tissue as possible.
2. Avoid inflicting additional neurologic damage.
3. Try to protect healthy pituitary tissue.

Several factors play a major role in fulfilling these objectives.

1. Experience of the surgeon. It has been amply demonstrated that experienced pituitary surgeons (those who perform > 50 operations per year) have a twofold to threefold higher success rate in hormonally active tumors [1] and a twofold to fourfold lower incidence of surgical complications [2] than less experienced surgeons.
2. Size and location of the tumor. Pituitary lesions smaller than 10 mm in diameter (microadenomas) can be grossly totally removed in 80% to 90% of cases. The outcome of surgery for so-called "macroadenomas" (ie, lesions > 10 mm in diameter) is less favorable. Overall, only about 50% to 60% of these can be completely removed by the most experienced surgeons [3]. Because the term macroadenoma refers to any tumor larger than 1 cm, it is important to keep in mind that the larger the tumor within this category, the more difficult total removal becomes. As an approximate guideline, tumors larger than 2 cm can be completely removed only in about 20% of cases [4]. The location of the lesion also determines the outcome. Intrasellar tumors or those with minor infrasellar extension can be removed with relative ease. Invasion of the cavernous sinuses generally prevents complete removal. Some suprasellar tumors adhere to the optic chiasm, the hypothalamus, or both, and an attempt at complete removal may result in diminished vision or hypothalamic damage.

3. Consistency of the tumor. Most tumors have a soft consistency and can be curetted easily. In contrast, some tumors are very fibrous and only limited resection is possible. This variable is unpredictable because it can be discovered only during surgery.
4. Other variables. Abundant vascularity of some pituitary lesions or large venous sinuses may result in intraoperative bleeding that may force even highly experienced surgeons to abandon the attempt.

Interpretation of images

With rare exception, imaging of lesions within the sella and in the parasellar area is done with MRI. Occasionally, CT is needed to look for calcification. Some type of angiography (MRI, CT, or conventional) is useful in evaluating a vascular lesion such as an aneurysm. The authors outline the interpretation of images of common sellar lesions.

Normal pituitary

Fig. 1 shows the coronal and sagittal views of a normal pituitary gland. The size of the gland varies and may fill only the bottom third of the sella or may be robust and fill the entire sella. The gland is often larger in young women. The stalk should be in the midline on the coronal view and the gland should be symmetric from side to side. On the non–contrast-enhanced T1 views, there is often a hyperintense (bright) spot in the posterior pituitary. This is normal and represents increased lipid content in this portion of the pituitary. The gland should enhance uniformly with contrast relative to the brain because it is outside the blood-brain barrier.

Adenomas

Figs. 2 and 3 are examples of large and small pituitary adenomas, respectively. Because these tumors arise from within the gland, they tend to cause

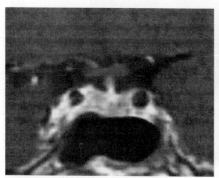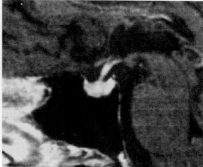

Fig. 1. MRI of normal pituitary, T1 with contrast. Coronal view (*left*). Sagittal view (*right*).

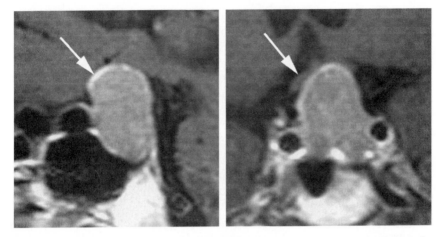

Fig. 2. MRI of macroadenoma, T1 with contrast. Sagittal view (*left*): arrow shows pituitary tissue draped over tumor. Coronal view (*right*): arrow shows optic chiasm elevated by tumor.

the expected compression and distortion of the gland. A small tumor located laterally will cause a shift of the gland and stalk to the opposite side, often associated with elevation of the diaphragma sellae on the side of the tumor (see Fig. 3). A macroadenoma will usually enlarge the bony sella turcica and may grow inferiorly, superiorly, or both. Because adenomas typically do not enhance as much as the pituitary itself, it is usually possible to identify the hyperintense gland draped over the surface of the tumor on T1 images with contrast (see Fig. 2). It is important to look for the optic chiasm to see whether it is being elevated by the adenoma. The optic chiasm is always found just superior to the tumor and will not enhance with contrast. Often, very large tumors invade the cavernous sinus on one side or both sides.

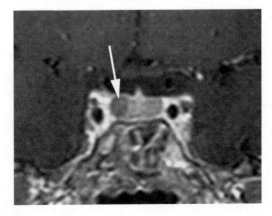

Fig. 3. MRI of microadenoma, T1 with contrast. Coronal view: arrow points to less enhancing tumor.

Although this invasion rarely results in loss of cranial nerve function, it makes it impossible to surgically resect the entire tumor.

Sometimes adenomas are cystic, and fluid-filled cysts can be identified as being dark on T1 images (with or without contrast) and bright on T2 images. Hemorrhage within an adenoma (pituitary apoplexy) appears bright on T1 imaging without contrast. This type of hemorrhage almost always occurs within a sizable macroadenoma. Any material that is bright on T1 without contrast is blood or fat.

Meningiomas

The most common location of parasellar meningiomas is the tuberculum sella, which is the midline bony surface along the anterior aspect of the sella. These meningiomas typically compress the optic nerves and cause posterior displacement of the pituitary gland. Unlike adenomas, they generally enhance uniformly with intravenous gadolinium (Fig. 4). This characteristic makes it difficult to identify the displaced pituitary tissue.

Another common location for meningiomas to arise is the dura of the cavernous sinuses. These tumors are unilateral to the sella and often cause cranial nerve dysfunction but not loss of pituitary function or vision.

Craniopharyngiomas

Craniopharyngiomas may arise anywhere along the pituitary-hypothalamic axis from within the sella itself to within the third ventricle. The most common location is at the level of the pituitary stalk, just above the sella. On imaging, they are usually a mixture of solid tumor that enhances with contrast on T1 and cysts of varying size that are bright on T2 (Fig. 5). They may be entirely cystic or virtually entirely solid and

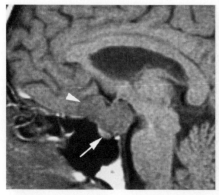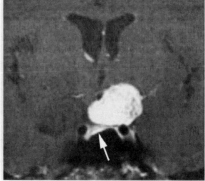

Fig. 4. MRI of meningioma. T1 noncontrast, sagittal view (*left*): arrow points to normal pituitary; arrowhead defines anterior border of tumor. T1 with contrast, coronal view (*right*): tumor enhances brightly and the arrow points to the pituitary.

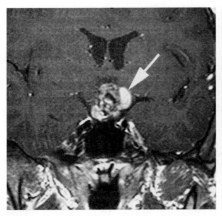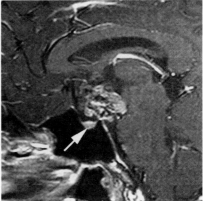

Fig. 5. MRI of craniophayngioma, T1 with contrast. Coronal view (*left*): arrow points to cystic component of tumor. Sagittal view (*right*): arrow points to normal pituitary.

enhancing. A plain CT scan is often helpful to show tumor calcification. Such a finding strongly supports the diagnosis of craniopharyngioma, although it may not be present in nearly half of these tumors.

Stalk and hypothalamic lesions

Lesions that occur primarily within the pituitary stalk and the hypothalamus include tumors and inflammatory lesions. Inflammatory lesions include sarcoidosis and Langerhans histiocytosis. Hypothalamic gliomas may occur in the median eminence of the hypothalamus and upper stalk. Choristomas (granular cell tumors) are rare tumors that arise from the pituitary stalk. Germinomas may arise in the stalk but are often associated with a similar lesion in the pineal region.

Cysts

Primary cysts occur within the sella and are usually referred to as Rathke's cysts. They contain material that is often thin like CSF but may be thick and mucinous. These cysts do not enhance with contrast and are usually darker than an adenoma on T1 images. They are often bright on T2 (Fig. 6), but when the fluid is thick and proteinacous, they may not be bright. Abscesses may occur in the pituitary and present as an isointense nonenhancing mass and are often confused with an adenoma.

Dermoid and epidermoid cysts present as complex, often heterogeneous lesions on MRI, usually with some hyperintense fatty material seen on T1 imaging.

A so-called "empty sella" can be differentiated from an arachnoid cyst, in that the pituitary stalk can be seen entering the sella and coursing to the compressed pituitary tissue at the bottom of the sella. In both of these situations, an enlarged sella is seen as filled with CSF (bright on T2).

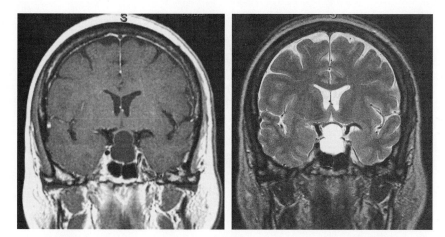

Fig. 6. MRI of Rathke's cyst. T1 with contrast (*left*): hypointense mass with elevation of optic chiasm. T2 without contrast (*right*): hyperintense (same as CSF in ventricles).

Carcinomas

It is fortunate that malignant adenomas are extremely rare. It is possible, however, for a malignant tumor to metastasize to the pituitary. These tumors cause rapid erosion of the surrounding skull base and often invade the cavernous sinus, causing ophthalmoplegia. Nasopharyngeal carcinomas may appear in the parasellar area but cause erosion from outside the sella and can usually be distinguished from primary pituitary tumors.

Chordomas

Chordomas arise from the clivus, directly beneath the sella, and should not be confused with intrasellar tumor. They erode the bone of the clivus and provide mixed signal with contrast enhancement on T1 imaging. They invade the skull base and often present with cranial nerve palsies.

Surgical approaches

Although most tumors in the region of the sella are approached by way of the sphenoid sinus, selected tumors require a different trajectory to maximize tumor removal and minimize the risk of the surgical procedure (Fig. 7). A number of these approaches can be combined.

Transsphenoidal approaches

The sublabial and transnasal transseptal approaches were used in the past but involved significant surgery involving the nasal septum. These approaches could be complicated by septal perforation or by anesthesia of

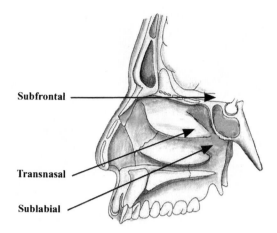

Fig. 7. Diagram of skull base and nasal region demonstrating the approaches to the sellar region.

the incisors. They also required bilateral postoperative nasal packing for several days. These approaches have largely been supplanted by the direct transnasal approach.

Direct transnasal transsphenoidal microscope approach

Griffith and Veerapen [5] in 1987 and Cooke and Jones [6] in 1994 described a transnasal approach involving placing a long narrow speculum directly into the nostril all the way back to the sphenoid ostia on one side. By making the mucosal incision at the very back of the nasal airway passage, there is no disruption of the midline septum of the nose and, therefore, less discomfort and no chance of a postoperative septal perforation. After the sphenoid sinus is entered, an excellent view of the anterior wall of the sella is obtained. The sella is opened under microscopic vision and the dura is opened with a small scalpel. The tumor is removed under direct microscopic view. Lateral fluoroscopy is used to localize the sella in all cases, and frameless stereotactic navigation is used in all microadenomas and repeat surgeries. This approach generally allows gross total removal of macroadenomas and complete removal of microadenomas.

Intraoperative complications are rare but may include injury to the carotid artery, injury to the optic pathways, injury to the contents of the cavernous sinuses (cranial nerves III, IV, V, and VI), intracranial bleeding, and major CSF leakage. Early postoperative complications are uncommon but include hematoma formation in the tumor cavity (with compression of cranial nerves II, III, or IV), CSF rhinorrhea, and epistaxis.

Although the authors perform this approach without the assistance of an ears, nose, and throat (ENT) surgeon, many neurosurgeons who do fewer transsphenoidal procedures use the skills of a trained ENT nasal surgeon to assist with the approach to the sella.

Direct transnasal transsphenoidal endoscopic approach

The entire procedure just described using the operating microscope can be duplicated by using the endoscope. This method has the potential advantage of using smaller instruments but has the significant disadvantage that only two-dimensional visualization is possible. The operator looks at a flat screen monitor while manipulating instruments in the surgical field. Although it is true that a 30° to 45° angled endoscope sees further laterally in the sphenoid sinus, it does not provide three-dimensional imaging of the sella and the pituitary tumor.

The usefulness of an endoscope is in examining the skull base anatomy lateral and superior to the sella and occasionally in looking within a tumor bed for residual. With small microadenomas such as in Cushing's disease, the authors would question whether the view afforded by the endoscope is adequate to perform careful dissection within the pituitary gland.

Extended transsphenoidal approach

The transsphenoidal approach can be extended into the parasellar areas for more extensive tumor resection. Jho [7] and Dusick and colleagues [8] used the transnasal route for resection of meningiomas of the planum sphenoidale region. Mason and colleagues [9] and Dumont and colleagues [10] described a more extensive procedure in which the bone of the planum sphenoidale is removed and underlying dura and the diaphragma sellae are opened widely to expose the entire infundibulum and the optic chiasm. This procedure is used for cases in which there is a relatively small but hormonally active portion of the tumor attached to the pituitary stalk.

Transcranial approaches

Unilateral subfrontal approach

The right-sided unilateral subfrontal approach to the sella is the method most commonly used for a midline or eccentric right suprasellar lesion (Fig. 8). When the lesion is clearly eccentric to the left, a left subfrontal approach may be appropriate. The classic subfrontal approach involves a transcoronal scalp incision to avoid a visible forehead scar and allows the elevation of a frontal bone flap.

The frontal lobe is gently elevated and the optic nerve identified. Microdissection around the optic nerve is performed, and the tumor is usually evident beneath and medial to the optic nerve. Intrasellar lesions may be approached in the window between the optic nerves and in the window between the optic nerve and the ipsilateral carotid artery. Tumor can also be removed by way of the lamina terminalis if it has grown into the third ventricle or if the chiasm is prefixed. Care must be taken to avoid injury to the pituitary stalk and to the undersurface of the optic chiasm. After decompression of the optic pathways and maximum tumor removal, the retractors are removed and the craniotomy closed in the standard fashion.

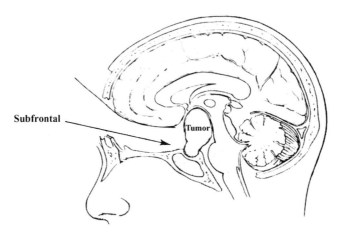

Fig. 8. Diagram showing subfrontal approach to a large sellar region tumor.

Pterional approach

The pterional approach involves adding a temporal exposure to the frontal approach described previously. This approach is not usually used for standard adenomas but can be particularly useful for the resection of complex craniopharyngiomas. This approach allows a more lateral exposure of the space between the ipsilateral optic nerve and the carotid artery and the space lateral to the carotid artery. It allows a view all the way back to the basilar artery, if needed. This approach is useful for choristomas, which tend to arise more posteriorly and extend back to the brainstem.

Choice of approach

Well over 90% of sellar and parasellar tumors can be approached transsphenoidally. The transcranial approaches described earlier should be used only for lesions that extend well into the middle fossa or have a large complex suprasellar component. When it is clear that a tumor is based above the pituitary, such as a craniopharyngioma or meningioma, the authors prefer the subfrontal or pterional approach.

How aggressive the surgeon should be is always a matter of judgment, both of the anatomy and the biology of the tumor. Because all macroadenomas are invasive of the surrounding dura, it is rarely, if ever, possible to obtain a 100% tumor removal. The goal is maximum safe removal—usually well over 95% of the tumor. Attempts to remove intracavernous portions of the tumor or strip tumor fragments from the optic nerves are likely to result in neurologic morbidity.

A few institutions have a magnetic resonance scanner available in the operating room. Because it is technically impossible for the MRI to clearly demarcate the residual tumor from the background of operative changes, the intraoperative MRI is limited. This intraoperative imaging technique may result in slightly greater tumor removal in a few patients, but it is not clear whether this changes short- or long-term results.

The decision to use an endoscope during tumor removal is entirely up to the judgment and bias of the surgeon. The authors prefer to rely primarily on the three-dimensional view of the operating microscope, but others are satisfied with the two-dimensional view afforded by the endoscope. The rigid endoscope is a handy adjunct to the microscope during surgery for tumors that are lateral in the sphenoid sinus. The authors keep it available during surgery but do not use it routinely.

The decision to use frameless stereotactic guidance during surgery also depends on the comfort and experience of the surgeon in combination with the size and location of the tumor. An experienced pituitary surgeon needs this guidance less often, but it is a tremendous help when the sella is small and the anatomy of the sphenoid sinus is complex. It is recommended for routine use by surgeons who perform this operation only occasionally.

Indications for surgery

Ideally, every individual considered for surgery would be evaluated by an endocrinologist and a neurosurgeon trained in pituitary surgery. Although there are always a few patients who fall in the "gray areas" and can be followed carefully or undergo tumor resection, most patients provide clear indications to their physicians as to whether they need surgery. Sometimes, surgery is necessary just to reach a diagnosis. The authors have seen situations in which metastatic tumors, craniopharyngiomas, meningiomas, and abscesses have mimicked pituitary adenomas.

Pituitary adenomas

Pituitary adenomas are, with rare exception, benign lesions. At the initial encounter, it is important to reassure the patient that the tumor they have is not cancerous and not a tumor within the brain.

As a rule, pituitary adenomas are slow-growing tumors. Although no exact data are available, the average doubling rate of these rumors is around 1 to 2 years. The indications for surgical treatment and the aggressiveness of surgery are determined by a number of factors, including the functional nature of the tumor.

Nonfunctioning adenomas

The main reason to remove a nonfunctioning adenoma is to alleviate or prevent its mass effects, which can be neurologic (eg, compression of the optic chiasm) or endocrinologic (hypopituitarism). Even when the latter effect is present, it is important to weigh the potential surgical risks in a given patient (including even further worsening of hypopituitarism) versus the benefits of restoring the pituitary function because replacement therapy is usually easy.

Headache is believed to be due to the stretching of the diaphragma sellae by an intrasellar mass. Thus, a small tumor, not distorting the upper contour of the pituitary gland, is unlikely to cause headaches.

Invasion of the cavernous sinus by a pituitary adenoma rarely produces ophthalmoplegia. Injury to the cranial nerves of the cavernous sinuses is more likely to happen with sudden pituitary apoplexy or may suggest a meningioma or metastasis as an etiology. Unless a schwannoma of cranial nerve V is suspected, no attempt should be made to remove tissue from within the cavernous sinus because it will likely lead to permanent ophthalmoplegia.

Thus, the strongest indication for surgical decompression of a nonfunctioning pituitary adenoma is threatened vision. This situation usually requires a suprasellar expansion of the tumor in excess of 1 to 1.5 cm above the level of the diaphragma sella.

Although gross total removal of tumor is always a goal, significant debulking of the tumor is usually sufficient to decompress the optic chiasm, thus achieving the major objective of surgical intervention.

Incidentally found asymptomatic tumors often pose a treatment dilemma. The decision to operate depends on the size of the tumor, the function of the pituitary, and the age of the patient.

In all instances, avoidance of surgically induced neurologic complications is paramount, even at the expense of incomplete tumor removal.

Functional adenomas

Cushing's disease

Virtually all patients with proven or suspected pituitary-dependent hypercortisolism need to have exploration of their pituitary. It is fortunate that most of these patients have microadenomas. Interventions for these microadenomas require the highest degree of surgical skills. Because there is no reliable medical therapy for Cushing's disease and the mortality and the morbidity of incompletely controlled disease are very high, it is ideal that the surgeon removes the entire tumor during the first operation. Approximately 20% to 30% of patients have tumors that are too small to be detected by MRI and that require multiple careful sections of the gland and a keen understanding of which small areas look and feel different from normal pituitary tissue.

Residual hypercortisolism justifies repeat surgical intervention to the point of total hypophysectomy. The development of drugs capable of inhibiting tumorous corticotropin secretion may alter the existing treatment paradigm.

Acromegaly

Most acromegalic patients have macroadenomas. Although surgery only results in complete endocrine remission in less than 50% of patients, it provides a very significant fall in growth hormone and insulin-like growth factor-I levels in all patients. Even a partial fall in hormone levels improves subsequent response to other treatments [11]. Primary medical therapy with somatostatin analogs can normalize growth hormone hypersecretion and effect tumor shrinkage [12,13] and can be used in selected cases such as when a patient refuses surgery or is in poor general health, precluding anesthesia.

The authors believe that surgery must be recommended as a first-line treatment to virtually all patients who have newly diagnosed acromegaly. A surgeon should strive for an as complete resection of the tumor as possible, without risking neurologic damage.

Prolactinoma

Careful history and clinical examination are mandatory to exclude non-tumorous causes of hyperprolactinemia (medications, severe primary hypothyroidism, chest wall lesions, and so forth).

It is important to establish a correct diagnosis of true prolactinomas because these tumors should not, as a general rule, be treated surgically. Instead, medical therapy with dopamine agonists should be offered. The authors prefer to recommend initial treatment with dopamine agonists, even in patients who have microadenomas, because the recurrence rate is high after surgery.

Surgery, however, may be indicated in patients who are unresponsive to or intolerant of dopamine agonists. Some prolactinomas may contain large cystic or hemorrhagic areas that are unlikely to respond to medications with a degree of shrinkage that is sufficient to decompress the optic chiasm.

Thyrotropinomas

Hyperthyroidism due to a thyroid-stimulating hormone secreting adenoma is a rare disease. Thus, there are no universal agreed-on standards of care of these lesions. Thyrotropinomas are sensitive to somatostatin analogs, and this medication can be used as a primary or postoperative modality. In general, when the tumor is surgically accessible, it should be removed or at least debulked. Most of these tumors are macroadenomas and need postoperative medical therapy.

Pituitary apoplexy

Pituitary apoplexy refers to acute infarction (and often associated hemorrhage) of a pituitary adenoma. As a rule, tumors undergoing apoplexy are substantial macroadenomas, and the acute expansion of tumor size is frequently accompanied by severe headache, vomiting, altered consciousness, visual-field defects to the point of blindness, and ophthalmoplegia. Most of these patients have severe hypopituitarism on admission. In some patients, initial CT or MRI reveals massive intratumoral hemorrhage (bright on noncontrast studies), whereas in other patients, the tumor appears ischemic (iso- or hypointense on noncontrast studies).

The appropriate management requires urgent administration of steroids in stress doses, fluid administration, and pain control. The role of urgent surgery is controversial: some studies found better neurologic recovery after pituitary decompression done within hours to days after the onset of clinical symptoms [14–16], whereas other studies did not [17,18]. Taking into account potential dire consequences of apoplexy (permanent visual compromise) and the low risk of transsphenoidal decompression, it is prudent to evacuate the accessible part of the tumor to relieve the intrasellar pressure as soon as medically possible in patients who have obvious (especially rapidly progressing) cranial nerve deficits.

Craniopharyngioma

When a craniopharyngioma is suggested by MRI, most patients require surgery and are operated on with an intracranial approach to their tumor. Often, these tumors are very adherent to the undersurface of the optic chiasm or the third ventricle, and attempt at complete removal may result in additional loss of vision or a significant neurologic deficit.

Some craniopharyngiomas may be approached surgically by way of the transsphenoidal approach, especially when they are largely cystic and have extended down into the sella. It is also possible to use the "extended transsphenoidal" approach described earlier to remove tumors that are partially solid and even extend up into the region of the third ventricle. The same guidelines apply to being cautious about adherence to the chiasm and third ventricular wall.

Most patients need a course of radiation after incomplete removal of a craniopharyngioma. In children, it is wise to postpone radiation as long as possible, even if repeated surgery is needed.

Meningioma

Meningiomas are benign tumors and can be followed with serial imaging if they are not large and are not causing symptoms. It is unfortunate that many tumors in the parasellar area cause significant compression of the optic pathways and require surgery to decompress these structures. Most meningiomas are approached intracranially, again usually by the subfrontal or pterional approach. Most of these tumors can be removed in a gross total fashion because they are dural based and do not protrude into the third ventricle. The goal of surgery is to reach a diagnosis and safely decompress the visual pathways. Some of these tumors invade the optic foramina and compress the optic nerves in this area. It is often necessary to carefully drill away the overlying bone of the canal to remove the entire tumor.

Meningiomas that arise from within the dura of the cavernous sinus region are usually radiated without a biopsy. Modern MRI can provide an extremely accurate diagnosis, and radiation is effective in controlling tumor growth in most cases.

Cysts

A number of patients have purely cystic lesions within the sella. When these lesions are small and the pituitary function is normal, they should be followed with MRI. If they enlarge or cause symptoms, then transsphenoidal surgery is usually effective in draining the cyst fluid and in reaching a diagnosis. It is important to keep in mind that when a craniopharyngioma or abscess is suspected, surgery is indicated irrespective of the size of the lesion.

Stalk and hypothalmic lesions

These lesions can be approached only through an intracranial approach, with panhypopituitarism being an almost inevitable consequence. Thus, the decision to operate on such lesions should never be reached lightly. Only tumors that are strongly suspected to be malignant or are severely affecting vision should be considered for surgical intervention. Small stalk lesions are often found incidentally and rarely progress. Close follow-up with MRI is mandatory.

Metastasis

Metastases are rare and often not suspected until surgery has been performed. Any unknown progressive or symptomatic lesion must undergo biopsy, usually transsphenoidally. When a frozen section during surgery suggests a metastatic malignant tumor, surgery is usually terminated and adjunctive treatments are considered.

Reoperation

A decision to reoperate on a pituitary tumor requires careful integration of all the available information. If an experienced surgeon did not accomplish complete tumor removal because of its invasiveness, fibrotic consistency, or excessive vascularity, then further aggressive surgery is unlikely to be successful and may result in significant morbidity.

Modest recurrence of a nonfunctional macroadneoma in the years following initial surgery favors radiation therapy [19]. Large recurrence, especially with visual impairment, requires repeat tumor debulking before radiation therapy.

Patients who have failed surgery for Cushing's disease or have recurrence of the disease are often candidates for repeat surgery. If hyperplasia is diagnosed and the patient is not in remission, then complete hypophysectomy may be indicated. Cushing's disease patients who have had successful resection of a microadenoma and experience a recurrence often benefit from reoperation.

The authors rarely reoperate for treatment of continued biochemical evidence of acromegaly and rely on medical treatment or radiation therapy.

Likewise, most patients who have persistent prolactinomas may benefit from adjustment of medical therapy or occasionally from radiation.

References

[1] Ahmed S, Elsheikh M, Stratton IM, et al. Outcome of transphenoidal surgery for acromegaly and its relationship to surgical experience. Clin Endocrinol (Oxf) 1999;50(5):557–9.

[2] Ciric I, Ragin A, Baumgartner C, et al. Complications of transsphenoidal surgery: results of a national survey, review of the literature, and personal experience. Neurosurgery 1997; 40(2):225–36.

[3] Lüdecke DK, Abe T. Transsphenoidal microsurgery for newly diagnosed acromegaly: a personal view after more than 1,000 operations. Neuroendocrinology 2006;83:230–9.

[4] Shimon I, Cohen ZR, Ram Z, et al. Transsphenoidal surgery for acromegaly: endocrinological follow-up of 98 patients. Neurosurgery 2001;48:1239–45.

[5] Griffith HB, Veerapen R. A direct transnasal approach to the sphenoid sinus. Technical note. J Neurosurg 1987;66:140–2.

[6] Cooke RS, Jones RA. Experience with the direct transnasal transsphenoidal approach to the pituitary fossa. Br J Neurosurg 1994;8:193–6.

[7] Jho HD. Endoscopic endonasal approach to the optic nerve: a technical note. Minim Invasive Neurosurg 2001;44(4):190–3.

[8] Dusick JR, Esposito F, Kelly DF, et al. The extended direct endonasal transsphenoidal approach for nonadenomatous suprasellar tumors. J Neurosurg 2005;102(5):832–41.

[9] Mason RB, Nieman LK, Doppman JL, et al. Selective excision of adenomas originating in or extending into the pituitary stalk with preservation of pituitary function. J Neurosurg 1997; 87:343–51.

[10] Dumont AS, Kanter AS, Jane JA Jr, et al. Extended transsphenoidal approach. Front Horm Res 2006;34:29–45.

[11] Jallad RS, Musolino NR, Kodaira S, et al. Does partial surgical tumour removal influence the response to octreotide-LAR in acromegalic patients previously resistant to the somatostatin analogue? Clin Endocrinol (Oxf) 2007;67(2):310–5.

[12] Barkan AL, Lloyd RV, Chandler WF, et al. Preoperative treatment of acromegaly with long-acting somatostatin analog SMS 201-995: shrinkage of invasive pituitary macroadenomas and improved surgical remission rate. J Clin Endocrinol Metab 1988;67(5):1040–8.

[13] Bevan JS, Atkin SL, Atkinson AB, et al. Primary medical therapy for acromegaly: an open, prospective, multicenter study of the effects of subcutaneous and intramuscular slow-release octreotide on growth hormone, insulin-like growth factor-I, and tumor size. J Clin Endocrinol Metab 2002;87(10):4554–63.

[14] Khaldi M, Ben Hamouda K, Jemel H, et al. Pituitary apoplexy. Report of 25 patients. Neurochirurgie 2006;52(4):330–8.

[15] Chuang CC, Chang CN, Wei KC, et al. Surgical treatment for severe visual compromised patients after pituitary apoplexy. J Neurooncol 2006;80(1):39–47.

[16] Dubuisson AS, Beckers A, Stevenaert A. Classical pituitary tumour apoplexy: clinical features, management and outcomes in a series of 24 patients. Clin Neurol Neurosurg 2007; 109(1):63–70.

[17] Gruber A, Clayton J, Kumar S, et al. Pituitary apoplexy: retrospective review of 30 patients—is surgical intervention always necessary? Br J Neurosurg 2006;20(6):379–85.

[18] Sibal L, Ball SG, Connolly V, et al. Pituitary apoplexy: a review of clinical presentation, management and outcome in 45 cases. Pituitary 2004;7(3):157–63.

[19] Park P, Chandler WF, Barkan AL, et al. The role of radiation therapy after surgical resection of nonfunctional pituitary macroadenomas. Neurosurgery 2004;55(1):100–7.

ELSEVIER
SAUNDERS

Endocrinol Metab Clin N Am
37 (2008) 67–99

ENDOCRINOLOGY
AND METABOLISM
CLINICS
OF NORTH AMERICA

Hyperprolactinemia and Prolactinomas

Tatiana Mancini, MD[a],
Felipe F. Casanueva, MD, PhD[b],
Andrea Giustina, MD[c,d],*

[a]*Internal Medicine, San Marino Hospital, 47899, Republic of San Marino*
[b]*Department of Medicine, Endocrine Division,*
Complejo Hospitalario Universitario de Santiago, University of Santiago, and Centro de
Investigación Biomédica en Rede Obesity-Nutrition, Santiago de Compostela, Spain
[c]*Department of Medical and Surgical Sciences, University of Brescia, 25125 Brescia, Italy*
[d]*Endocrine Service, Montichiari Hospital, 25018 Montichiari, Italy*

Neuroregulation and physiology of prolactin

Prolactin (PRL) is a protein hormone secreted by the lactotroph cells of the pituitary [1,2]. The gene encoding for PRL is unique; in people, it is located on chromosome 6. After removal of the signal peptide, the mature form of the protein contains 199 residues (199 kilodaltons [kDa]) [1,3]. We now know that PRL physiology is not as simple as previously described. In fact, PRL is not only synthesized in the pituitary gland but by the central nervous system (CNS), the immune system, the uterus, the placenta, and the mammary gland. Biochemically, PRL appears in several posttranslational forms ranging from size variants to chemical modification, such as phosphorylation or glycosylation. Phosphorylated PRL constitutes 5% to 30% of the PRL released by the pituitary, but its function is still debated. In fact, it seems to be able to have agonistic and antagonistic properties [4,5]. It has also been described that there may be some proteolytic cleavage of PRL by means of cathepsin D (6–16-kDa fragments) or by means of kallikrein (22-kDa fragments) [2,6]. Recently, an antiangiogenic 16-kDA PRL has been described [7].

PRL is secreted in a pulsatile manner, but it also has a circadian fluctuation because its levels are high during non–rapid eye movement (REM) sleep [8]. The most important physiologic stimuli are suckling, stress, and increased levels of ovarian steroids, primarily estrogens [2]. In response, the hypothalamus elaborates a host of prolactin-releasing factors (PRFs)

* Corresponding author.
E-mail address: a.giustina@libero.it (A. Giustina).

0889-8529/08/$ - see front matter © 2008 Elsevier Inc. All rights reserved.
doi:10.1016/j.ecl.2007.10.013

and prolactin-inhibiting factors (PIFs). Lactotrophs are also regulated by PRFs and PIFs released from neighboring cells (paracrine regulation) or from the lactotrophs themselves (autocrine regulation) [2]. The general view is that lactotrophs have spontaneously high secretory activity. Therefore, pituitary PRL secretion is under a tonic and predominantly inhibitory control exerted by the hypothalamus. Dopamine, the most important PIF, is present in the portal blood in sufficient concentrations to inhibit PRL release. Dopamine suppresses PRL synthesis and secretion by means of the D_2 subtype dopamine receptors. These actions constitute the physiologic basis for the therapeutic effect of dopamine agonists in hyperprolactinemia [9].

As shown in Fig. 1, the regulation of PRL secretion is quite complex because it involves many substances, including neurotransmitters, neurohormones, neuropeptides, metabolic substrates, and systemic hormonal signals. The physiologic relevance of most of these reported mechanisms, which have been demonstrated in vitro or in experimental animals, is uncertain.

Neurotransmitters regulate PRL secretion through the CNS, particularly at the hypothalamic level, and at the level of the tuberoinfundibular dopaminergic system (TIDA) in most cases. The inhibitory neurotransmitters, such as serotonin and norepinephrine, increase PRL secretion by means of a decrease in TIDA activity. Adrenergic modulation, mediated at the β-receptors by norepinephrine and epinephrine, plays an important role in stress-induced PRL secretion [10]. Acetylcholine, conversely, causes a decrease in serum PRL levels through the TIDA stimulation [11]. Among hypothalamic neurohormones, thyrotropin-releasing hormone (TRH), oxytocin, and vasoactive intestinal peptide (VIP) are well-known PRFs, whereas dopamine is a well-known PIF. Some "lactotroph responsiveness factors" have been described and can be defined as substances that alter the response of lactotrophs to PIFs or PRFs: α-melanocyte-stimulating hormone (MSH), for example, decreases the response of lactotrophs to high dopamine dose [12]. Neuropeptides, such as galanin, which are largely present in hypothalamic neurons, are also abundantly expressed in the anterior lobe of the pituitary, determining an increase in PRL secretion. Galanin is regulated by dopamine and somatostatin (inhibition), and TRH (stimulation) and estrogens have a positive effect on galanin gene expression in the hypothalamus [13,14]. Finally, it is well known that somatostatin inhibits not only growth hormone (GH) but the baseline and induced PRL secretion in vitro in PRL-producing cell lines [15]. Somatostatin neurons receive abundant efferent connections from galanin, neurotensin, neuropeptide Y, γ-aminobutyric acid (GABA), serotonin, enkephalin, substance P, TRH, and the catecholaminergic system [16]. Estradiol upregulates SST2 receptor gene expression in rat prolactinoma cells [2]. Conversely, GABA is partially responsible for the nondopaminergic PIF activity. The activity of GABAergic neurons is strongly affected by gonadal steroids [17]. Finally, relative to metabolic substrates, hypoglycemia and arginine stimulate PRL secretion [2].

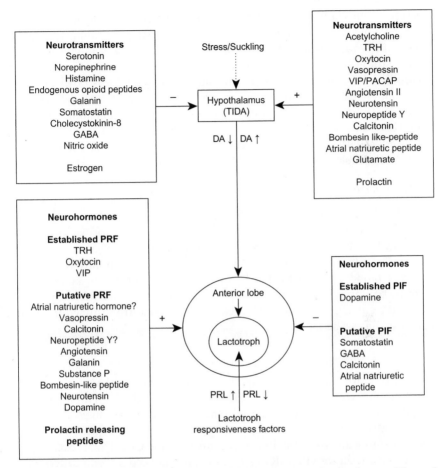

Fig. 1. Regulation of PRL secretion. The most important physiologic stimuli are suckling and stress (*broken arrow*) and the increased levels of ovarian steroids, primarily estrogens. The inhibitory agents, such as serotonin, norepinephrine, endogenous opioids, galanin, and estrogens, promote an increase of PRL secretion as a result of diminishing tuberoinfundibular dopaminergic system (TIDA) activity. Conversely, the stimulatory neurotransmitters tend to decrease PRL secretion as a result of increasing output of TIDA neurons. The final common pathways are the production of PRL-inhibiting factors (PIFs), such as dopamine, and PRL-releasing factor (PRFs), such as thyrotropin-releasing hormone (TRH), oxytocin, and vasoactive intestinal peptide (VIP). The lactotroph response depends on the action of "lactotroph responsiveness factors," which are substances that alter lactotrophs' response to PIF or PRF. DA, dopamine; PACAP, pituitary adenylate cyclase-activating polypeptide.

Glucocorticoids seem to have an inhibitory role on PRL and GH [18] secretion. These hormones stimulate the differentiation of somatotrophs but suppress that of lactotrophs in the fetal rat pituitary gland [19]. In rats, plasma levels of PRL increase significantly after adrenalectomy, whereas the effect of adrenalectomy can be reversed by the administration of corticosteroids [20]. Long-term elevation of the serum glucocorticoid levels by chronic administration of corticotropin (ACTH) or hydrocortisone or by prolonged stress decreases opioid-induced PRL secretion [21]. Estrogens and thyroid hormones have opposite effects on PRL synthesis and release. Estradiol acts at the pituitary level by increasing the secretion of PRL, controlling PRL gene expression, and modifying its sensitivity to physiologic stimuli but also within the hypothalamus by inhibiting the activity of all three populations of hypothalamic neuroendocrine dopaminergic neurons [22]. Low thyroxine (T_4) and triiodothyronine (T_3) levels increase TRH-induced PRL secretion, whereas high T_4 and T_3 levels inhibit PRL mRNA accumulation and release [23].

Prolactin feedback

PRL affects its own secretion by regulating its own hypothalamic control through a short-loop feedback mechanism. Elevation of serum PRL increases hypothalamic dopamine synthesis and its concentration in portal blood. The rate of dopamine synthesis is reduced by hypophysectomy or lowering blood levels of PRL by bromocriptine. Neurotensin and GABA seem to be implicated in PRL feedback. It seems also that PRL, together with VIP, galanin, and endothelin, can regulate lactotroph function in an autocrine/paracrine manner [2].

Prolactin receptors

PRL receptors are present in the mammary gland and the ovary, two of the best-characterized sites of PRL action but also in multiple tissues, including the pituitary gland, heart, lung, thymus, spleen, liver, pancreas, kidney, adrenal gland, uterus, skeletal muscle, and skin [24]. Interestingly, PRL receptors are also found in several areas of the CNS [2,25]. Activation of prolactin receptor (PRL-R) involves ligand-induced sequential receptor dimerization driven by the PRL molecule containing two binding sites. The formation of the initial hormone-receptor complex induces the interaction of binding site 2 on the same PRL molecule with a second PRL-R. Then, the tyrosine kinase termed *Janus kinase 2* (Jak 2), which is associated with the intracellular domain of PRL-R, is activated. Jak 2 kinases transphosphorylate each other and phosphorylate the Tyr residue of the PRL-R itself. At this point, the phosphotyrosine of Jak 2 can serve as a docking site for stat-1, a member of the signal transducer and activator of transcription (STAT) protein family. The activation of PRL-R also induces the activation of the mitogen-activated protein kinase (MAPK) and Src kinase [2].

Causes of hyperprolactinemia

The causes of hyperprolactinemia can be divided simply into physiologic, pharmacologic, and pathologic causes. Normal PRL levels are less than

25 µg/L in women and less than 20 µg/L in men, but the normal range should be adjusted for the specific assay used [26]. For the initial determination, to avoid the effect of pulsatile secretion and venipuncture stress, two to three samples separated by at least 15 to 20 minutes should be drawn after obtaining venous access. The sampling should be performed at least 1 hour after awakening or eating, with the patient in a recumbent position [26,27].

Pregnancy is the most common cause of hyperprolactinemic amenorrhea, and there is a 10-fold increase in PRL during the third trimester. Normal lactation is also associated with a marked elevation of serum PRL. PRL levels increase after exercise, meals, and stimulation of the chest wall. Physical and psychologic stress increases the secretion of PRL, even if the levels rarely exceed 40 µg/L [27,28]. As predicted from the physiologic dopaminergic inhibition of PRL secretion, treatment with dopamine receptor antagonist drugs commonly induce hyperprolactinemia, with levels rarely exceeding 150 µg/L. These drugs include antipsychotics (phenothiazines, butyrophenones, and atypical antipsychotics), antidepressants (tricyclic, monoamine oxidase [MAO] inhibitors, and selective serotonin reuptake inhibitors [SSRIs]), opiates, cocaine, gastrointestinal medication (metoclopramide, domperidone, and ranitidine), and antihypertensives (verapamil, methyldopa, and reserpine) [29,30]. PRL levels may also be mildly elevated after the administration of estrogens. Similarly, occupational exposure to heavy metals and some over-the-counter herbal or alternative remedies may cause an increase in PRL (Box 1) [30–38]. For this reason, a comprehensive drug history of the hyperprolactinemic patient is essential. To determine if treatment with a given drug is the cause of hyperprolactinemia, it has been suggested to withdraw it for at least 72 hours if this can be done safely or to switch to an alternative drug.

When the drug cannot be stopped, MRI of the sella should be performed, especially in patients who have neurologic disturbances, to exclude a mass lesion [26,39].

To rule out pathologic causes of hyperprolactinemia, it is important to evaluate kidney and liver function and exclude hypothyroidism and polycystic ovary syndrome [26,27]. After excluding these causes, MRI of the sella should be performed. Hyperprolactinemia in the presence of a pituitary adenoma is consistent but not unequivocally diagnostic of a prolactinoma, because any hypothalamic-pituitary lesion that compresses the pituitary stalk may increase PRL levels (disconnection hyperprolactinemia). Mixed GH- and PRL-secreting tumors are well recognized. Rarely, cosecretion of thyroid-stimulating hormone (TSH) or ACTH is observed. Occasionally, prolactinomas may be a component of MEN 1. Hyperprolactinemia may be also found in the empty sella syndrome [40]. Other rare pituitary masses, such as primary pituitary lymphoma [41], may cause hyperprolactinemia. Hypothalamic lesions (eg, sarcoidosis, histiocytosis) are also rare causes of hyperprolactinemia (see Box 1) [28]. Subjects in whom a cause of hyperprolactinemia is not identified are defined as having idiopathic hyperprolactinemia. In one third of these

Box 1. Causes of hyperprolactinemia

Hypothalamic diseases
Tumors (craniopharyngioma, meningioma, dysgerminoma, third
    ventricle tumor, cyst, glioma, hamartoma, and metastasis)
Infiltrative diseases (sarcoidosis, tuberculosis, Langerhans' cell
    histiocytosis, and eosinophilic granuloma)
Cranial irradiation
Vascular abnormalities
Pseudotumor cerebri
Genetic syndromes (multiple endocrine neoplasia syndrome
    [MEN], Carney complex, McCune-Albright syndrome)

Pituitary diseases
Functioning and nonfunctioning adenomas, MEN 1
Empty sella syndrome
Lymphocytic hypophysitis
Primitive tumors (meningioma, germinoma, metastasis,
    and lymphoma) and metastasis
Infiltrative diseases (giant cell granuloma and sarcoidosis)

Drugs
Neuroleptics (phenothiazines, butyrophenones, and atypical
    antipsychotics)
Antidepressants (tricyclic and tetracyclic antidepressants, MAO
    inhibitors, SSRIs, and others)
Antihypertensive medications (verapamil, methyldopa,
    and reserpine)
Gastrointestinal medications (metoclopramide, domperidone,
    and H_2 blockers)
Opiates
Cocaine
Estrogens
Protease inhibitors

Heavy metals and other chemical substances
Manganese
Organic mercury
Lead
Cadmium
Uranium
Arsenic
Barium
Chemicals (styrene and perchloroethylene)
Anesthetic gases

Medicinal herbs
Echinacea purpurea
Hypericum perforatum
Purariae isoflavone
Cimicifuga racemosa
Acacia nilotica ssp *adansonii*

Neurogenic
Chest wall lesions
Spinal cord lesions
Breast stimulation
Physical or psychologic stress

Other
Hypothyroidism
Chronic renal failure
Cirrhosis
Adrenal insufficiency
Pseudocyesis
Polycystic ovary syndrome

patients, during a follow-up period of 5 to 6 years, the levels of PRL return to the normal range, whereas they remain unchanged in nearly half of these patients [42,43]. In one study, a pituitary adenoma was observed only in 10% of patients who had idiopathic hyperprolactinemia during a follow-up period of 6 years [42]. In the past, TRH and other dynamic tests have been used for the differential diagnosis of idiopathic versus pathologic hyperprolactinemia; however, because of their low diagnostic power, they are now predominantly considered research tools.

Prolactinoma

Epidemiology

The prevalence of hyperprolactinemia in women with secondary amenorrhea or oligoamenorrhea is estimated to be 10% to 25%. Hyperprolactinemia is noted in approximately 30% of women with galactorrhea or infertility and in 75% of those with both amenorrhea and galactorrhea [44,45].

At the same time, pituitary tumors seem to be common in the general population, as observed not only in autopsy series but in radiologic imaging studies. In autopsy series, the generally accepted mean prevalence is approximately 10%, and a similarly high rate has been reported by Hall and colleagues [46] in a cohort of healthy individuals submitted to MRI evaluation.

Prolactinomas are the most common pituitary adenomas and account for approximately 40% of pituitary tumors, with an estimated prevalence in the adult population of 100 per million [27]. Recently, however, Daly and colleagues [47] found a much higher prevalence of 775 per million in a tightly defined geographic area in Liege, Belgium. In contrast to autopsy and radiologic studies, the study by Daly and colleagues [47] included only patients who had a previous definitive diagnosis of pituitary adenoma (Table 1).

The prevalence of prolactinoma varies with age and gender, occurring most frequently in women between 20 and 50 years old, with a gender ratio of 10:1. Microprolactinomas are more frequent than macroprolactinomas in women, whereas macroprolactinomas are more frequent in men. One possible explanation for the increased prevalence of microprolactinomas in women may be related to the fact that the clinical presentation is more evident. Women, in fact, present with the classic amenorrhea-galactorrhea syndrome, whereas men frequently ignore the symptoms of impotence and decreased libido caused by hyperprolactinemia and the diagnosis is often based on signs of compression. A more aggressive course of prolactinoma in men has been hypothesized but not definitively demonstrated [50].

After the fifth decade of life, the prevalence of prolactinomas is similar in both genders [52]. In the pediatric and adolescent years, prolactinomas are rare but represent approximately half of all pituitary adenomas. Rarely, young subjects with hyperprolactinemia may be affected by the McCune-Albright syndrome, characterized by the clinical triad of polystotic or monostotic fibrous dysplasia, café-au-lait macules, and endocrine abnormalities, such as GH hypersecretion [53,54]. The female preponderance seen in adults is maintained in children.

Pituitary carcinomas are rare. Only approximately 140 cases have been reported in the literature to date, and 47 of these are prolactinomas. Malignant prolactinomas should not be confused with aggressive prolactinomas, which are a more frequent finding; the differential diagnosis between the two is based on the presence of metastatic lesions. The prognosis of malignant prolactinoma is poor, with only 50% of patients described in the literature surviving more than 1 year [55].

Table 1
Epidemiologic data concerning prevalence, gender, and dimensional distribution of prolactinomas among pituitary tumors

Type of study [reference]	Prevalence prolactinoma/pituitary tumors	Gender (F/M)	Dimension (micro/macro)
Cross-sectional [47]	45/68	36/9	30/10 (5 not available)
Retrospective [48]	182/504	—	—
Retrospective [49]	11/75	9/2	—
Prospective [50]		130/74	97/107
Retrospective [51]	96/371	66/30	46/46 (4 not available)
Retrospective [52]	39%	F > M	—

Abbreviations: F, female; M, male.

Genetically, prolactinoma may present in the setting of MEN 1. Overall, 22% of patients who have MEN-1 develop a prolactinoma. Macroadenomas seem to be more frequent (84% versus 24%), and normalization of PRL levels is less frequent than in sporadic cases (44% versus 90%) [56,57]. Asymptomatic hyperprolactinemia associated with elevations of GH and insulin-like growth factor-I (IGF-I) is present in up to 75% of patients who have Carney complex, an autosomal dominant syndrome characterized by the complex of spotty skin pigmentation, myxomas, endocrine overactivity, and schwannomas [58]. Familiar prolactinomas unrelated to MEN-1 and Carney complex have been also described [58–60]. Germline aryl hydrocarbon receptor interacting protein (AIP) gene mutations have been described in familial isolated pituitary adenoma (FIPA). These mutations are less frequent in prolactinomas or mixed GH/PRL-secreting tumors than in pure GH-secreting tumors [61].

Pathogenesis

Although prolactinomas are the most frequent pituitary tumors, they are rarely surgically removed; therefore, the few published molecular biology studies mainly describe aggressive and atypical prolactinomas. Several clinical observations suggest the existence of a multistep process in prolactinoma pathogenesis. Long-term follow-up of patients who have microprolactinoma suggest that these tumors have a low, if any, tendency for growth over time. Conversely, some macroprolactinomas that seem to be resistant to any therapeutic approach are characterized by a tendency to rapid growth [62].

Few proto-oncogenes have been found to be mutated or overexpressed in prolactinoma. The exception is represented by the point mutation (Gly12Val) in the RAS gene, a gene coding for guanosine triphosphate (GTP)–binding proteins, which was identified in one lethal prolactinoma [63]. Pituitary tumor-transforming gene (PTTG), a novel oncogene that is expressed at high levels in most pituitary tumors as compared with normal pituitary samples, is increased only in animal prolactinoma generated by estrogen treatment [64]. More interesting for the pathogenesis of human prolactinoma is the mutation at the C-terminal peptide of the PTTG1, the human PPTG homologue that inactivates PRL gene suppression [65].

Different growth factors and receptors have been studied in the pathogenesis of pituitary tumors. Experimental work in animals has shown that estradiol exposure leads to prolactinoma formation through events involving dopamine D_2 receptors, transforming growth factor-β (TGFβ) isoforms and their receptors and factors secondary to TGFβ action. These studies also demonstrate that TGF-β and basic fibroblast growth factor interact to facilitate the communication between lactotrophs and folliculostellate cells that is necessary for the mitogenic action of estradiol. The downstream signaling that governs lactotroph cell proliferation involves activation of the MAPK p44/42-dependent pathway [66]. No direct relation between the exposure to estrogens, even at high doses, and the occurrence of prolactinoma has been clearly demonstrated, however [62]. Several in vitro and in vivo studies suggest that lactotroph cells secrete nerve growth factor (NGF) together with PRL. The decrease of NGF with the normalization of PRL levels induced by cabergoline, its absence in resistant prolactinomas, and the restoration of the responsiveness to dopamine agonists in resistant prolactinomas through NGF administration suggest a role of the NGF loop in the pathogenesis of prolactinoma with different degrees of malignancy [67,68]. Finally, the aberrant expression of an N-terminally truncated FGF receptor-4 has been also reported in prolactinoma [69]. High-mobility group A nonhistone chromosomal proteins (HMGAs), which are involved in the determination of chromatin structure, have been found to be overexpressed in human prolactinoma, especially in the "non–drug responders" [70].

Diagnosis

Once the diagnosis of hyperprolactinemia is established, secondary causes should be ruled out by a careful clinical history (with particular attention to drug treatment), physical examination, pregnancy test, routine biochemical analysis (kidney and liver function), and TSH determination [26]. There are two potential pitfalls in the biochemical diagnosis of hyperprolactinemia: the presence of macroprolactin and the so-called "hook effect." Macroprolactin is a complex of PRL with, generally, an IgG antibody. Hyperprolactinemia results from a reduced clearance of this complex that is a cause of potential "false-positive" results [71]. Macroprolactin presents reduced bioactivity and is not detected by all PRL assays. For confirmation of macroprolactinemia, polyethylene glycol precipitation and, recently, ultrafiltration are the most practical methods. Alternatively, gel filtration chromatography can be used but is not suitable for routine use [72,73]. Whether macroprolactin should be measured in patients with signs or symptoms of hyperprolactinemia is still controversial, but it seems reasonable to ascertain its presence in patients with moderately elevated PRL levels and less typical symptoms, such as headaches or diminished libido in the presence of regular menses [26,74]. The hook effect can be observed in some cases of giant prolactinomas. The extremely high PRL levels cause antibody saturation in the two-site assays, resulting in an artifactually low reported value. This artifact can be eliminated by 1:100 dilution of serum samples. It has been recommended to exclude the hook effect in all new patients who have a large macroadenoma with normal to mildly elevated PRL levels [75]. Dynamic tests have been largely abandoned in the differential diagnosis of hyperprolactinemia (Fig. 2) [28].

After excluding potential secondary causes of hyperprolactinemia, gadolinium-enhanced MRI should be performed to confirm the diagnosis of prolactinoma. CT with intravenous contrast enhancement may be used if MRI is unavailable or contraindicated, even if is less effective than MRI

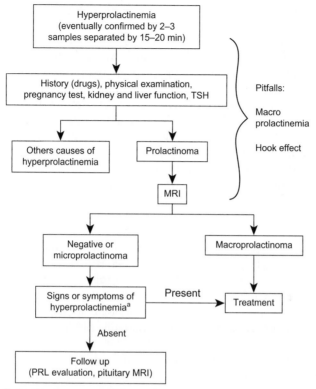

Fig. 2. Diagnosis and management of prolactinoma: algorithm. Once the diagnosis of hyperprolactinemia is established (keeping in mind the two potential pitfalls in the biochemical diagnosis, which are the stress effect and macroprolactinemia), secondary causes should first be ruled out by a careful clinical history (with particular attention to drugs), physical examination, pregnancy test, routine biochemical analysis (kidney and liver function), and thyroid-stimulating hormone (TSH) determination. Subsequently, gadolinium-enhanced MRI should be performed to confirm the diagnosis of prolactinoma (in the presence of a macroadenoma with low PRL levels, the presence of the so-called "hook effect" should be ruled out). Therapy is always advisable for all macroadenomas, whereas indications for treatment of microadenomas include infertility, bothersome galactorrhea, long-lasting hypogonadism, alteration in pubertal development, and prevention of bone loss. Premenopausal women with normal cycles and tolerable galactorrhea and postmenopausal women with tolerable galactorrhea who have a microprolactinoma should be reassured and not treated. These women must be followed clinically and with periodic PRL measurements and MRI only if PRL levels increase or symptoms of mass effect develop. (*Adapted from* Casanueva FF, Molitch ME, Schlechte JA, et al. Guidelines of the Pituitary Society for the diagnosis and management of prolactinoma. Clin Endocrinol (Oxf) 2006;65:265–73; with permission.)

in diagnosing small adenomas and in defining the extension of large tumors. Two important points should be noted, however: microadenomas are present in 10% of the normal population, and a normal MRI scan does not completely exclude a microadenoma [74,76]. One potential additional problem is represented by the differential diagnosis between a large nonsecreting tumor causing modest PRL elevations and a true prolactinoma. In this situation, unequivocal diagnosis requires pathologic evaluation, but an empiric confirmation should be obtained by the response to dopamine agonist treatment. Normalization of PRL levels associated with a substantial reduction of adenoma size confirms the diagnosis of prolactinoma. Patients who have macroadenomas that extend beyond the sella should undergo visual field examination (Goldman perimetry) and testing of anterior pituitary function [26,27]. Some groups routinely perform initial determination of all pituitary and peripheral hormones plus IGF-1 (to exclude co-GH hypersecretion) [77]. Moreover, anterior pituitary function could be usefully re-evaluated in the follow-up of patients who have prolactinomas.

Clinical picture

PRL initiates and maintains lactation. After delivery, the rapid decline in estrogen and progesterone concentrations enables PRL to initiate lactation. Moreover, PRL acts in the hypothalamus to regulate dopamine turnover and influence gonadotrophin secretion. Physiologic hyperprolactinemia during pregnancy and lactation and pathologic hyperprolactinemia are associated with suppression of the hypothalamic-pituitary gonadal axis [2] through the inhibition of the pulsatile secretion of gonadotropin-releasing hormone (GnRH). Moreover, PRL inhibits the release of luteinizing hormone (LH) and follicle-stimulating hormone (FSH) and directly impairs gonadal steroidogenesis. Collectively, these actions lead to various forms of primary or secondary hypogonadism in both genders. Women present with the classic amenorrhea-galactorrhea syndrome, whereas men frequently ignore the symptoms of impotence, decreased libido, and gynecomastia caused by hyperprolactinemia, and the diagnosis is often made with signs of compression. Hyperprolactinemia is present in 16% of patients who have erectile dysfunction and in approximately 11% of patients who have oligospermia [78]. Neurologic symptoms (headache and visual impairment) are common in patients who have macroadenomas or giant adenomas, whereas atypical clinical manifestations (eg, diplopia, cranial nerve paralysis) are most frequent in aggressive or malignant forms.

Another well-known clinical feature of patients who have prolactinoma is osteopenia, which has recently been considered a new indication for early treatment of prolactinoma [26]. In fact, a significant increase of markers of bone turnover associated with a significant decrease of bone mineral density (BMD) at various sites can be observed [79]. These negative effects seem to be more prominent on the trabecular bone of the spine than on cortical bone of the wrist in both gender [80]. The relative contributions of hyperprolactinemia-induced hypogonadism and the PRL excess, per se, to bone damage have still not been completely clarified, even if in vitro and in vivo studies suggest a predominant role for estrogen deficiency [81].

An additional possible clinical manifestation of hyperprolactinemia is insulin resistance independent of the association with polycystic ovary syndrome. In fact, PRL affects metabolic homeostasis by regulating key enzymes and transporters that are associated with glucose and lipid metabolism in several target organs. Interestingly, short-term therapy with dopamine agonists ameliorates various components of the metabolic syndrome in obese women [82].

Moreover, because of its role in the activation of many immunologic responses, PRL enhances the progression of the immune process in autoimmune diseases. Hyperprolactinemia has often been observed in some non–organ-specific and organ-specific autoimmune diseases, suggesting an immunomodulatory role of PRL itself. Several human and experimental studies on systemic lupus erythematosus (SLE) show a relation between hyperprolactinemia and the activity of SLE, as confirmed by the remission of active SLE in patients treated with bromocriptine [83].

Treatment

General considerations

The primary goals of therapy in patients who have prolactinoma are (1) reduction of tumor size and (2) normalization of PRL, with complete restoration of gonadal and sexual function (including fertility) (Fig. 3). In the decision to treat or not to treat, an important element to consider is that approximately 90% of microprolactinomas do not enlarge over 4 to 6 years of follow-up [42,84,85]. Therefore, therapy is always advisable for all macroadenomas, whereas in microadenoma, indications for treatment include infertility, bothersome galactorrhea, long-lasting hypogonadism, alteration in pubertal development, and prevention of bone loss [26,28,86]. According to current guidelines (see Fig. 2), premenopausal women with normal cycles and tolerable galactorrhea and postmenopausal women with tolerable galactorrhea who have microprolactinomas may be reassured and not treated. These women must be followed clinically with periodic PRL measurements. An MRI study may be ordered only if PRL levels increase or symptoms of mass effect develop. In fact, it is unlikely for a prolactinoma to grow significantly without an increase in PRL levels [26,28,86]. In any case, some clinicians prefer to perform periodic pituitary MRI to verify the absence of tumor growth [84,86]. Hypogonadal women with microprolactinoma may be treated with oral contraceptives [26,27,87]. In fact, no substantial risk for tumor growth was described in amenorrheic patients who had idiopathic hyperprolactinemia or microprolactinomas treated with oral contraceptives [88–90]. Case reports of prolactinoma growth during estrogen administration have, however, been described [91,92]. Although this may depend on the natural history of a given tumor, it is, nevertheless, advisable to monitor patients on treatment with oral contraceptives carefully through periodic measurement of PRL levels and pituitary MRI, particularly if PRL increases or in case of clinical signs of tumor growth [26,86,87].

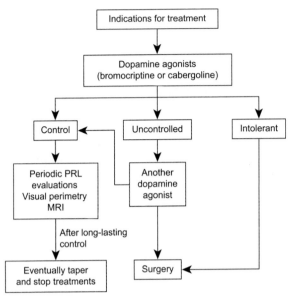

Fig. 3. Treatment of prolactinoma: algorithm. Dopamine agonists, such as bromocriptine and cabergoline, are the primary therapy for patients who have prolactinomas. Patients who are resistant to or cannot tolerate a particular dopamine agonist should be switched to an alternative one or, finally, undergo surgery. Dopamine agonists should be withdrawn in patients with long-term normalization of PRL levels and a marked reduction or disappearance of the tumor on MRI. (*Adapted from* Casanueva FF, Molitch ME, Schlechte JA, et al. Guidelines of the Pituitary Society for the diagnosis and management of prolactinoma. Clin Endocrinol (Oxf) 2006;65:265–73; with permission.)

Treatment should aim to normalize PRL levels, but many investigators suggest aiming for reaching as low a PRL level as possible to maximize the chances of reduction or disappearance of the tumor. After achieving tumor shrinkage, the dopamine agonist dose should be slowly decreased to maintain PRL in the normal range. In fact, it has been suggested that fertility may be more effectively restored with normal and not suppressed PRL levels [26].

The greatest experience in treating prolactinoma to date has been obtained with bromocriptine and cabergoline. In head-to-head randomized prospective comparisons and general clinical experience, cabergoline has been shown to be more effective and to have fewer adverse effects: most patients found to be resistant to bromocriptine subsequently responded to cabergoline [86]. Thus, in general, cabergoline is preferable as an initial therapeutic agent; however, bromocriptine has been used satisfactorily for years, and because it is less expensive, it should be considered in medical settings with limited budgets [26].

Relative to the possibility of withdrawal from medical therapy, in the past, a greater incidence of recurrent hyperprolactinemia with tumor expansion has been described as compared with that observed after surgery

[86,93]. In a large prospective study [94], prevalence of persistent normoprolactinemia in more than 60% of the patients after cabergoline withdrawal independent of baseline tumor size was reported. Other studies confirm that dopamine agonists can be safely withdrawn in patients with long-term normalization of PRL levels [95,96]. In a recent study, Biswas and colleagues [97] confirmed that abrupt withdrawal of chronic dopamine agonist therapy after 2 to 3 years of treatment is safe and associated with long-term remission in 30% to 40% of subjects with microprolactinoma. If the treatment is stopped in patients who have macroprolactinomas, a higher recurrence rate could be anticipated and a more careful follow-up is essential, including MRI at 6 months after withdrawal and yearly thereafter [98]. In fact, systematic prospective studies after long-term (>2 years) dopamine agonist withdrawal in patients who have macroprolactinomas are needed [98]. Moreover, it is still unclear whether this persistent PRL normalization is attributable to the cytocidal effect of prolonged dopamine agonist treatment or is part of the natural history of prolactinoma itself [99]. Because menopause may be associated with remission of hyperprolactinemia, the possibility of drug withdrawal should be carefully evaluated during this period [100–102], but prospective studies are still required [98]. Patients who are resistant or intolerant to a particular dopamine agonist should be switched to an alternative one [26]. Generally, resistant prolactinoma might require surgery, but this treatment may not be curative, particularly if the tumor is large; radiotherapy could still be necessary in such cases [26].

Medical therapy

Dopaminergic agonists are the primary therapy for patients who have prolactinomas. Among these, bromocriptine and cabergoline are the most commonly used. The other dopamine agonists are ergot (pergolide) and nonergot (quinagolide, lisuride, and terguride) derivatives. Several studies [103,104] report the efficacy of metergoline, a serotonin receptor antagonist, in normalizing gonadal function and restoring fertility in women, but there are no data with this drug in macroprolactinoma and hyperprolactinemia in men. Several new potential pharmacologic approaches have been suggested based on experimental evidence, which may be particularly attractive in patients who have prolactinomas resistant to dopamine agonists.

Dopamine receptors may be subdivided into D_1 receptors, which stimulate adenylyl cyclase activity, and D_2 receptors, which inhibit this enzyme. Three further receptor subtypes have been described (D_3, D_4, and D_5) with an apparent minor role in the regulation of PRL secretion. Dopamine inhibition of PRL secretion is mediated by D_2 receptors expressed by normal and tumoral lactotrophs [105]. Dopamine agonists reduce the number and size of intracellular PRL secretory granules, inhibiting PRL synthesis and then PRL release. Chronic dopamine agonist treatment may also have a cytocidal effect on the tumor [106].

Bromocriptine. The first medical treatment for prolactinoma, introduced more than 25 years ago, was bromocriptine, a D_2 agonist and D_1 antagonist. Pharmacokinetically, the drug nadir is observed at 7 hours after oral ingestion, and only a little bromocriptine remains detectable in the circulation after 11 to 14 hours. Therefore, it is usually taken two to three times daily, although once daily may be effective in some patients. Generally, the therapeutic doses are in the range of 2.5 to 15 mg/d. Because of frequent side effects, it is usually recommended at a low starting dose (0.625–1.25 mg/d) with a gradual increase by 1.25 mg at weekly intervals until a dose of approximately 7.5 mg/d is achieved [26,86]. In patients who have microprolactinomas, bromocriptine is successful in 80% to 90% of cases in normalizing PRL levels, restoring gonadal function, and shrinking tumor mass [87]. For macroprolactinoma, the rate of success is 70% [86]. Visual field improvement occurs in 80% to 90% of cases and generally parallels and often precedes the change seen on MRI. In most patients, headache and visual field defects improve dramatically within days after the first administration of bromocriptine and gonadal and sexual function improve even before complete PRL level normalization [107,108]. Data from a multicenter study show that tumor shrinkage does not correlate with basal PRL levels or nadir PRL levels achieved or the percentage of decline in PRL [107]. Bromocriptine treatment is also associated with an increase in BMD in both genders [109,110] and with improvement of semen quality [111].

Bromocriptine can cause gastrointestinal, cardiovascular, and neurologic side effects [112]. Usually, symptoms occur at the beginning of treatment and with dosage increases but can be minimized by an incremental dosage schedule and taking tablets with a snack before retiring. Up to 12% of patients are unable to tolerate therapeutic doses of bromocriptine [113]. Persistent nausea and vomiting are the most common gastrointestinal side effects, which can be observed in up to one third of the patients [112]. In approximately 25% of patients, postural hypotension develops at the beginning of treatment, which can result in dizziness and, rarely, syncope [113]. The most frequent neurologic adverse effects are headache and drowsiness. Signs and symptoms of psychosis or exacerbation of preexisting psychosis has also been described; thus, the safety of this drug in psychiatric patients remains to be established [114,115]. Moreover, dyskinesias are well-recognized effects of high-dose treatment. Rarely, cerebrospinal fluid (CSF) rhinorrhea related to tumor shrinkage has been observed in patients treated with bromocriptine [116]. Reversible pleuropulmonary changes and retroperitoneal fibrosis have been reported in patients treated with a high dose of bromocriptine for Parkinson's disease; however, because the effects seem to depend on dose, they are unlikely to occur at the low doses used for prolactinoma [113].

Cabergoline. Cabergoline is different from bromocriptine in that it has a long half-life, is better tolerated, and can be given orally once or twice weekly. After oral administration, PRL-lowering effects are initially detectable at 3 hours and gradually increase with a plateau between 48 and 120 hours [117,118]. Cabergoline (0.5-mg tablets) therapy is begun at a dose of 0.25 to 0.5 mg administered once or twice weekly, and the dose is increased monthly until PRL levels normalize [26]. Large comparative studies of cabergoline and bromocriptine have convincingly demonstrated the superiority of cabergoline in patient tolerability and compliance, in PRL reduction, in restoration of gonadal function, and in tumor shrinkage [119,120]. In a multicenter, randomized, 24-week trial conducted in 459 hyperprolactinemic women [120], cabergoline induced normal PRL levels in 83% versus 59% with bromocriptine; ovulatory cycles or pregnancies were reported in 72% versus 52%. Three percent of the women stopped taking cabergoline and 12% stopped taking bromocriptine because of the side effects [120]. Several studies [119–127] have assessed the effect of cabergoline on macroadenoma size, and a greater than 50% tumor size reduction has been observed in approximately 30% of patients. These data are also more relevant considering that many of these patients had been previously treated with other dopamine agonists, with some patients intolerant and others resistant [28]. Moreover, cabergoline treatment induced further tumor shrinkage in 60% of patients previously treated with other dopamine agonists compared with 82.3% of naive patients [123]. Finally, in a recent study, Shimon and colleagues [125] demonstrated the efficacy of cabergoline in 12 men with giant prolactinoma, who displayed a mean maximal decrease of the tumor diameter of 47% ± 21%.

Side effects of cabergoline are similar to those reported for other dopamine agonists but are generally less frequent, less severe, and of shorter duration; in fact, withdrawal of this drug because of side effects is reported in less than 3% of patients [87,113,126]. The most common adverse event is nausea or vomiting, followed by headache and dizziness [113,126]. Recently, several studies have been published describing the occurrence of cardiac valve (mitral, aortic, and tricuspid) insufficiency in patients who were treated with high dose of cabergoline (~4-mg total daily dose) or pergolide for Parkinson's disease but not in patients taking non–ergot-derived dopamine agonists [128,129]. In one case [130], cardiac symptoms improved with discontinuation of the drug, whereas in another case [131], mitral valve replacement was required. Even if the dose used in Parkinson's disease is significantly higher than that used in hyperprolactinemia, these latter patients treated with high-dose cabergoline should be monitored for this potential adverse effect [86].

Other dopamine agonists. All dopamine agonists are effective in the treatment of prolactinoma, but pergolide and quinagolide are less commonly used. Patients who are resistant or intolerant to a particular dopamine agonist should be switched to an alternative one [26,132–134]. In a multicenter randomized controlled trial, Lamberts and Quik [135] reported that bromocriptine and pergolide were equally effective in lowering PRL levels and in inducing tumor shrinkage, but a high incidence of adverse effects was reported with both drugs. Data concerning the reduction of macroadenoma size by pergolide are limited [136,137]. In a recent study on 22 de novo patients who had macroprolactinomas, Orrego and colleagues [138] reported normalization of PRL in 15 patients and tumor shrinkage by at least 75% in 10 patients. In general, the nature and incidence of most side effects reported with pergolide are similar to those of bromocriptine [135]. As already discussed, cases of pergolide-associated valvular heart disease have been reported in Parkinson's disease with much higher doses than those used for hyperprolactinemia treatment [128,129].

Quinagolide is a nonergot dopamine agonist that can be given once daily. Approximately 50% of patients who are resistant to bromocriptine respond to quinagolide [139,140]. Crossover studies [141–143] comparing the outcome of quinagolide and cabergoline demonstrated similar clinical efficacy and side effects.

Resistance to dopamine agonists. Varying definitions of dopamine agonist resistance are used throughout the literature. Clinically, the definition of such resistance, such as that for GH-secreting adenoma [144], should be bimodal: "biochemical" resistance, which can be absolute or partial and is the failure to control PRL, and "mass" resistance, which is the absence of tumor skrinkage [26,145]. Failure to normalize PRL levels in patients who have microprolactinomas occurs in approximately 20% of patients treated with bromocriptine and in approximately 10% of patients treated with cabergoline. In macroprolactinoma, the percentage of resistance increases to approximately 30% and to approximately 20% with bromocriptine and cabergoline, respectively [145]. Resistance of the tumor to shrinkage is approximately 50% with bromocriptine versus 10% to 15% with cabergoline and pergolide [146]. The mechanism of resistance seems to be related to loss of D_2 receptors in lactotrophs [147,148]. Partial resistance is common, and a progressive increase in the dose or a switch to another dopamine-agonist might be effective in normalizing PRL levels or decreasing tumor size. Cabergoline is the most effective dopamine agonist, and tumors resistant to bromocriptine frequently respond to cabergoline. Some resistant patients normalize PRL levels after therapy with no change in tumor size and vice versa. In some cases, clinical goals are reached without normalization of PRL levels or without significant shrinkage. Transsphenoidal pituitary surgery should be reserved for patients in whom medical therapy has clinically failed, whereas fractionated radiation or radiosurgery should be reserved for patients in whom medical and surgical therapy have failed [26,27,86,144].

Perspective on new drugs
    Patients who have prolactinomas and have partial or absolute resistance (biochemical or mass) to dopamine may theoretically benefit from new

potential drugs that have recently been proposed for clinical use based on interesting experimental evidence.

Somatostatin analogues and chimeric compounds. All five somatostatin receptor (SSTR) subtypes have been found in human prolactinoma, with SSTR5 exhibiting the highest level of expression [149,150]. SSTR5 subtype-selective analogues, which have been recently developed [151], suppressed in vitro PRL secretion by 30% to 40% in four of six prolactinomas, including two that exhibited dopamine agonist resistance [152]. None of these tumors responded to the clinically available somatostatin analogues. SOM 230, which has a broad SSTR-binding profile, with a high binding activity to SSTR5, has been found to be more potent than octreotide in suppressing PRL release by mixed GH/PRL-secreting adenoma and prolactinoma cells [153]. Finally, chimeric compounds containing structural elements of somatostatin and dopamine in a single molecule have been shown in vitro to induce a maximal PRL suppression of 46% to 74% [154]. These studies support further investigations of the treatment of prolactinomas in human subjects with somatostatin analogues and chimeric compounds, especially if they are resistant to dopamine agonists.

Prolactin receptor antagonists. Several PRL-R antagonists have been developed by introducing various mutations into their natural ligands. For all but one of these analogues, the mechanism of action involves a competition with endogenous PRL for receptor binding. Such compounds are thus candidates to counteract the undesired actions of PRL at the peripheral level [155].

Surgery

Up to 10% of patients who have prolactinomas may require surgery because they do not respond to dopamine agonists or have persistent visual field defects. According to recently published guidelines, other indications for surgery include unstable pituitary apoplexy with neurologic signs; cystic macroprolactinomas (which generally do not shrink with medical therapy) causing neurologic symptoms; intolerance to dopamine agonists; personal choice, especially for women with macroadenomas who desire pregnancy; and symptomatic tumor enlargement during pregnancy that does not respond to dopamine agonist treatment [26,86]. A transsphenoidal approach represents the standard of care for microprolactinoma and most macroprolactinomas [156]. Interesting results have been recently published with the endoscopic endonasal unilateral approach [157]. The surgical success rates depend highly on the experience of the surgeon and the size of the tumor [158,159]. Analyzing data from 50 published series, 74.7% of microadenomas and 33.9% of macroadenomas were reported to be curatively resected: mean PRL levels normalized within 1 to 12 weeks after surgery [86]. From the same series, it seems that the recurrence rates are 18.2% and 22.8% for microadenomas and macroadenomas, respectively [86]. Giant prolactinomas and those with considerable cavernous sinus invasion cannot be cured by surgery [28,86]. Higher success rates have been observed in patients with PRL levels lower than 200 μg/L, small tumors, and amenorrhea of short duration. Low immediate postoperative PRL levels seem to be good predictors of long-term surgical cure [159,160]. Because medical therapy is now universally considered the first-line treatment in patients who have prolactinomas, the debate regarding the effects of pretreatment with dopamine agonists on surgical outcome has lost its clinical relevance. Previous reports of a better surgical cure rate in patients not previously exposed to dopamine agonists [161] have not been confirmed in the recent studies, however [162,163]. Complications from transsphenoidal surgery are quite infrequent, with the mortality rate being 0.6% for microadenomas and 0.9% for macroadenomas; the major morbidity rate is approximately 3.4% for microadenomas and 6.5% for macroadenomas; the incidence of CSF rhinorrhea is reported to be 1.9% for microadenomas and 3.3% for macroadenomas [164].

Radiotherapy

Considering the availability of highly effective medical and surgical therapy for most prolactinomas and the significant incidence of major side effects of conventional radiotherapy, this approach is not considered an acceptable primary therapy for prolactinoma and it is reserved for patients not responding to dopamine agonists and surgery or for malignant prolactinomas [26]. Today, several methodologies for the delivery of radiotherapy other than conventional fractionated external beam radiotherapy are available, such as stereotactic conformal radiotherapy and single-dose radiotherapy (gamma knife and linear accelerator [LINAC]). The normalization rate of PRL with conventional radiotherapy alone or after medical or surgical therapy is approximately 34%, and normalization frequently occurs after a long latency period [165,166]. With single-dose stereotactic radiotherapy alone or after failure of medical or surgical therapy, an overall normalization rate of approximately 31% has been reported, even if the number of patients treated with this technique and the length of follow-up are still limited [86,167,168]. The major side effects related to conventional radiotherapy include hypopituitarism, damage to the optic nerve, neurologic dysfunction, and increased risk for stroke and secondary brain tumors [26]. Whether stereotactic radiosurgery may minimize these side effects is not yet known.

Aggressive or malignant prolactinomas

Macroprolactinomas, particularly in men, may occasionally exhibit an aggressive clinical course, as evidenced by accelerated growth and invasion through bone into the sphenoid sinus, cavernous sinus, suprasellar region, or nasopharynx. Some may even progress to pituitary carcinoma with craniospinal or systemic metastases. Generally, malignant prolactinomas are indistinguishable from invasive macroadenomas at presentation. The diagnosis of pituitary carcinoma can only be made on the demonstration of metastatic spread [169,170]. Invasive prolactinoma may be associated with an increase in known histologic markers of aggressiveness (eg, high Ki-67/MIB-1 labeling index, increased expression of the polysialylated neural cell adhesion molecule [NCAM], loss of tumor suppressor genes), but only reduced E-cadherin/catenin expression and overexpression of *hst* gene seem to be relatively specific markers for prolactinoma invasiveness as compared with other pituitary adenomas [171]. Typically, there is a long latent period (years) between the initial medical, surgical, or radiotherapy treatment of the original tumor and recurrence or progression and the appearance of metastatic spread. Once metastases are diagnosed, the length of survival is usually short and neither radiotherapy nor chemotherapy prolongs it significantly [170]. Recently [55], epidemiologic, clinical, and histopathologic characteristics of the 47 malignant prolactinomas reported in the literature have been reviewed. From this analysis, the investigators conclude that, in case of an invasive macroprolactinoma, atypical clinical manifestations (eg, diplopia, nerve paralysis) together with the development of resistance to dopamine agonists should prompt the clinician to obtain histologic information. The presence of atypical histologic aspects (nuclear pleomorphism, numerous mitosis, and increased Ki-67 index) may then indicate the potential for malignant transformation [55,171].

Prolactinoma and pregnancy

During pregnancy, estrogens stimulate PRL synthesis and secretion and promote lactotroph cell hyperplasia. Moreover, a gradual increase in pituitary volume beginning in the second month of pregnancy with a peak on the first week postpartum has been observed. After delivery, the volume of the gland rapidly decreases, and normalization of the size of the gland occurs within 6 months postpartum [172]. Conversely, the decrease of PRL levels or even normalization after pregnancy is a well-known possible event in patients who have prolactinomas [100,173,174]. Reduction or regression of the tumor up to "empty" sella has been observed [175]. The paradoxical "curative" effect of pregnancy on prolactinoma could be explained by necrosis or microinfarctions of the adenoma induced by estrogens [176].

Effects of pregnancy on prolactinoma growth

The risk for enlargement of prolactinoma during pregnancy is correlated to two factors: its size and the patient's history of prior radiotherapy or surgery. In fact, the overall risk for clinically significant growth of microprolactinoma is low (2.6%). It is similarly low for macroprolactinoma surgically resected before gestation (5%). Conversely, the risk is higher (31%) for macroadenomas that have only been treated with dopamine agonists before pregnancy [26,86,173,177,178].

Safety of dopamine agonists

There is considerable experience with patients who become pregnant while taking bromocriptine and continue it for the first few weeks of gestation [26–28,176]. The incidence of spontaneous abortions, ectopic pregnancies, trophoblastic disease, multiple pregnancies, or congenital malformations is not higher than that in the general population [87,179,180]. No adverse effects on childhood development have been described in a long-term study of 64 children who were born to mothers who took bromocriptine in early pregnancy [181]. There are fewer data on the effects of continuing bromocriptine throughout gestation on fetal or infant development. Experience in 100 women who used bromocriptine throughout gestation revealed abnormalities in two infants [28,179].

Although the safety data for pergolide and quinagolide are limited, the number of associated abortions and malformations suggests that these drugs should not be used if pregnancy is desired [113,182,183].

Experience with cabergoline in pregnancy is accumulating. Outcome data on more than 350 cases in which cabergoline was administered in the first several weeks of pregnancy have not shown increased risk for preterm, ectopic, or multiple birth deliveries or malformations [121,176]. Short-term follow-up studies of babies born to mothers who used cabergoline during pregnancy (approximately 100 cases) thus far indicate normal physical and mental development [184,185]. Nevertheless, considering the long duration of cabergoline action, which is associated with fewer outcome data (approximately 350 versus 6000 pregnancies for cabergoline and bromocriptine, respectively), when fertility is the major reason for treatment or during pregnancy, current guidelines suggest that bromocriptine is still the treatment of choice, even if cabergoline can be given in women who are intolerant to bromocriptine and doing well with cabergoline [26,28,86,176]. Because there are no data suggesting that breastfeeding may lead to an increase in tumor size, it should be allowed in women with prolactinoma and dopamine agonists should not be given because they may impair lactation [26,27]. Patients presenting with signs of tumor growth during pregnancy must be carefully assessed, however; in case of mass effect, breastfeeding must be interrupted and dopamine agonists reinstated [176].

Management of prolactinoma in pregnancy

The management of prolactinoma in a woman who desires pregnancy depends on the tumor size (Fig. 4). For the hyperprolactinemic woman with microadenoma or intrasellar or inferiorly extending macroadenoma, dopamine agonists are preferred as primary treatment because of their efficacy in restoring ovulation and low risk for clinically significant tumor enlargement. Women must be warned that restoration of fertility may be immediate, such that mechanical contraception should eventually be advised. Because the risk for tumor growth is low, dopamine agonists can

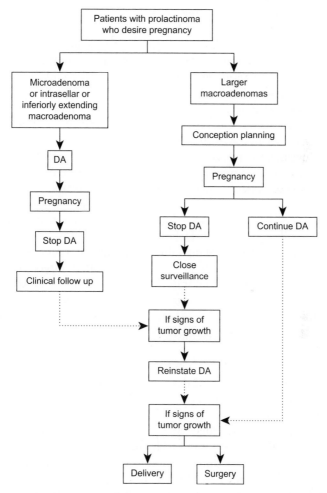

Fig. 4. Management of prolactinoma in pregnancy: algorithm. For the hyperprolactinemic woman with a microadenoma or intrasellar or inferiorly extending macroadenoma who desires pregnancy, a dopamine agonist (DA) is preferred as the primary treatment. With the risk for tumor growth being low in these cases, dopamine agonists can be safely stopped as soon as pregnancy has been confirmed. Serial PRL determinations are not necessary because PRL levels may also not increase with tumor enlargement. The patients should be advised to report for urgent assessment (MRI without gadolinium) in case of headache or visual disturbance, and dopamine agonists should be restarted if the tumor has grown significantly. For patients who have larger macroadenomas, because of the greater risk for tumor enlargement, it is necessary to plan conception to occur after significant tumor shrinkage so as to reduce the risk for compression of the optic chiasm during pregnancy. Dopamine agonists should be stopped but with close surveillance, or they can be continued throughout the pregnancy. Whenever signs of tumor growth are observed (*dotted arrows*), treatment with dopamine agonists should be reinstated. If the tumor enlarges despite continuing or reinstating dopamine agonists (*dotted arrows*), options include delivery if the pregnancy is advanced enough or transsphenoidal surgery.

be safely stopped as soon as pregnancy is confirmed [26,186]. Serial PRL determinations are not necessary because PRL levels may sometimes not increase in case of tumor enlargement [187]. The patients should be advised to refer for urgent assessment (MRI without gadolinium) in case of headache or visual disturbances, and dopamine agonists should be restarted if the tumor has grown significantly [188].

For patients who have larger macroadenomas, because of the higher risk for tumor enlargement, it is necessary to plan conception after the occurrence of significant tumor shrinkage to reduce the risk for compression of the optic chiasm during pregnancy [26]. As for microprolactinoma, serum PRL monitoring during pregnancy does not add information on tumor status [176]. In these patients, there are different therapeutic approaches that should be individualized and discussed with the patient. Dopamine agonists should be stopped but with close surveillance, or they may be continued throughout the pregnancy [26]. Debulking surgery before pregnancy is less preferable, because medical therapy during pregnancy is probably less harmful than surgery and massive tumor re-expansion after surgery has been reported [189]. If the enlarged tumor does not respond to reinstated dopamine agonists, options include delivery if the pregnancy is advanced enough or transsphenoidal surgery [26].

Summary

Hyperprolactinemia is one of the most frequently diagnosed clinical disorders in routine endocrine practice. Once the diagnosis of hyperprolactinemia is established, secondary causes should initially be ruled out by a careful clinical history (with particular attention to drug treatments), physical examination, pregnancy test, routine biochemical analysis (kidney and liver function), and TSH determination. Subsequently, gadolinium-enhanced MRI should be performed to confirm the diagnosis of prolactinoma (in the presence of a macroadenoma with low PRL levels, the presence of the hook effect should be ruled out).

Medical therapy with dopamine agonists is the treatment of choice because it allows successful treatment of most prolactinomas. Cabergoline is the first-line treatment because it is more effective and better tolerated than the other available dopamine agonists, even if bromocriptine has the largest safety database for pregnancy to date. Transsphenoidal surgery remains an option when medical therapy is ineffective, whereas radiotherapy represents the last option because of the high incidence of major side effects. A small proportion of prolactinomas that are aggressive or, rarely, malignant are often associated with a poor response to all commonly used treatments. Early diagnosis and treatment of these atypical forms currently represent the two major open issues in the management of prolactinoma.

References

[1] Bachelot A, Binart N. Reproductive role of PRL. Reproduction 2007;133(2):361–9.

[2] Freeman ME, Kanyicska B, Lerant A, et al. PRL: structure, function, and regulation of secretion. Physiol Rev 2000;80(4):1523–631.

[3] Horseman ND, Yu-Lee LY. Transcriptional regulation by the helix bundle peptide hormones: growth hormone, PRL, and hematopoietic cytokines. Endocr Rev 1994;15(5): 627–49.

[4] Bernichtein S, Kinet S, Jeay S, et al. S179D-human PRL, a pseudophosphorylated human PRL analog, is an agonist and not an antagonist. Endocrinology 2001;142(9):3950–63.

[5] Wu W, Coss D, Lorenson MY, et al. Different biological effects of unmodified PRL and a molecular mimic of phosphorylated PRL involve different signaling pathways. Biochemistry 2003;42(24):7561–70.

[6] Sinha YN. Structural variants of PRL: occurrence and physiological significance. Endocr Rev 1995;16(3):354–69.

[7] Piwnica D, Fernandez I, Binart N, et al. A new mechanism for PRL processing into 16K PRL by secreted cathepsin D. Mol Endocrinol 2006;20(12):3263–78.

[8] Sassin JF, Frantz AG, Weitzman ED, et al. Human prolactin: 24-hour pattern with increased release during sleep. Science 1972;177(55):1205–7.

[9] Neill JD. Neuroendocrine regulation of PRL secretion. In: Martini L, Ganong WF, editors. Frontiers in neuroendocrinology. New York: Raven; 1980. p. 129–55.

[10] Haanwinckel MA, Antunes-Rodrigues J, De Castro e Silva E. Role of central beta-adreno-ceptors on stress-induced PRL release in rats. Horm Metab Res 1991;23(7):318–20.

[11] Wojcikiewicz RJ, Dobson PR, Brown BL. Muscarinic acetylcholine receptor activation causes inhibition of cyclic AMP accumulation, PRL and growth hormone secretion in GH3 rat anterior pituitary tumor cells. Biochim Biophys Acta 1984;805(1):25–9.

[12] Hill JB, Nagy GM, Frawley LS. Suckling unmasks the stimulatory effect of dopamine on PRL release: possible role for alpha-melanocyte-stimulating hormone as a mammotrope responsiveness factor. Endocrinology 1991;129(2):843–7.

[13] Giustina A, Licini M, Schettino M, et al. Physiological role of galanin in the regulation of anterior pituitary function in humans. Am J Physiol 1994;266(1 Pt 1):E57–61.

[14] De Marinis L, Mancini A, Valle D, et al. Effects of galanin on growth hormone and PRL secretion in anorexia nervosa. Metabolism 2000;49(2):155–9.

[15] Enjalbert A, Epelbaum J, Arancibia S, et al. Reciprocal interactions of somatostatin with thyrotropin-releasing hormone and vasoactive intestinal peptide on PRL and growth hormone secretion in vitro. Endocrinology 1982;111(1):42–7.

[16] Giustina A, Veldhuis JD. Pathophysiology of the neuroregulation of growth hormone secretion in experimental animals and the human. Endocr Rev 1998;19(6):717–97.

[17] Racagni G, Apud JA, Cocchi D, et al. Regulation of PRL secretion during suckling: involvement of the hypothalamo-pituitary GABAergic system. J Endocrinol Invest 1984; 7(5):481–7.

[18] Giustina A, Wehrenberg WB. The role of glucocorticoids in the regulation of growth hormone secretion. Trends Endocrinol Metab 1992;3:306–11.

[19] Sato K, Watanabe YG. Corticosteroids stimulate the differentiation of growth hormone cells but suppress that of PRL cells in the fetal rat pituitary. Arch Histol Cytol 1998; 61(1):75–81.

[20] Brann DW, Putnam CD, Mahesh VB. Corticosteroid regulation of gonadotropin and PRL secretion in the rat. Endocrinology 1990;126(1):159–66.

[21] Hubina E, Nagy GM, Toth BE, et al. Dexamethasone and adrenocorticotropin suppress PRL secretion in humans. Endocrine 2002;18(3):215–9.

[22] DeMaria JE, Livingstone JD, Freeman ME. Ovarian steroids influence the activity of neuroendocrine dopaminergic neurons. Brain Res 2000;879(1–2):139–47.

[23] Snyder PJ, Jacobs LS, Utiger RD, et al. Thyroid hormone inhibition of the prolactin response to thyrotropin-releasing hormone. J Clin Invest 1973;52(9):2324–9.

[24] Bole-Feysot C, Goffin V, Edery M, et al. PRL (PRL) and its receptor: actions, signal transduction pathways and phenotypes observed in PRL receptor knockout mice. Endocr Rev 1998;19(3):225–68.

[25] Bakowska JC, Morrell JI. Atlas of the neurons that express mRNA for the long form of the PRL receptor in the forebrain of the female rat. J Comp Neurol 1997;386(2):161–77.

[26] Casanueva FF, Molitch ME, Schlechte JA, et al. Guidelines of the Pituitary Society for the diagnosis and management of prolactinoma. Clin Endocrinol (Oxf) 2006;65(2): 265–73.

[27] Schlechte JA. Clinical practice. Prolactinoma. N Engl J Med 2003;349(21):2035–41.

[28] Molitch ME. Disorders of PRL secretion. Endocrinol Metab Clin North Am 2001;30(3): 585–610.

[29] Molitch ME. Medication-induced hyperprolactinemia. Mayo Clin Proc 2005;80(8):1050–7.

[30] Romeo JH, Dombrowski R, Kwak YS, et al. Hyperprolactinemia and verapamil: prevalence and potential association with hypogonadism in men. Clin Endocrinol (Oxf) 1996; 45(5):571–5.

[31] de Burbure C, Buchet JP, Leroyer A, et al. Renal and neurologic effects of cadmium, lead, mercury, and arsenic in children: evidence of early effects and multiple interactions at environmental exposure levels. Environ Health Perspect 2006;114(4):584–90.

[32] Lafuente A, Gonzalez-Carracedo A, Romero A, et al. Toxic effects of cadmium on the regulatory mechanism of dopamine and serotonin on PRL secretion in adult male rats. Toxicol Lett 2005;155(1):87–96.

[33] Niu Q, Shuchang H, Sheng W, et al. Neurobehavioral functions, serum PRL and plasma renin activity of manganese-exposed workers. Int J Immunopathol Pharmacol 2004; 17(Suppl 2):17–24.

[34] Carta P, Flore C, Alinovi R, et al. Sub-clinical neurobehavioral abnormalities associated with low level of mercury exposure through fish consumption. Neurotoxicology 2003; 24(4–5):617–23.

[35] Lucchini R, Albini E, Cortesi I, et al. Assessment of neurobehavioral performance as a function of current and cumulative occupational lead exposure. Neurotoxicology 2000;21(5): 805–11.

[36] Alessio L, Lucchini R. Prolactin changes as a consequence of chemical exposure. Environ Health Perspect 2006;114(10):A573–4.

[37] Waschek JA, Dave JR, Eskay RL, et al. Barium distinguishes separate calcium targets for synthesis and secretion of peptides in neuroendocrine cells. Biochem Biophys Res Commun 1987;146(2):495–501.

[38] Schule C, Baghai T, Ferrera A, et al. Neuroendocrine effects of Hypericum extract WS 5570 in 12 healthy male volunteers. Pharmacopsychiatry 2001;34(Suppl 1):S127–33.

[39] Haddad PM, Wieck A. Antipsychotic-induced hyperprolactinemia: mechanisms, clinical features and management. Drugs 2004;64(20):2291–314.

[40] De Marinis L, Bonadonna S, Bianchi A, et al. Primary empty sella. J Clin Endocrinol Metab 2005;90(9):5471–7.

[41] Giustina A, Gola M, Doga M, et al. Clinical review 136: primary lymphoma of the pituitary: an emerging clinical entity. J Clin Endocrinol Metab 2001;86(10):4567–75.

[42] Schlechte J, Dolan K, Sherman B, et al. The natural history of untreated hyperprolactinemia: a prospective analysis. J Clin Endocrinol Metab 1989;68(2):412–8.

[43] Sluijmer AV, Lappohn RE. Clinical history and outcome of 59 patients with idiopathic hyperprolactinemia. Fertil Steril 1992;58(1):72–7.

[44] Ciccarelli A, Daly AF, Beckers A. The epidemiology of prolactinoma. Pituitary 2005;8(1): 3–6.

[45] Bevan JS. Prolactinoma. In: Wass JAH, Shalet SM, editors. Oxford textbook of endocrinology and diabetes. New York: Oxford University Press; 2002. p. 172–81.

[46] Hall WA, Luciano MG, Doppman JL, et al. Pituitary magnetic resonance imaging in normal human volunteers: occult adenomas in the general population. Ann Intern Med 1994; 120(10):817–20.
[47] Daly AF, Rixhon M, Adam C, et al. High prevalence of pituitary adenomas: a cross-sectional study in the province of Liege, Belgium. J Clin Endocrinol Metab 2006;91(12): 4769–75.
[48] Vrkljan M, Matovinovic M, Maric A, et al. Incidence of pituitary tumors in the human population of Croatia. Coll Antropol 2006;30(1):157–61.
[49] Zargar AH, Laway BA, Masoodi SR, et al. Clinical and endocrine aspects of pituitary tumors. Saudi Med J 2004;25(10):1428–32.
[50] Colao A, Sarno AD, Cappabianca P, et al. Gender differences in the prevalence, clinical features and response to cabergoline in hyperprolactinemia. Eur J Endocrinol 2003;148(3): 325–31.
[51] Drange MR, Fram NR, Herman-Bonert V, et al. Pituitary tumor registry: a novel clinical resource. J Clin Endocrinol Metab 2000;85(1):168–74.
[52] Mindermann T, Wilson CB. Age-related and gender-related occurrence of pituitary adenomas. Clin Endocrinol (Oxf) 1994;41(3):359–64.
[53] Fideleff HL, Boquete HR, Sequera A, et al. Peripubertal prolactinoma: clinical presentation and long-term outcome with different therapeutic approaches. J Pediatr Endocrinol Metab 2000;13(3):261–7.
[54] Mindermann T, Wilson CB. Pituitary adenomas in childhood and adolescence. J Pediatr Endocrinol Metab 1995;8(2):79–83.
[55] Kars M, Roelfsema F, Romijn JA, et al. Malignant prolactinoma: case report and review of the literature. Eur J Endocrinol 2006;155(4):523–34.
[56] Burgess JR, Shepherd JJ, Parameswaran V, et al. Prolactinoma in a large kindred with multiple endocrine neoplasia type 1: clinical features and inheritance pattern. J Clin Endocrinol Metab 1996;81(5):1841–5.
[57] Verges B, Boureille F, Goudet P, et al. Pituitary disease in MEN type 1 (MEN1): data from the France-Belgium MEN1 multicenter study. J Clin Endocrinol Metab 2002;87(2):457–65.
[58] Stratakis CA, Kirschner LS, Carney JA. Clinical and molecular features of the Carney complex: diagnostic criteria and recommendations for patient evaluation. J Clin Endocrinol Metab 2001;86(9):4041–6.
[59] Berezin M, Karasik A. Familial prolactinoma. Clin Endocrinol (Oxf) 1995;42(5):483–6.
[60] Daly AF, Jaffrain-Rea ML, Ciccarelli A, et al. Clinical characterization of familial isolated pituitary adenomas. J Clin Endocrinol Metab 2006;91(9):3316–23.
[61] Daly AF, Vanbellinghen JF, Khoo SK, et al. Aryl hydrocarbon receptor interacting protein gene mutations in familial isolated pituitary adenomas: analysis in 73 families. J Clin Endocrinol Metab 2007;92(5):1891–6.
[62] Spada A, Mantovani G, Lania A. Pathogenesis of prolactinoma. Pituitary 2005;8(1):7–15.
[63] Karga HJ, Alexander JM, Hedley-Whyte ET, et al. Ras mutations in human pituitary tumors. J Clin Endocrinol Metab 1992;74(4):914–9.
[64] Cristina C, Diaz-Torga GS, Goya RG, et al. PTTG expression in different experimental and human prolactinoma in relation to dopaminergic control of lactotropes. Mol Cancer 2007; 6:1–10.
[65] Horwitz GA, Miklovsky I, Heaney AP, et al. Human pituitary tumor-transforming gene (PTTG1) motif suppresses PRL expression. Mol Endocrinol 2003;17(4):600–9.
[66] Sarkar DK. Genesis of prolactinoma: studies using estrogen-treated animals. Front Horm Res 2006;35:32–49.
[67] Sigala S, Martocchia A, Missale C, et al. Increased serum concentration of nerve growth factor in patients with microprolactinoma. Neuropeptides 2004;38(1):21–4.
[68] Fiorentini C, Guerra N, Facchetti M, et al. Nerve growth factor regulates dopamine D(2) receptor expression in prolactinoma cell lines via p75(NGFR)-mediated activation of nuclear factor-kappaB. Mol Endocrinol 2002;16(2):353–66.

[69] Ezzat S, Zheng L, Zhu XF, et al. Targeted expression of a human pituitary tumor-derived isoform of FGF receptor-4 recapitulates pituitary tumorigenesis. J Clin Invest 2002;109(1): 69–78.

[70] Finelli P, Pierantoni GM, Giardino D, et al. The High Mobility Group A2 gene is amplified and overexpressed in human prolactinoma. Cancer Res 2002;62(8):2398–405.

[71] Smith TP, Kavanagh L, Healy ML, et al. Technology insight: measuring PRL in clinical samples. Nat Clin Pract Endocrinol Metab 2007;3(3):279–89.

[72] Gibney J, Smith TP, McKenna TJ. The impact on clinical practice of routine screening for macroprolactin. J Clin Endocrinol Metab 2005;90(7):3927–32.

[73] Quinn AM, Rubinas TC, Garbincius CJ, et al. Determination of ultrafilterable PRL: elimination of macroprolactin interference with a monomeric PRL-selective sample pretreatment. Arch Pathol Lab Med 2006;130(12):1807–12.

[74] Hauache OM, Rocha AJ, Maia AC, et al. Screening for macroprolactinaemia and pituitary imaging studies. Clin Endocrinol (Oxf) 2002;57(3):327–31.

[75] Barkan AL, Chandler WF. Giant pituitary prolactinoma with falsely low serum PRL: the pitfall of the "high-dose hook effect": case report. Neurosurgery 1998;42(4):913–5.

[76] Naidich MJ, Russell EJ. Current approaches to imaging of the sellar region and pituitary. Endocrinol Metab Clin North Am 1999;28(1):45–79.

[77] Giustina A, Barkan A, Casanueva FF, et al. Criteria for cure of acromegaly: a consensus statement. J Clin Endocrinol Metab 2000;85(2):526–9.

[78] Ambrosi B, Gaggini M, Moriondo P, et al. PRL and sexual function. JAMA 1980;244(23): 2608.

[79] Klibanski A, Neer RM, Beitins IZ, et al. Decreased bone density in hyperprolactinemic women. N Engl J Med 1980;303(26):1511–4.

[80] Schlechte J, el-Khoury G, Kathol M, et al. Forearm and vertebral bone mineral in treated and untreated hyperprolactinemic amenorrhea. J Clin Endocrinol Metab 1987;64(5): 1021–6.

[81] Adler RA, Evani R, Mansouri A, et al. Relative effects of PRL excess and estrogen deficiency on bone in rats. Metabolism 1998;47(4):425–8.

[82] Kok P, Roelfsema F, Frolich M, et al. Activation of dopamine D2 receptors simultaneously ameliorates various metabolic features of obese women. Am J Physiol Endocrinol Metab 2006;291(5):1038–43.

[83] Alvarez-Nemegyei J, Cobarrubias-Cobos A, Escalante-Triay F, et al. Bromocriptine in systemic lupus erythematosus: a double-blind, randomized, placebo-controlled study. Lupus 1998;7(6):414–9.

[84] March CM, Kletzky OA, Davajan V, et al. Longitudinal evaluation of patients with untreated PRL-secreting pituitary adenomas. Am J Obstet Gynecol 1981;139(7):835–44.

[85] Weiss MH, Teal J, Gott P, et al. Natural history of microprolactinoma: six-year follow-up. Neurosurgery 1983;12(2):180–3.

[86] Gillam MP, Molitch ME, Lombardi G, et al. Advances in the treatment of prolactinoma. Endocr Rev 2006;27(5):485–534.

[87] Molitch ME. Medical treatment of prolactinoma. Endocrinol Metab Clin North Am 1999; 28(1):143–69.

[88] Corenblum B, Donovan L. The safety of physiological estrogen plus progestin replacement therapy and with oral contraceptive therapy in women with pathological hyperprolactinemia. Fertil Steril 1993;59(3):671–3.

[89] Fahy UM, Foster PA, Torode HW, et al. The effect of combined estrogen/progestogen treatment in women with hyperprolactinemic amenorrhea. Gynecol Endocrinol 1992; 6(3):183–8.

[90] Testa G, Vegetti W, Motta T, et al. Two-year treatment with oral contraceptives in hyperprolactinemic patients. Contraception 1998;58(2):69–73.

[91] Garcia MM, Kapcala LP. Growth of a microprolactinoma to a macroprolactinoma during estrogen therapy. J Endocrinol Invest 1995;18(6):450–5.

[92] Kovacs K, Stefaneanu L, Ezzat S, et al. PRL-producing pituitary adenoma in a male-to-female transsexual patient with protracted estrogen administration. A morphologic study. Arch Pathol Lab Med 1994;118(5):562–5.

[93] Orrego JJ, Chandler WF, Barkan AL. Rapid re-expansion of a macroprolactinoma after early discontinuation of bromocriptine. Pituitary 2000;3(3):189–92.

[94] Colao A, Di Sarno A, Cappabianca P, et al. Withdrawal of long-term cabergoline therapy for tumoral and nontumoral hyperprolactinemia. N Engl J Med 2003;349(21):2023–33.

[95] Johnston DG, Hall K, Kendall-Taylor P, et al. Effect of dopamine agonist withdrawal after long-term therapy in prolactinoma. Studies with high-definition computerised tomography. Lancet 1984;2(8396):187–92.

[96] Passos VQ, Souza JJ, Musolino NR, et al. Long-term follow-up of prolactinoma: normoPRLemia after bromocriptine withdrawal. J Clin Endocrinol Metab 2002;87(8): 3578–82.

[97] Biswas M, Smith J, Jadon D, et al. Long-term remission following withdrawal of dopamine agonist therapy in subjects with microprolactinoma. Clin Endocrinol (Oxf) 2005;63(1):26–31.

[98] Wass JA. When to discontinue treatment of prolactinoma? Nat Clin Pract Endocrinol Metab 2006;2(6):298–9.

[99] Bronstein MD. Potential for long-term remission of microprolactinoma after withdrawal of dopamine-agonist therapy. Nat Clin Pract Endocrinol Metab 2006;2(3):130–1.

[100] Crosignani PG, Mattei AM, Severini V, et al. Long-term effects of time, medical treatment and pregnancy in 176 hyperprolactinemic women. Eur J Obstet Gynecol Reprod Biol 1992; 44(3):175–80.

[101] Jeffcoate WJ, Pound N, Sturrock ND, et al. Long-term follow-up of patients with hyperprolactinemia. Clin Endocrinol (Oxf) 1996;45(3):299–303.

[102] Karunakaran S, Page RC, Wass JA. The effect of the menopause on PRL levels in patients with hyperprolactinemia. Clin Endocrinol (Oxf) 2001;54(3):295–300.

[103] Crosignani PG, Peracchi M, Lombroso GC, et al. Antiserotonin treatment of hyperprolactinemic amenorrhea: long-term follow-up with metergoline, methysergide, and cyproheptadine. Am J Obstet Gynecol 1978;132(3):307–12.

[104] Bohnet HG, Kato K, Wolf AS. Treatment of hyperprolactinemic amenorrhea with Metergoline. Obstet Gynecol 1986;67(2):249–52.

[105] Wood DF, Johnston JM, Johnston DG. Dopamine, the dopamine D2 receptor and pituitary tumors. Clin Endocrinol (Oxf) 1991;35(6):455–66.

[106] Gen M, Uozumi T, Ohta M, et al. Necrotic changes in prolactinoma after long term administration of bromocriptine. J Clin Endocrinol Metab 1984;59(3):463–70.

[107] Molitch ME, Elton RL, Blackwell RE, et al. Bromocriptine as primary therapy for PRL-secreting macroadenomas: results of a prospective multicenter study. Clin Endocrinol Metab 1985;60(4):698–705.

[108] Weiss MH, Wycoff RR, Yadley R, et al. Bromocriptine treatment of PRL-secreting tumors: surgical implications. Neurosurgery 1983;12(6):640–2.

[109] Di Somma C, Colao A, Di Sarno A, et al. Bone marker and bone density responses to dopamine agonist therapy in hyperprolactinemic males. J Clin Endocrinol Metab 1998;83(3): 807–13.

[110] Klibanski A, Greenspan SL. Increase in bone mass after treatment of hyperprolactinemic amenorrhea. N Engl J Med 1986;315(9):542–6.

[111] De Rosa M, Colao A, Di Sarno A, et al. Cabergoline treatment rapidly improves gonadal function in hyperprolactinemic males: a comparison with bromocriptine. Eur J Endocrinol 1998;138(3):286–93.

[112] Kissner DG, Jarrett JC. Side effects of bromocriptine. N Engl J Med 1980;302(13):749–50.

[113] Webster J. A comparative review of the tolerability profiles of dopamine agonists in the treatment of hyperprolactinaemia and inhibition of lactation. Drug Saf 1996;14(4):228–38.

[114] Pearson KC. Mental disorders from low-dose bromocriptine. N Engl J Med 1981;305(3): 173.

[115] Turner TH, Cookson JC, Wass JA, et al. Psychotic reactions during treatment of pituitary tumors with dopamine agonists. Br Med J (Clin Res Ed) 1984;289(6452):1101–3.

[116] Baskin DS, Wilson CB. CSF rhinorrhea after bromocriptine for prolactinoma. N Engl J Med 1982;306(3):178.

[117] Andreotti AC, Pianezzola E, Persiani S, et al. Pharmacokinetics, pharmacodynamics, and tolerability of cabergoline, a PRL-lowering drug, after administration of increasing oral doses (0.5, 1.0, and 1.5 milligrams) in healthy male volunteers. J Clin Endocrinol Metab 1995;80(3):841–5.

[118] Ferrari C, Barbieri C, Caldara R, et al. Long-lasting PRL-lowering effect of cabergoline, a new dopamine agonist, in hyperprolactinemic patients. J Clin Endocrinol Metab 1986; 63(4):941–5.

[119] Ferrari CI, Abs R, Bevan JS, et al. Treatment of macroprolactinoma with cabergoline: a study of 85 patients. Clin Endocrinol (Oxf) 1997;46(4):409–13.

[120] Webster J, Piscitelli G, Polli A, et al. A comparison of cabergoline and bromocriptine in the treatment of hyperprolactinemic amenorrhea. Cabergoline Comparative Study Group. N Engl J Med 1994;331(14):904–9.

[121] Verhelst J, Abs R, Maiter D, et al. Cabergoline in the treatment of hyperprolactinemia: a study in 455 patients. J Clin Endocrinol Metab 1999;84(7):2518–22.

[122] Ciccarelli E, Giusti M, Miola C, et al. Effectiveness and tolerability of long term treatment with cabergoline, a new long-lasting ergoline derivative, in hyperprolactinemic patients. J Clin Endocrinol Metab 1989;69(4):725–8.

[123] Colao A, Di Sarno A, Landi ML, et al. Macroprolactinoma shrinkage during cabergoline treatment is greater in naive patients than in patients pretreated with other dopamine agonists: a prospective study in 110 patients. J Clin Endocrinol Metab 2000;85(6):2247–52.

[124] Colao A, Di Sarno A, Landi ML, et al. Long-term and low-dose treatment with cabergoline induces macroprolactinoma shrinkage. J Clin Endocrinol Metab 1997;82(11):3574–9.

[125] Shimon I, Benbassat C, Hadani M. Effectiveness of long-term cabergoline treatment for giant prolactinoma: study of 12 men. Eur J Endocrinol 2007;156(2):225–31.

[126] Rains CP, Bryson HM, Fitton A. Cabergoline. A review of its pharmacological properties and therapeutic potential in the treatment of hyperprolactinemia and inhibition of lactation. Drugs 1995;49(2):255–79.

[127] Melis GB, Gambacciani M, Paoletti AM, et al. Reduction in the size of PRL-producing pituitary tumor after cabergoline administration. Fertil Steril 1989;52(3):412–5.

[128] Zanettini R, Antonini A, Gatto G, et al. Valvular heart disease and the use of dopamine agonists for Parkinson's disease. N Engl J Med 2007;356(1):39–46.

[129] Schade R, Andersohn F, Suissa S, et al. Dopamine agonists and the risk of cardiac-valve regurgitation. N Engl J Med 2007;356(1):29–38.

[130] Horvath J, Fross RD, Kleiner-Fisman G, et al. Severe multivalvular heart disease: a new complication of the ergot derivative dopamine agonists. Mov Disord 2004;19(6):656–62.

[131] Pinero A, Marcos-Alberca P, Fortes J. Cabergoline-related severe restrictive mitral regurgitation. N Engl J Med 2005;353(18):1976–7.

[132] Colao A, Di Sarno A, Sarnacchiaro F, et al. Prolactinoma resistant to standard dopamine agonists respond to chronic cabergoline treatment. J Clin Endocrinol Metab 1997;82(3): 876–83.

[133] Ferrari C, Mattei A, Melis GB, et al. Cabergoline: long-acting oral treatment of hyperprolactinemic disorders. J Clin Endocrinol Metab 1989;68(6):1201–6.

[134] Ferrari C, Paracchi A, Mattei AM, et al. Cabergoline in the long-term therapy of hyperprolactinemic disorders. Acta Endocrinol (Copenh) 1992;126(6):489–94.

[135] Lamberts SW, Quik RF. A comparison of the efficacy and safety of pergolide and bromocriptine in the treatment of hyperprolactinemia. J Clin Endocrinol Metab 1991;72(3):635–41.

[136] Franks S, Horrocks PM, Lynch SS, et al. Treatment of hyperprolactinaemia with pergolide mesylate: acute effects and preliminary evaluation of long-term treatment. Lancet 1981; 2(8248):659–61.

[137] Kleinberg DL, Boyd AE 3rd, Wardlaw S, et al. Pergolide for the treatment of pituitary tumors secreting PRL or growth hormone. N Engl J Med 1983;309(12):704–9.

[138] Orrego JJ, Chandler WF, Barkan AL. Pergolide as primary therapy for macroprolactinoma. Pituitary 2000;3(4):251–6.

[139] Vance ML, Cragun JR, Reimnitz C, et al. CV 205–502 treatment of hyperprolactinemia. J Clin Endocrinol Metab 1989;68(2):336–9.

[140] Vance ML, Lipper M, Klibanski A, et al. Treatment of PRL-secreting pituitary macroadenomas with the long-acting non-ergot dopamine agonist CV 205–502. Ann Intern Med 1990;112(9):668–73.

[141] Di Sarno A, Landi ML, Marzullo P, et al. The effect of quinagolide and cabergoline, two selective dopamine receptor type 2 agonists, in the treatment of prolactinoma. Clin Endocrinol (Oxf) 2000;53(1):53–60.

[142] De Luis DA, Becerra A, Lahera M, et al. A randomized cross-over study comparing cabergoline and quinagolide in the treatment of hyperprolactinemic patients. J Endocrinol Invest 2000;23(7):428–34.

[143] Giusti M, Porcella E, Carraro A, et al. A cross-over study with the two novel dopaminergic drugs cabergoline and quinagolide in hyperprolactinemic patients. J Endocrinol Invest 1994;17(1):51–7.

[144] Gola M, Bonadonna S, Mazziotti G, et al. Resistance to somatostatin analogs in acromegaly: an evolving concept? J Endocrinol Invest 2006;29(1):86–93.

[145] Olafsdottir A, Schlechte J. Management of resistant prolactinoma. Nat Clin Pract Endocrinol Metab 2006;2(10):552–61.

[146] Molitch ME. Pharmacologic resistance in prolactinoma patients. Pituitary 2005;8(1): 43–52.

[147] Pellegrini I, Rasolonjanahary R, Gunz G, et al. Resistance to bromocriptine in prolactinoma. J Clin Endocrinol Metab 1989;69(3):500–9.

[148] Caccavelli L, Feron F, Morange I, et al. Decreased expression of the two D2 dopamine receptor isoforms in bromocriptine-resistant prolactinoma. Neuroendocrinology 1994;60(3): 314–22.

[149] Tulipano G, Schulz S. Novel insights in somatostatin receptor physiology. Eur J Endocrinol 2007;156(Suppl 1):S3–11.

[150] Jaquet P, Ouafik L, Saveanu A, et al. Quantitative and functional expression of somatostatin receptor subtypes in human prolactinoma. J Clin Endocrinol Metab 1999;84(9):3268–76.

[151] Tulipano G, Bonfanti C, Milani G, et al. Differential inhibition of growth hormone secretion by analogs selective for somatostatin receptor subtypes 2 and 5 in human growth-hormone-secreting adenoma cells in vitro. Neuroendocrinology 2001;73(5):344–51.

[152] Shimon I, Yan X, Taylor JE, et al. Somatostatin receptor (SSTR) subtype-selective analogues differentially suppress in vitro growth hormone and PRL in human pituitary adenomas. Novel potential therapy for functional pituitary tumors. J Clin Invest 1997;100(9): 2386–92.

[153] Hofland LJ, van der Hoek J, van Koetsveld PM, et al. The novel somatostatin analog SOM230 is a potent inhibitor of hormone release by growth hormone- and PRL-secreting pituitary adenomas in vitro. J Clin Endocrinol Metab 2004;89(4):1577–85.

[154] Jaquet P, Gunz G, Saveanu A, et al. Efficacy of chimeric molecules directed towards multiple somatostatin and dopamine receptors on inhibition of GH and PRL secretion from GH-secreting pituitary adenomas classified as partially responsive to somatostatin analog therapy. Eur J Endocrinol 2005;153(1):135–41.

[155] Goffin V, Bernichtein S, Touraine P, et al. Development and potential clinical uses of human PRL receptor antagonists. Endocr Rev 2005;26(3):400–22.

[156] Losa M, Mortini P, Barzaghi R, et al. Surgical treatment of PRL-secreting pituitary adenomas: early results and long-term outcome. J Clin Endocrinol Metab 2002;87(7):3180–6.

[157] Cappabianca P, Cavallo LM, de Divitiis E. Endoscopic endonasal transsphenoidal surgery. Neurosurgery 2004;55(4):933–40.

[158] Thomson JA, Davies DL, McLaren EH, et al. Ten year follow up of microprolactinoma treated by transsphenoidal surgery. BMJ 1994;309(6966):1409–10.

[159] Amar AP, Couldwell WT, Chen JC, et al. Predictive value of serum PRL levels measured immediately after transsphenoidal surgery. J Neurosurg 2002;97(2):307–14.

[160] Nelson AT Jr, Tucker HS Jr, Becker DP. Residual anterior pituitary function following transsphenoidal resection of pituitary macroadenomas. J Neurosurg 1984;61(3):577–80.

[161] Landolt AM, Keller PJ, Froesch ER, et al. Bromocriptine: does it jeopardise the result of later surgery for prolactinoma? Lancet 1982;2(8299):657–8.

[162] Bevan JS, Adams CB, Burke CW, et al. Factors in the outcome of transsphenoidal surgery for prolactinoma and non-functioning pituitary tumor, including pre-operative bromocriptine therapy. Clin Endocrinol (Oxf) 1987;26(5):541–56.

[163] Fahlbusch R, Buchfelder M, Rjosk HK, et al. Influence of preoperative bromocriptine therapy on success of surgery for microprolactinoma. Lancet 1984;2(8401):520.

[164] Sudhakar N, Ray A, Vafidis JA. Complications after trans-sphenoidal surgery: our experience and a review of the literature. Br J Neurosurg 2004;18(5):507–12.

[165] Johnston DG, Hall K, Kendall-Taylor P, et al. The long-term effects of megavoltage radiotherapy as sole or combined therapy for large prolactinoma: studies with high definition computerized tomography. Clin Endocrinol (Oxf) 1986;24(6):675–85.

[166] Tsagarakis S, Grossman A, Plowman PN, et al. Megavoltage pituitary irradiation in the management of prolactinoma: long-term follow-up. Clin Endocrinol (Oxf) 1991;34(5): 399–406.

[167] Kuo JS, Chen JC, Yu C, et al. Gamma knife radiosurgery for benign cavernous sinus tumors: quantitative analysis of treatment outcomes. Neurosurgery 2004;54(6):1385–93.

[168] Landolt AM, Lomax N. Gamma knife radiosurgery for prolactinoma. J Neurosurg 2000; 93(Suppl 3):14–8.

[169] Popadic A, Witzmann A, Buchfelder M, et al. Malignant prolactinoma: case report and review of the literature. Surg Neurol 1999;51(1):47–54.

[170] Kaltsas GA, Nomikos P, Kontogeorgos G, et al. Clinical review: diagnosis and management of pituitary carcinomas. J Clin Endocrinol Metab 2005;90(5):3089–99.

[171] Gurlek A, Karavitaki N, Ansorge O, et al. What are the markers of aggressiveness in prolactinoma? Changes in cell biology, extracellular matrix components, angiogenesis and genetics. Eur J Endocrinol 2007;156(2):143–53.

[172] Elster AD, Sanders TG, Vines FS, et al. Size and shape of the pituitary gland during pregnancy and post partum: measurement with MR imaging. Radiology 1991;181(2):531–5.

[173] Molitch ME. Pregnancy and the hyperprolactinemic woman. N Engl J Med 1985;312(21): 1364–70.

[174] Rjosk HK, Fahlbusch R, von Werder K. Influence of pregnancies on prolactinoma. Acta Endocrinol (Copenh) 1982;100(3):337–46.

[175] Ahmed M, al-Dossary E, Woodhouse NJ. Macroprolactinoma with suprasellar extension: effect of bromocriptine withdrawal during one or more pregnancies. Fertil Steril 1992;58(3): 492–7.

[176] Bronstein WD. Prolactinoma and pregnancy. Pituitary 2005;8:31–8.

[177] Gemzell C, Wang CF. Outcome of pregnancy in women with pituitary adenoma. Fertil Steril 1979;31(4):363–72.

[178] Rossi AM, Vilska S, Heinonen PK. Outcome of pregnancies in women with treated or untreated hyperprolactinemia. Eur J Obstet Gynecol Reprod Biol 1995;63(2):143–6.

[179] Konopka P, Raymond JP, Merceron RE, et al. Continuous administration of bromocriptine in the prevention of neurological complications in pregnant women with prolactinoma. Am J Obstet Gynecol 1983;146(8):935–8.

[180] Krupp P, Monka C. Bromocriptine in pregnancy: safety aspects. Klin Wochenschr 1987; 65(17):823–7.

[181] Raymond JP, Goldstein E, Konopka P, et al. Follow-up of children born of bromocriptine-treated mothers. Horm Res 1985;22(3):239–46.

[182] De Mari M, Zenzola A, Lamberti P. Antiparkinsonian treatment in pregnancy. Mov Disord 2002;17(2):428–9.

[183] Morange I, Barlier A, Pellegrini I, et al. Prolactinoma resistant to bromocriptine: long-term efficacy of quinagolide and outcome of pregnancy. Eur J Endocrinol 1996;135(4):413–20.

[184] Robert E, Musatti L, Piscitelli G, et al. Pregnancy outcome after treatment with the ergot derivative, cabergoline. Reprod Toxicol 1996;10(4):333–7.

[185] Ricci E, Parazzini F, Motta T, et al. Pregnancy outcome after cabergoline treatment in early weeks of gestation. Reprod Toxicol 2002;16(6):791–3.

[186] Molitch ME. Pituitary disorders during pregnancy. Endocrinol Metab Clin North Am 2006;35(1):99–116.

[187] Divers WA Jr, Yen SS. PRL-producing microadenomas in pregnancy. Obstet Gynecol 1983;62(4):425–9.

[188] Kupersmith MJ, Rosenberg C, Kleinberg D. Visual loss in pregnant women with pituitary adenomas. Ann Intern Med 1994;121(7):473–7.

[189] Belchetz PE, Carty A, Clearkin LG, et al. Failure of prophylactic surgery to avert massive pituitary expansion in pregnancy. Clin Endocrinol (Oxf) 1986;25(3):325–30.

ELSEVIER
SAUNDERS

Endocrinol Metab Clin N Am
37 (2008) 101–122

ENDOCRINOLOGY
AND METABOLISM
CLINICS
OF NORTH AMERICA

Acromegaly

Anat Ben-Shlomo, MD[a,b,*],
Shlomo Melmed, MBChB, FRCP[a,b]

[a]Cedars-Sinai Medical Center, 8700 Beverly Boulevard, Los Angeles, CA, 90048, USA
[b]David Geffen School of Medicine at UCLA, Los Angeles, CA, USA

Acromegaly is a disease of exaggerated somatic growth and distorted proportion arising from hypersecretion of growth hormone (GH) and insulin-like growth factor 1 (IGF-1). The condition was described more than 120 years ago [1] and later ascribed to pituitary secretion and adenomas [2,3]. Acromegaly is a rare condition with a prevalence less than or equal to 70 cases per million and annual incidence of 3 to 4 cases per million [4,5]. The condition in children where there is accelerated growth of epiphyseal plates is referred to as gigantism rather than acromegaly.

Pathogenesis

Hypersecretion of GH or GH-releasing hormone (GHRH) can lead to acromegaly. Pituitary GH-secreting adenomas are responsible for 98% of acromegaly and almost exclusively are benign. The tumors usually are comprised of cells with sparsely or densely granulated cytoplasm secreting GH alone or a mixture of cells secreting either GH or prolactin (PRL). Less commonly, the tumor is composed of mammosomatotroph cells or the more aggressive acidophilic stem cell adenoma secreting GH and PRL. Plurihormonal adenomas secreting GH and many other hormones (PRL, thyrotropin, corticotropin, gonadotropins [follicle-stimulating hormone (FSH) and luteinizing hormone (LH)], and α subunit) are rare. Metastatic pituitary carcinoma secreting GH is extremely rare. Some clinically silent somatotroph adenomas are described as associated with high GH and IGF-1 levels [6].

---

* Corresponding author. Cedars-Sinai Medical Center, 8700 Beverly Boulevard, Davis Building, Room 3021, Los Angeles, CA 90048.
E-mail address: benshlomoa@cshs.org (A. Ben-Shlomo).

0889-8529/08/$ - see front matter © 2008 Elsevier Inc. All rights reserved.
doi:10.1016/j.ecl.2007.10.002

Familial syndromes associated with GH hypersecretion include multiple endocrine neoplasia type 1 (germ cell inactivation of the *MENIN* tumor suppressor gene, which includes pituitary, parathyroid, and pancreatic tumors) [7,8], McCune-Albright syndrome ($G_s\alpha$ mutation; clinical appearance includes polyostotic fibrous dysplasia, cutaneous pigmentation, and pituitary hypersecretion) [9], and Carney complex (*PRKAR1A* gene mutations; clinical appearance includes skin pigmentation, mucocutaneous mixomatosis, cardiac myxoma, thyroid and breast lesions, and GH-secreting pituitary adenoma) [10]. Isolated familial acromegaly is described with loss of heterozygosity in chromosome 11q13 [11] and, recently, low-penetrance germline mutations in the aryl hydrocarbon receptor–interacting protein gene were found in individuals who had familial pituitary adenoma predisposition [12,13].

Other rare causes of GH hypersecretion are extrapituitary pancreatic islet cell tumors [14] and central (hypothalamic hamartoma, choristoma, and ganglioneuroma) [15] or peripheral (neuroendocrine tumors) GHRH oversecretion [16–18].

Exogenous administration of GH to non-GH deficient subjects as an athletic performance enhancer [19] or anti-aging treatment [20] has been a growing phenomenon during the last decade, exposing GH recipients to pathologies similar to those of patients who have endogenous GH hypersecretion.

Diagnosis

Signs and symptoms

Insidious clinical manifestation of GH excess resulting from a GH-secreting pituitary adenoma renders acromegaly a disease with typically delayed diagnosis, approximately 10 years from symptoms onset [21]. Changes in appearance bring only 13% of patients who have acromegaly to seek medical care [22], even though these changes account for 98% of presenting features [23].

Changes in appearance derive from skeletal growth, and soft tissue enlargement is subtle early in the course of the disease. Facial changes include large lips and nose, frontal skull bossing and cranial ridges, mandibular overgrowth with prognathism, maxillary widening with teeth separation, jaw malocclusion, and overbite. Increased shoe and ring size often are reported [22].

Large joint arthropathy is a common feature of the disease, occurring in approximately 70% of patients [24], resulting from cartilaginous and periarticular fibrous tissue thickening, causing joint swelling, pain, and hypomobility followed by narrowing of joint spaces, osteophytosis, and features of osteoarthritis with chronic disease [25]. Axial involvement is present in up to 60% of patients at presentation and includes disk space widening, vertebral enlargement, and osteophyte formation. Kyphoscoliosis occurs in 21%, cervical or lumbar linearization in 37%, and diffuse idiopathic skeletal hyperostosis in 20% of patients who have active acromegaly [26].

Skin thickening that is noticed mainly in the face, hands, and feet is the result of accumulation of glycosaminoglycans. Oversecretion and hypertrophy of sebaceous and sweat glands result in oily and sweaty skin, respectively. Pigmented skin tags and hypertrichosis are common features of the disease [27].

Upper airways obstruction is the consequence of macroglossia, prognathism, thick lips, and laryngeal mucosal and cartilage hypertrophy; it can cause sleep apnea and excessive snoring and can complicate tracheal intubation during anesthesia. Hypoventilation and hypoxemia also can arise from central respiratory depression [28] and kyphoscoliosis. Lungs show increased distensibility with normal diffusion capacity, suggesting an increase in alveolar size [29] or number [30].

The most common cardiovascular manifestation of acromegaly is biventricular cardiac hypertrophy that develops independently of hypertension and manifests early during the disease course. Approximately 90% of autopsied older patients who have longstanding acromegaly [31] and approximately 20% of young patients who have short disease duration [32] have biventricular cardiac hypertrophy. Diastolic dysfunction at rest or systolic dysfunction on effort can ensue and are exacerbated by exercise. If acromegaly is uncontrolled, diastolic heart failure follows exacerbated by the coexistence of hypertension, diabetes, and aging. The frequency of overt congestive heart failure in patients presenting with acromegaly ranges from less than 1% [33] to 10% [34]. Using highly sensitive angiography, postexercise ejection fraction increase was insufficient in 73% of patients who had active acromegaly [35] and in 40% of patients under age 40 [36]. Cardiac dysrhythmias [37–39] and late potentials [40] are more frequent and exacerbated by exercise. Arterial blood pressure (systolic and diastolic) is higher with loss of normal daily circadian variability [41]. Hypertension was reported in approximately one third of patients who had acromegaly [42,43]; however, whether or not hypertension is more common than in the general population as yet is unclear. When the risk for coronary atherosclerosis was calculated based on clinical risk assessment and measurements of coronary arterial calcifications [44], 41% of patients were at intermediate to high risk for coronary atherosclerosis.

Peripheral paresthesias, symmetric peripheral sensory and motor neuropathy, proximal myopathy, myalgia, and cramps are encountered. Carpal tunnel syndrome develops with medial nerve compression resulting from wrist synovial edema and ligament and tendon growth [45]. Exophthalmos [46] and open-angle glaucoma [47] may develop with hypertrophy of extraoccular tissue and around Schlemm's canal.

Hyperprolactinemia with or without galactorrhea develops in approximately 30% of patients [48] because of pituitary stalk compression or mixed tumor secretion of GH and PRL. Hypopituitarism ensues by mass compression of normal pituitary tissue in approximately 40% [49] of patients; amenorrhea or impotence [50] or secondary thyroid [51] or adrenal failure can develop. Goiter and thyroid abnormalities are common [52,53], potentially as a result of IGF-1–stimulating effects on thyrocyte growth. Hyperthyroidism rarely develops because of high levels of serum thyrotropin secreted from plurihormonal pituitary tumors [53]. Rarely, Cushing's disease develops when the pituitary tumor cosecretes GH and corticotropin [54] or as part of the McCune-Albright syndrome [55].

Insulin resistance and diabetes mellitus occur as a result of direct anti-insulin effects of GH [56,57]. GH stimulation of 1α-hydroxylase activity increases levels of serum 1,25-dihydroxycholecalciferol, resulting in intestinal calcium absorption and hypercalciuria [58]. Osteoporosis may occur as a consequence of secondary gonadal failure [59,60]. A recent cross-sectional study showed that postmenopausal women who had acromegaly develop vertebral fractures in relation to disease activity (IGF-1 and duration). Moreover, vertebral fractures occur even in the presence of normal bone mass density [61].

A direct cause-effect association between acromegaly and cancer initiation has not been proved [62,63] and the controversy as to whether or not the risk for developing cancer in patients who have acromegaly differs from that of the general population is ongoing [64]. Cancer incidence in patients who had acromegaly was not increased in a critical analysis of nine retrospective reports (1956–1998; 21,470 person-years at risk) [63]. Benign colon polyps (adenomatous and hyperplastic) have been reported in 45% of 678 acromegalic patients in 12 prospective studies [63]; however, this incidence seen in patients who had acromegaly is similar to that of the general population [65]. The prevalence of recurrent colon adenomas (but not hyperplastic polyps) correlated with serum IGF-1 levels [66]. Three or more skin tags is a reliable screen for colon polyps in patients over age 50 who have 10 or more years of active disease [67]. In a large literature review, colon cancer was reported in 2.5% of 678 patients who had acromegaly [63]. In 1362 patients who had acromegaly in the United Kingdom, colon cancer mortality but not incidence was higher than in the general population and correlated with GH serum levels [68]. Patients who had active acromegaly should be screened by colonoscopy at baseline and than every 3 to 5 years depending on coexisting risks factors [69].

Mortality ratio in acromegaly calculated from retrospective analysis over the past 30 years is increased significantly compared with healthy subjects [70–73]. Age- and gender-adjusted standardized mortality ratio (SMR) in patients from Finland who had acromegaly and basal serum GH concentration greater than 2.5 μg/L approximately 5 years from beginning of treatment was 1.63 (CI, 1.1–2.35; $P<.001$) with post-treatment IGF-1 plasma levels not affecting mortality [72]. In a study from New Zealand, observed to expected mortality ratios were 2.6 (95% CI, 1.9–3.6), 2.5 (1.6–3.8), 1.6 (0.9–3), and 1.1 (0.5–2.1) for patients who had 5 or more, less than 5, less than 2, and less than 1 μg/L last follow-up baseline serum GH levels, respectively ($P < .001$). Also serum IGF-1 levels (SD score) correlated with mortality ratios. Independent predictors of survival by multivariate analysis were last serum GH level ($P < .001$), last IGF-1 SD score ($P < .02$), age, duration of symptoms before diagnosis ($P < .03$), and hypertension ($P < .04$) [71]. In the West Midlands pituitary database, age- and gender-adjusted SMR of 1.26 (CI, 1.03–1.54; $P < .046$) was calculated for patients who had acromegaly. Post-treatment basal GH levels greater than or equal to 2 μg/L increased ratio of mortality rates to 1.55 (CI, 0.97–2.50; $P < .068$) and radiotherapy to 1.67 (CI, 1.09–2.56; $P < .018$). In this study, IGF-1 was not a predicting factor. Leading causes of death were cerebrovascular and cardiovascular and respiratory disease [70]. Whether or not GH, IGF-1, or both can be independent predictors of mortality requires further assessment as the assays used to measure them increase in sensitivity and specificity.

Biochemical markers

Considering the limitations of GH and IGF-1 biochemical assays currently available and the nonstandardized reporting of results gathered in different studies [74–76], the cutoff defining acromegaly from normalcy is unclear. From an international consensus point of view, however, absolute numbers are used when discussing disease control rather than cure.

Nadir GH serum levels should be below 1 μg/L, preferably less than 0.4μg/ L, in the 2 hours after 75-g oral glucose load (oral glucose tolerance test [OGTT]) [69,77]. This criterion often is used for diagnosis of acromegaly and for follow-up during treatment. Serum GH concentrations are affected by circadian periodicity, pulsatile secretion, exercise, starvation, and blood glucose levels. This cutoff is based on the sensitivity of recent sandwich-type immunometric assays with a sensitivity of 0.2 μg/L and even 0.001 μg/L. These assays have replaced competitive radioimmunoassays with detection sensitivity of 0.3 to 0.5 μg/L. Trials conducted for assays' external quality assessment schemes show lack of standardization and method dependent variability, in many cases of up to 100%. Assay imperfections are the result of a variety of factors, including the use of monoclonal versus polyclonal antibody, sensitivity of the antibody to different GH isoforms (that also may change between patients), the inability to apply a linear "conversion factor," the use of more than one standardization international reference GH preparation (currently preferred is the 22-kd GH International Reference Preparation (IRP) 98/574) [78], and whether or not plasma GH-binding proteins interfere in the antibody and specific epitope interaction. Efforts currently are underway to overcome these challenges. For now, these confounding factors should be taken into consideration with regard to agreement on a cutoff value to determine disease activity, especially with borderline GH values [75,79]. GH measurements after an OGTT are unreliable in patients who have uncontrolled diabetes mellitus or liver or renal diseases, in patients receiving estrogens, or in patients who are pregnant and during late adolescence [69].

Age and gender serum IGF-1 levels should be within normal ranges. The long half-life and stable (as compared with GH) serum levels of IGF-1 allow for assessment of disease activity. Several factors affect serum IGF-1 levels and need to be taken into account for interpretation. IGF-1 is affected dramatically by age; however, a uniform standard for optimal age ranges has not been established; moreover, body mass index and racial differences currently are not accounted for in most assays. Methods used for removal of IGF binding proteins that interfere with sensitivity and reproducibility differ in their efficiency; IGF-1 standard references differ between laboratories as do the affinity and specificity of the antibodies used. Other physiologic factors that influence IGF-1 concentrations include circadian rhythm, nutrition, insulin, thyroxine, and steroid levels [76].

Ideally, GH and IGF-1 values should be obtained to complement evidence for assessing disease activity; however, a discrepancy between abnormal GH levels coexisting with normal IGF-1 serum levels is not encountered uncommonly [80].

Imaging

Pituitary MRI with contrast material is most sensitive for determining a pituitary source of GH oversecretion, detecting tumors as small as 2 mm. MRI also can visualize tumor dimensions, invasiveness, and proximity to the optic chiasm. When the GH source is extrapituitary, CT, MRI, or both can be used to localize the ectopic source [77].

Treatment

Treatment should aim at managing the tumor mass and GH hypersecretion to prevent morbidity and increased mortality while preserving normal pituitary function (Table 1).

Surgery currently is the preferred approach for treating most patients. Serum GH levels are controlled within an hour after complete removal of the GH-secreting adenoma. Transsphenoidal microsurgical adenomectomy approach is used most commonly and, in the hands of experienced neurosurgeons, cures the majority of patients who are harboring a well-circumscribed microadenoma and who have serum GH levels less than 40 μg/L [81–83]. In general, approximately 80% of patients who have microadenoma and approximately 50% of those who have macroadenoma normalize serum IGF-1 levels after transsphenoidal adenomectomy [84,85]. In a recent retrospective study of 506 patients in one center, during 19 years, who underwent transsphenoidal surgery, cure rates (as defined by basal GH serum levels less than or equal to 2.5 μg/L, post-OGTT GH serum levels less than or equal to 1 μg/L, and normal IGF-1) were 75% for microadenomas and 50% for macroadenomas. These tests used different biomarker assays, affecting biochemical remission definition and, therefore, the reported percentage of patients in remission. Remission rate in patients who have intrasellar macroadenomas, suprasellar macroadenomas without visual field impairment or visual field impairment, tumors with parasellar or sphenoidal expansion, or giant adenomas were 74%, 45%, 33%, 42%, and 1%, respectively [86]. Transsphenoidal surgery was required for recurrent tumor in 0.4% of patients; however, approximately 6% is reported in a previous literature review [69] and usually is the result of incomplete resection. Presurgical hypopituitarism improved in 30% of patients after transsphenoidal adenomectomy, did not change in 50%, and worsened in 2% [86].

Post-transsphenoidal surgical mortality is rare and most side effects are transient. Permanent diabetes insipidus, cerebrospinal fluid leak, hemorrhage, and meningitis develop in up to 5% [69], and their frequency correlates with tumor size, invasiveness, and neurosurgical experience [81]. Other approaches include endoscopic transsphenoidal and transnasal pituitary surgery, which can be undertaken with intraoperative MRI. These approaches maximize the extent of tumor resection; however, whether or not they improve remission rates is yet to be assessed [87,88].

Somatostatin receptor ligands

Somatostatin receptor ligands (SRLs) are the first-choice pharmacotherapy for treating patients who have acromegaly. Two formulas are available for treatment of acromegaly octreotide (Novartis) and lanreotide (Ipsen). Short- and long-acting derivatives of these molecules have been developed. Both bind to somatostatin receptor subtype 2 (SST2) with high affinity and, to a lesser extent, SST5, whereas octreotide also exhibits some SST3 affinity [89]. For clinical use only, octreotide compounds are approved in the United States. Octreotide acetate (Sandostatin) is a cyclic octapeptide administered by deep subcutaneous or intravenous injections. The typical starting dose is 100 to 250 μg thrice daily up to 1500 μg daily [90,91]. Sandostatin LAR Depot is a long-acting octreotide compound. Octreotide acetate encapsulated within microspheres is administered as an intramuscular injection every 4 weeks. Starting dose is 20-mg monthly increasing up to 40 mg depending on clinical and biochemical responses. Lanreotide (Somatulin SR) contains lanreotide (30 or 60 mg) incorporated into a biodegradable polymer microparticle, allowing prolonged release after intramuscular injection every 7 to 14 days. Somatulin Autogel is a depot preparation of lanreotide delivered as an aqueous, small-volume mixture (60, 90, or 120 mg) in prefilled syringes for deep subcutaneous administration every 28 days [92].

Most studies assessing SRLs efficacy in acromegaly define disease control by mean fasting random serum GH levels less than 2.5 μg/L or normalization of age- and gender-matched IGF-1 plasma levels [93]. Sandostatin LAR suppressed GH and IGF-1 levels in 65% and 63% of patients, respectively

Table 1
Results of acromegaly treatment

Type of therapy or dose of drug	Surgery	Somatostatin receptor ligands	Growth hormone receptor antagonist	Dopamine agonist	Radiotherapy
	Transsphenoidal resection	Octreotide (50–400 µg every 8 hours) Octreotide LAR (10–40 mg IM every 4 weeks) Lanreotide SR (30 or 60 mg IM every 10 or 14 or 21 days) Lanreotide gel (60, 90, or 120 mg deep SC every 4 weeks)	Pegvisomant (10–40 mg SC daily)	Bromocriptine (up to 20 mg daily) Cabergoline (1–4 mg orally weekly)	Conventional or radiosurgery
Biochemical control					
Mean fasting serum GH level <2.5 µg/L	Macroadenomas <50% Microadenomas >80%	Approximately 65%	Increases	<15%	60% in 10 years
Serum IGF-1 level normalization	Macroadenomas <50% Microadenomas >80%	Approximately 65%	>90%	<15%	60% in 10 years
Onset of response	Rapid	Rapid	Rapid	Slow (weeks)	Slow (years)
Patient compliance	One-time consent	Must be sustained	Must be sustained	Good	Good

	Debulked or resected	Growth constrained or shrinkage	Unknown	Unchanged	Ablated
Tumor mass					
Disadvantages					
Cost	One time charge	Ongoing	Ongoing	Ongoing	One-time charge
Hypopituitarism	10%	None	Very low IGF-1 if overtreated	None	>50%
Other	Tumor persistence or recurrence: 6%	Gallstones 20%	Elevated liver enzymes	Nausea 30%	Local nerve damage
	Diabetes insipidus: 3%	Nausea; diarrhea		Sinusitis	Visual and CNS disorders, 2% cerebrovascular risk
	Local complications: 5%			High dose required	

Goals of acromegaly management include controlling GH and IGF-1 secretion and tumor growth, relieving central compressive effects, preserving or restoring pituitary function, treating co-existing illnesses, preventing premature death, and preventing disease recurrence. Percentages denote an approximation of patients having the result after treatment.

Abbreviations: CNS, central nervous system; IM, intramuscular; LAR, long-acting release; SC, subcutaneous; SR, slow release.

Modified from Melmed S. Medical progress: acromegaly. N Engl J Med 2006;355(24):2558–73; with permission. Copyright © 2006, Massachusetts Medical Society. All rights reserved.

[70,93–106], whereas Somatulin SR (30 mg every 7 to 14 days) suppressed GH and IGF-1 levels in 55% and 54% of patients, respectively [100,102,107–111]. Treatment with Somatulin SR (60 mg every 21 or 28 days) reduced GH less than 2.5 μg/L in 76% of patients [96,112]. Somatulin Autogel (up to 120 mg every 21 or 28 days) is not shown superior to the other lanreotide compounds [113–116]. If mean fasting baseline serum GH levels less than 1 μg/L are the cutoff for remission, 33% of patients treated with Sandostatin LAR [96,100,103,106] and 25% those treated with of Somatulin SR [96,100] are controlled. Biochemical control improves with longer treatment duration as IGF-1 plasma levels continue to decrease over the years [70,94–96,99,104,117,118]. Primary pharmacotherapy is used for selected patients [94,119]. Approximately 65% of patients receiving either primary or adjuvant SRLs treatment exhibit serum GH levels less than or equal to 2.5 μg/L (64%) or normalization of IGF-1 [70,94,96–99,107], even though treatment-naive patients exhibit higher pretreatment GH and IGF-1 levels than those treated previously with surgery or radiotherapy [96,99]. These studies also demonstrate tumor shrinkage with SRL treatment. Seventy percent tumor shrinkage was demonstrated with Sandostatin LAR, 26% with Somatulin SR (30 mg), and 39% with Somatulin SR (60 mg), and data are not yet reported for Somatulin Autogel [93]. With primary SRLs pharmacotherapy, 79% tumor shrinkage was evident with Sandostatin LAR [94,96,99], 50% with Somatulin (60 mg) [96], and 25% with Somatulin (30 mg) [107,109].

Sandostatin LAR [96,109,120] and Somatulin SR [120–122] reduced left ventricular hypertrophy, improved diastolic dysfunction, improved sleep apnea [70], and improved lipid profile [96,123,124]. Improvement in headache, perspiration, paresthesias, fatigue, osteoarthralgia, and carpal tunnel syndrome and reduction in soft tissue enlargement are reported [94,99,103,106,114,116].

Side effects are documented extensively for Sandostatin LAR, according to manufacturer reports [95,96,99,103–106,125,126], Somatulin Autogel [95,113,114,116] and Somatulin SR [96,100,108,110,111,115,127–130] usually are mild to moderate in severity and transient. Most common side effects include gastrointestinal symptoms, such as abdominal discomfort, flatulence, diarrhea or constipation, and nausea. Biliary tract abnormalities, including gallstones, microlithiasis, sediment, sludge, and dilatation, are reported in up to 50% of patients and develop during the first 2 years of treatment and tend not to progress thereafter. Asymptomatic cholelithiasis is described in 20% to 40% of patients and approximately 1% of these patients require cholecystectomy. Injection site irritation and pain usually is mild and dose dependent. Asymptomatic sinus bradycardia is described in up to 25% and conduction abnormalities in up to 10% of patients treated with subcutaneous octreotide acetate. Abnormal glucose metabolism is described with the use of SRLs, as activation of SST2 and SST5 in the pancreatic insulin-secreting beta cells likely inhibits insulin secretion and counter-regulatory hormones, such as glucagon. Mild hyperglycemia and, rarely, hypoglycemia [131], manifest mostly in patients who have pre-existing glucose abnormalities. Octreotide alters nutrient absorption and may alter gastrointestinal drug absorption. Blood levels of cyclosporine may be attenuated, resulting in transplant rejection. Altered absorption of oral hypoglycemic agents, β-blockers, calcium channel blockers, or agents to control fluid and electrolyte balance may ensue; hence, patient monitoring is required and dose adjustments of these therapeutic agents is recommended. Somatostatin might decrease cytochrome P450 enzyme action; therefore, drugs metabolized mainly by CYP3A4 and that have a low therapeutic index (eg, quinidine, terfenadine, and warfarin) should be used cautiously [126]. SRLs should be avoided in patients treated with drugs known to commonly prolong QT interval, such as cisapride [123].

Growth hormone receptor antagonist

Pegvisomant (Somavert, Pfizer) is a pegylated GH receptor (GHR) antagonist approved for treatment of acromegaly that interferes with the signaling of the GH receptor, inhibiting subsequent IGF-1 generation. Pegvisomant binds through a high affinity site 1 to one GHR dimer subunit but cannot bind through a mutated site 2 to the second GHR dimer subunit, resulting in failure to initiate subsequent GH signal transduction pathways [132–136]. Pegvisomant is more potent than SRLs for inhibition of peripheral IGF-1 levels. Daily pegvisomant (20 mg) given for 12 weeks, normalized IGF-1 levels in 82% of patients who had acromegaly [137]. Daily doses (up to 40 mg given for 12 months) normalized IGF-1 levels in 97% of patients [138]. Open-label, prospective, 1-year treatment with pegvisomant (10–40 mg) in 12 patients resistant to high-dose SRLs reduced IGF-1 serum levels in all patients, with normalization achieved in 75%. In another multicenter, open-label, 32-week trial, 53 patients who had acromegaly, treated previously with octreotide LAR, were switched to pegvisomant (10–40 mg, adjusted based on serum IGF-1 concentrations). At the end of the study, IGF-1 levels were normalized in 78% of patients [139].

Dose-dependent regression of soft tissue swelling, excessive perspiration, and fatigue were observed [137]. Pegvisomant also improves insulin sensitivity and glucose tolerance, reducing fasting serum insulin and glucose levels [138–142]. Glycated hemoglobin (HgA1C) was not decreased in patients treated for 12 [140,142] or 18 months [138]; however, in a multicenter, open-label trial, 53 patients who had acromegaly who were switched from octreotide LAR to pegvisomant reported decreased HgA1C levels after 32 weeks' treatment [139]. Serum GH levels are increased as much as 76% over baseline levels and persistent tumor growth is reported [138], even though, in most cases, GH-secreting adenoma volumes do not change [138–140,143]. Current recommendations are to perform a pituitary MRI every 6 months in all patients [69]. Elevation of serum transaminases are reported, which, at times, may necessitate drug discontinuation

[138,140,144]. Idiosyncratic chronic active hepatitis, with elevated transaminases more than 3 times above the upper normal range, was reported in 9% of patients receiving pegvisomant for more than a year. Liver biopsy in a single patient revealed chronic mild hepatitis with mixed portal inflammation, including eosinophilic granulocytes [145]. Current recommendations are to assess liver function tests before and monthly during the first 6 months' treatment and, thereafter, every 6 months [69].

Pegvisomant should be considered in patients resistant to SRLs and also can be administered in combination with octreotide. This offers improved serum IGF-1 levels and improved control of altered glucose metabolism and permits the use of lower doses of a costly drug [146,147]. Because serum GH levels are elevated during pegvisomant treatment, serum IGF-1 levels are the only marker to be used for follow-up. Recurrent pegvisomant injections in one area of the abdominal wall produced lipohypertrophy at injection sites. Therefore, the drug is recommended for injection in different body areas [148]. Possible overtreatment with pegvisomant causes GHR resistance-GH deficiency similar to features of adult GH deficiency and doses of pegvisomant should be monitored carefully during treatment to avoid IGF-1 deficiency.

Dopamine analogs

Bromocriptine and carbegoline have been used as adjuvant therapy for acromegaly [149]. Bromocriptine suppresses serum GH level to less than 5 µg/L in less than 15% of patients who have acromegaly when used in high doses (up to 20 mg per day), and patients report reduced soft tissue swelling, perspiration, fatigue, and headache. Carbegoline is a long-acting dopamine agonist that reduced serum GH levels to less than 2 µg/L and normalized IGF-1 in approximately 30% of patients [150,151]. Side effects include gastrointestinal discomfort, transient nausea and vomiting, nasal congestion, dizziness, postural hypotension, headache, and mood disorders [150]. In light of recent studies demonstrating increased incidence of valvular heart disease with high doses of carbegoline [131,152], this mode of treatment should be undertaken with caution.

Radiotherapy

Radiotherapy usually is reserved for patients who have postoperative persistent or recurrent tumors that are resistant or intolerant to medical treatment. Conventional external deep X-ray therapy usually is given over 5 to 7 weeks in 1.8-cGy doses to a maximum accumulating dose of 40 to 50 cGy. In a multicenter retrospective study encompassing 884 irradiated patients, investigators report a gradual decrease in basal serum GH levels over 20 years correlating with preirradiation basal serum GH levels. Basal GH serum levels were less than 2.5 µg/L in 22% of patients after 2 years,

60% by 10 years, and 77% by 20 years [153]. IGF-1 levels were attenuated in parallel to GH levels in 63% of patients achieving normal ranges after 10 years. Ten years after irradiation, 27% of patients developed thyrotropin deficiency, 18% FSH/LH deficiency, and 15% corticotropin deficiency. Secondary intracranial tumor formation or visual impairment was not observed [153]. Similar results were observed previously, showing that conventional megavoltage irradiation of GH-secreting tumors prevented tumor growth in 99% of patients with a predictable fall in GH serum levels reaching 90% 15 years post irradiation, without evidence of side effects other than pituitary axes deficiencies [154].

Stereotactic radiosurgery using gamma knife delivers a single tumor-focused radiation fraction. A recent study retrospectively analyzed 96 patients who had acromegaly 12 to 120 months after gamma knife radiosurgery (mean follow-up 53 months). Serum IGF-1 levels normalized within 54 months and post-OGTT serum GH levels were less than 1 μg/L after 66 months in 50% of patients. Adenoma growth arrest was observed in all, and shrinkage occurred in 62% of patients. Hypopituitarism developed in 26% of patients only when irradiated by 15 Gy or more [155]. Gamma knife radiosurgery requires precise delineation of the tumor target to allow exact focusing with minimal surrounding tissue exposure, especially to the optic tract.

Treatment approach

For patients who have newly diagnosed acromegaly and a microadenoma or a well-defined intrasellar adenoma, a surgical approach is preferred, as cure is highly probable in the hands of experienced neurosurgeons (Fig. 1). Because surgery may not be curative for patients who have macroadenomas, especially if invasive, other treatment approaches can be undertaken. Tumor debulking is necessary if there is evidence for pressure on the optic chiasm or other vital organs. There is insufficient scientific evidence to support tumor debulking in other instances; however, this approach is taken commonly and there is evidence for enhancement of SRLs action if 75% of the mass adenoma is resected [94,156]. Surgery also should be considered if patients are anticipated to be noncompliant. Primary pharmacotherapy should be considered in newly diagnosed patients who have invasive macroadenoma, especially if patients are reluctant to undertake surgery or cannot endure the procedure. Primary pharmacotherapy usually is a long-acting SRL. The GH receptor antagonist should be considered in patients who have uncontrolled diabetes mellitus where SRLs may exacerbate glucose abnormalities or in patients resistant to or those who cannot tolerate SRLs treatment.

Patients who have persistent or recurrent GH-secreting pituitary adenoma usually are considered for pharmacotherapy, unless there are clear indications for second surgery. SRLs usually are the first choice, with pegvisomant as an alternative treatment or as an adjuvant with SRLs, providing a "sparing effect" on daily dose requirements. Increasing dosing

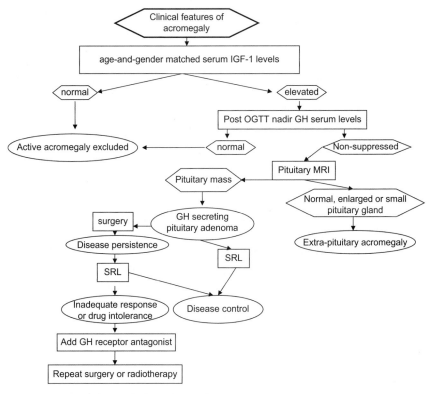

Fig. 1. Treatment approach to a patient with acromegaly. (*Modified from* Melmed S. Medical progress: acromegaly. N Engl J Med 2006;355(24):2558–73; with permission. Copyright © 2006, Massachusetts Medical Society. All rights reserved.)

frequency is more efficacious than increasing dosing per se. Radiotherapy usually is the last choice for adjuvant therapy when patients are resistant to other medications or cannot tolerate, cannot afford, or refuse long-term pharmacologic treatment. Pharmacotherapy, however, may be required for years after radiation for effective disease control.

Signs and symptoms of acromegaly and serum biomarkers should be monitored quarterly until biochemical control is achieved and the disease is inactive. Thereafter, regardless of the treatment used, annual clinical, biochemical, and MRI evaluations are suggested. Disease recurrence is unlikely if post-OGTT serum GH levels are less than 1 μg/L and IGF-1 is within the normal range. Subtle serum GH elevations can predict recurrence, however, even if serum IGF-1 levels are normal [80], and, conversely, increased serum IGF-1 levels indicate relapse even if serum GH levels are less than 1 μg/L [157]. Patients should be monitored for signs of local tumor growth, including deterioration in visual fields, increased headache, or other signs of mass effect, especially when treated with pegvisomant. Glucose abnormalities, liver function tests (with pegvisomant), endogenous pituitary reserve, cardiovascular function, pulmonary status, and rheumatologic complications should be assessed carefully. Mammography, colonoscopy, and prostate evaluation should be followed as for the general population. Gallbladder ultrasonogram should be performed for signs and symptoms indicating possible cholelithiasis or cholecystitis. Fertility and cosmetic treatments and psychologic support may be required. Patients should be taught about their disease, its complications, modes of therapy, and, if possible, to self-inject medications if so preferred.

Summary

Acromegaly is a rare disease caused by GH hypersecretion, mostly from a pituitary adenoma, driving IGF-1 overproduction. Manifestations include skeletal and soft tissue growth and deformities and cardiac, respiratory, neuromuscular, endocrine, and metabolic complications. Increased morbidity and mortality require early and tight disease control. Surgery is considered the treatment of choice for microadenomas and well-defined intrasellar macroadenomas. Complete resection of large and invasive macroadenomas rarely is achieved, however, hence their low rate of disease remission. Pharmacologic treatments, including long-acting somatostatin analogs, dopamine agonists, and GH receptor antagonists, have assumed more importance in achieving biochemical and symptomatic disease control.

References

[1] Marie P. On two cases of acromegaly: marked hypertrophy of the upper and lower limbs and head. Rev Med 1886;6:297–333.

[2] Cushing H. Partial hypophysectomy for acromegaly: with remarks on the function of the hypophysis. Ann Surg 1909;50:1002–17.

[3] Evans H, Long J. The effect of the anterior lobe of the pituitary administered intra-peritoneally upon growth, maturity and oestrus cycle of the rat. Anat Rev 1921;21:62.

[4] Alexander L, Appleton D, Hall R, et al. Epidemiology of acromegaly in the Newcastle region. Clin Endocrinol (Oxf) 1980;12(1):71–9.

[5] Ritchie CM, Atkinson AB, Kennedy AL, et al. Ascertainment and natural history of treated acromegaly in Northern Ireland. Ulster Med J 1990;59(1):55–62.

[6] Sakharova AA, Dimaraki EV, Chandler WF, et al. Clinically silent somatotropinomas may be biochemically active. J Clin Endocrinol Metab 2005;90(4):2117–21.

[7] Chandrasekharappa SC, Guru SC, Manickam P, et al. Positional cloning of the gene for multiple endocrine neoplasia-type 1. Science 1997;276(5311):404–7.

[8] Teh BT, Kytola S, Farnebo F, et al. Mutation analysis of the MEN1 gene in multiple endocrine neoplasia type 1, familial acromegaly and familial isolated hyperparathyroidism. J Clin Endocrinol Metab 1998;83(8):2621–6.

[9] Weinstein LS, Shenker A, Gejman PV, et al. Activating mutations of the stimulatory G protein in the McCune-Albright syndrome. N Engl J Med 1991;325(24):1688–95.

[10] Boikos SA, Stratakis CA. Carney complex: the first 20 years. Curr Opin Oncol 2007;19(1):24–9.

[11] Gadelha MR, Prezant TR, Une KN, et al. Loss of heterozygosity on chromosome 11q13 in two families with acromegaly/gigantism is independent of mutations of the multiple endocrine neoplasia type I gene. J Clin Endocrinol Metab 1999;84(1):249–56.

[12] Vierimaa O, Georgitsi M, Lehtonen R, et al. Pituitary adenoma predisposition caused by germline mutations in the AIP gene. Science 2006;312(5777):1228–30.

[13] Daly AF, Vanbellinghen JF, Khoo SK, et al. Aryl hydrocarbon receptor-interacting protein gene mutations in familial isolated pituitary adenomas: analysis in 73 families. J Clin Endocrinol Metab 2007;92(5):1891–6.

[14] Thorner MO, Perryman RL, Cronin MJ, et al. Somatotroph hyperplasia. Successful treatment of acromegaly by removal of a pancreatic islet tumor secreting a growth hormone-releasing factor. J Clin Invest 1982;70(5):965–77.

[15] Asa SL, Scheithauer BW, Bilbao JM, et al. A case for hypothalamic acromegaly: a clinico-pathological study of six patients with hypothalamic gangliocytomas producing growth hormone-releasing factor. J Clin Endocrinol Metab 1984;58(5):796–803.

[16] Wilson DM, Ceda GP, Bostwick DG, et al. Acromegaly and Zollinger-Ellison syndrome secondary to an islet cell tumor: characterization and quantification of plasma and tumor human growth hormone-releasing factor. J Clin Endocrinol Metab 1984;59(5): 1002–5.

[17] Ezzat S, Ezrin C, Yamashita S, et al. Recurrent acromegaly resulting from ectopic growth hormone gene expression by a metastatic pancreatic tumor. Cancer 1993;71(1):66–70.

[18] Melmed S. Acromegaly. N Engl J Med 1990;322(14):966–77.

[19] Nelson AE, Ho KK. Abuse of growth hormone by athletes. Nat Clin Pract Endocrinol Metab 2007;3(3):198–9.

[20] Perls TT, Reisman NR, Olshansky SJ. Provision or distribution of growth hormone for "antiaging": clinical and legal issues. JAMA 2005;294(16):2086–90.

[21] Jadresic A, Banks LM, Child DF, et al. The acromegaly syndrome. Relation between clinical features, growth hormone values and radiological characteristics of the pituitary tumours. Q J Med 1982;51(202):189–204.

[22] Nabarro JD. Acromegaly. Clin Endocrinol (Oxf) 1987;26(4):481–512.

[23] Molitch ME. Clinical manifestations of acromegaly. Endocrinol Metab Clin North Am 1992;21(3):597–614.

[24] Lieberman SA, Bjorkengren AG, Hoffman AR. Rheumatologic and skeletal changes in acromegaly. Endocrinol Metab Clin North Am 1992;21(3):615–31.

[25] Dons RF, Rosselet P, Pastakia B, et al. Arthropathy in acromegalic patients before and after treatment: a long-term follow-up study. Clin Endocrinol (Oxf) 1988;28(5):515–24.

[26] Scarpa R, De Brasi D, Pivonello R, et al. Acromegalic axial arthropathy: a clinical case-control study. J Clin Endocrinol Metab 2004;89(2):598–603.

[27] Ben-Shlomo A, Melmed S. Skin manifestations in acromegaly. Clin Dermatol 2006;24(4): 256–9.

[28] Grunstein RR, Ho KY, Berthon-Jones M, et al. Central sleep apnea is associated with increased ventilatory response to carbon dioxide and hypersecretion of growth hormone in patients with acromegaly. Am J Respir Crit Care Med 1994;150(2):496–502.

[29] Garcia-Rio F, Pino JM, Diez JJ, et al. Reduction of lung distensibility in acromegaly after suppression of growth hormone hypersecretion. Am J Respir Crit Care Med 2001;164(5): 852–7.

[30] Donnelly PM, Grunstein RR, Peat JK, et al. Large lungs and growth hormone: an increased alveolar number? Eur Respir J 1995;8(6):938–47.

[31] Lie JT. Pathology of the heart in acromegaly: anatomic findings in 27 autopsied patients. Am Heart J 1980;100(1):41–52.

[32] Minniti G, Jaffrain-Rea ML, Moroni C, et al. Echocardiographic evidence for a direct effect of GH/IGF-I hypersecretion on cardiac mass and function in young acromegalics. Clin Endocrinol (Oxf) 1998;49(1):101–6.

[33] Hayward RP, Emanuel RW, Nabarro JD. Acromegalic heart disease: influence of treatment of the acromegaly on the heart. Q J Med 1987;62(237):41–58.

[34] Damjanovic SS, Neskovic AN, Petakov MS, et al. High output heart failure in patients with newly diagnosed acromegaly. Am J Med 2002;112(8):610–6.

[35] Fazio S, Cittadini A, Cuocolo A, et al. Impaired cardiac performance is a distinct feature of uncomplicated acromegaly. J Clin Endocrinol Metab 1994;79(2):441–6.

[36] Colao A, Cuocolo A, Marzullo P, et al. Impact of patient's age and disease duration on cardiac performance in acromegaly: a radionuclide angiography study. J Clin Endocrinol Metab 1999;84(5):1518–23.

[37] Kahaly G, Olshausen KV, Mohr-Kahaly S, et al. Arrhythmia profile in acromegaly. Eur Heart J 1992;13(1):51–6.

[38] Rodrigues EA, Caruana MP, Lahiri A, et al. Subclinical cardiac dysfunction in acromegaly: evidence for a specific disease of heart muscle. Br Heart J 1989;62(3):185–94.

[39] Lombardi G, Colao A, Marzullo P, et al. Improvement of left ventricular hypertrophy and arrhythmias after lanreotide-induced GH and IGF-I decrease in acromegaly. A prospective multi-center study. J Endocrinol Invest 2002;25(11):971–6.

[40] Herrmann BL, Bruch C, Saller B, et al. Occurrence of ventricular late potentials in patients with active acromegaly. Clin Endocrinol (Oxf) 2001;55(2):201–7.

[41] Terzolo M, Matrella C, Boccuzzi A, et al. Twenty-four hour profile of blood pressure in patients with acromegaly. Correlation with demographic, clinical and hormonal features. J Endocrinol Invest 1999;22(1):48–54.

[42] Pietrobelli DJ, Akopian M, Olivieri AO, et al. Altered circadian blood pressure profile in patients with active acromegaly. Relationship with left ventricular mass and hormonal values. J Hum Hypertens 2001;15(9):601–5.

[43] Minniti G, Moroni C, Jaffrain-Rea ML, et al. Prevalence of hypertension in acromegalic patients: clinical measurement versus 24-hour ambulatory blood pressure monitoring. Clin Endocrinol (Oxf) 1998;48(2):149–52.

[44] Cannavo S, Almoto B, Cavalli G, et al. Acromegaly and coronary disease: an integrated evaluation of conventional coronary risk factors and coronary calcifications detected by computed tomography. J Clin Endocrinol Metab 2006;91(10):3766–72.

[45] Jenkins PJ, Sohaib SA, Akker S, et al. The pathology of median neuropathy in acromegaly. Ann Intern Med 2000;133(3):197–201.

[46] Zafar A, Jordan DR. Enlarged extraocular muscles as the presenting feature of acromegaly. Ophthal Plast Reconstr Surg 2004;20(4):334–6.

[47] Howard GM, English FP. Occurrence of glaucoma in acromegalics. Arch Ophthalmol 1965;73:765–8.

[48] Barkan AL, Stred SE, Reno K, et al. Increased growth hormone pulse frequency in acromegaly. J Clin Endocrinol Metab 1989;69(6):1225–33.

[49] Greenman Y, Tordjman K, Kisch E, et al. Relative sparing of anterior pituitary function in patients with growth hormone-secreting macroadenomas: comparison with nonfunctioning macroadenomas. J Clin Endocrinol Metab 1995;80(5):1577–83.

[50] Kaltsas GA, Mukherjee JJ, Jenkins PJ, et al. Menstrual irregularity in women with acromegaly. J Clin Endocrinol Metab 1999;84(8):2731–5.

[51] Eskildsen PC, Kruse A, Kirkegaard C. The pituitary-thyroid axis in acromegaly. Horm Metab Res 1988;20(12):755–7.

[52] Kasagi K, Shimatsu A, Miyamoto S, et al. Goiter associated with acromegaly: sonographic and scintigraphic findings of the thyroid gland. Thyroid 1999;9(8):791–6.

[53] Gasperi M, Martino E, Manetti L, et al. Prevalence of thyroid diseases in patients with acromegaly: results of an Italian multi-center study. J Endocrinol Invest 2002;25(3):240–5.

[54] Tahara S, Kurotani R, Ishii Y, et al. A case of Cushing's disease caused by pituitary adenoma producing adrenocorticotropic hormone and growth hormone concomitantly: aberrant expression of transcription factors NeuroD1 and Pit-1 as a proposed mechanism. Mod Pathol 2002;15(10):1102–5.

[55] Mantovani G, Bondioni S, Lania AG, et al. Parental origin of Gsalpha mutations in the McCune-Albright syndrome and in isolated endocrine tumors. J Clin Endocrinol Metab 2004;89(6):3007–9.

[56] Coculescu M, Niculescu D, Lichiardopol R, et al. Insulin resistance and insulin secretion in non-diabetic acromegalic patients. Exp Clin Endocrinol Diabetes 2007;115(5): 308–16.

[57] Kasayama S, Otsuki M, Takagi M, et al. Impaired beta-cell function in the presence of reduced insulin sensitivity determines glucose tolerance status in acromegalic patients. Clin Endocrinol (Oxf) 2000;52(5):549–55.

[58] Lund B, Eskildsen PC, Norman AW, et al. Calcium and vitamin D metabolism in acromegaly. Acta Endocrinol (Copenh) 1981;96(4):444–50.

[59] Ezzat S, Melmed S, Endres D, et al. Biochemical assessment of bone formation and resorption in acromegaly. J Clin Endocrinol Metab 1993;76(6):1452–7.

[60] Lesse GP, Fraser WD, Farquharson R, et al. Gonadal status is an important determinant of bone density in acromegaly. Clin Endocrinol (Oxf) 1998;48(1):59–65.

[61] Bonadonna S, Mazziotti G, Nuzzo M, et al. Increased prevalence of radiological spinal deformities in active acromegaly: a cross-sectional study in postmenopausal women. J Bone Miner Res 2005;20(10):1837–44.

[62] Jenkins PJ, Mukherjee A, Shalet SM. Does growth hormone cause cancer? Clin Endocrinol (Oxf) 2006;64(2):115–21.

[63] Melmed S. Acromegaly and cancer: not a problem? J Clin Endocrinol Metab 2001;86(7): 2929–34.

[64] Jenkins PJ, Besser M. Clinical perspective: acromegaly and cancer: a problem. J Clin Endocrinol Metab 2001;86(7):2935–41.

[65] Renehan AG, Bhaskar P, Painter JE, et al. The prevalence and characteristics of colorectal neoplasia in acromegaly. J Clin Endocrinol Metab 2000;85(9):3417–24.

[66] Jenkins PJ, Frajese V, Jones AM, et al. Insulin-like growth factor I and the development of colorectal neoplasia in acromegaly. J Clin Endocrinol Metab 2000;85(9):3218–21.

[67] Ezzat S, Strom C, Melmed S. Colon polyps in acromegaly. Ann Intern Med 1991;114(9): 754–5.

[68] Orme SM, McNally RJ, Cartwright RA, et al. Mortality and cancer incidence in acromegaly: a retrospective cohort study. United Kingdom Acromegaly Study Group. J Clin Endocrinol Metab 1998;83(8):2730–4.

[69] Melmed S. Medical progress: acromegaly. N Engl J Med 2006;355(24):2558–73.

[70] Ayuk J, Clayton RN, Holder G, et al. Growth hormone and pituitary radiotherapy, but not serum insulin-like growth factor-I concentrations, predict excess mortality in patients with acromegaly. J Clin Endocrinol Metab 2004;89(4):1613–7.

[71] Holdaway IM, Rajasoorya RC, Gamble GD. Factors influencing mortality in acromegaly. J Clin Endocrinol Metab 2004;89(2):667–74.

[72] Kauppinen-Makelin R, Sane T, Reunanen A, et al. A nationwide survey of mortality in acromegaly. J Clin Endocrinol Metab 2005;90(7):4081–6.

[73] Sheppard MC. GH and mortality in acromegaly. J Endocrinol Invest 2005;28(11 Suppl): 75–7.

[74] Pokrajac A, Wark G, Ellis AR, et al. Variation in GH and IGF-I assays limits the applicability of international consensus criteria to local practice. Clin Endocrinol (Oxf) 2007;67(1): 65–70.

[75] Bidlingmaier M, Strasburger CJ. Growth hormone assays: current methodologies and their limitations. Pituitary 2007;10(2):115–9.

[76] Clemmons DR. IGF-I assays: current assay methodologies and their limitations. Pituitary 2007;10(2):121–8.

[77] Melmed S, Casanueva F, Cavagnini F, et al. Consensus statement: medical management of acromegaly. Eur J Endocrinol 2005;153(6):737–40.

[78] Trainer PJ, Barth J, Sturgeon C, et al. Consensus statement on the standardisation of GH assays. Eur J Endocrinol 2006;155(1):1–2.

[79] Popii V, Baumann G. Laboratory measurement of growth hormone. Clin Chim Acta 2004; 350(1–2):1–16.

[80] Freda PU, Nuruzzaman AT, Reyes CM, et al. Significance of "abnormal" nadir growth hormone levels after oral glucose in postoperative patients with acromegaly in remission with normal insulin-like growth factor-I levels. J Clin Endocrinol Metab 2004;89(2):495–500.

[81] Gittoes NJ, Sheppard MC, Johnson AP, et al. Outcome of surgery for acromegaly—the experience of a dedicated pituitary surgeon. QJM 1999;92(12):741–5.

[82] Shimon I, Cohen ZR, Ram Z, et al. Transsphenoidal surgery for acromegaly: endocrinological follow-up of 98 patients. Neurosurgery 2001;48(6):1239–43 [discussion: 1244–5].

[83] Kreutzer J, Vance ML, Lopes MB, et al. Surgical management of GH-secreting pituitary adenomas: an outcome study using modern remission criteria. J Clin Endocrinol Metab 2001;86(9):4072–7.

[84] Ahmed S, Elsheikh M, Stratton IM, et al. Outcome of transphenoidal surgery for acromegaly and its relationship to surgical experience. Clin Endocrinol (Oxf) 1999;50(5):561–7.

[85] Laws ER, Vance ML, Thapar K. Pituitary surgery for the management of acromegaly. Horm Res 2000;53(Suppl 3):71–5.

[86] Fahlbusch R, Keller B, Ganslandt O, et al. Transsphenoidal surgery in acromegaly investigated by intraoperative high-field magnetic resonance imaging. Eur J Endocrinol 2005; 153(2):239–48.

[87] Schwartz TH, Stieg PE, Anand VK. Endoscopic transsphenoidal pituitary surgery with intraoperative magnetic resonance imaging. Neurosurgery 2006;58(1 Suppl):ONS44–51.

[88] Jho HD. Endoscopic transsphenoidal surgery. J Neurooncol 2001;54(2):187–95.

[89] Patel YC. Somatostatin and its receptor family. Front Neuroendocrinol 1999;20(3):157–98.

[90] Barnard LB, Grantham WG, Lamberton P, et al. Treatment of resistant acromegaly with a long-acting somatostatin analogue (SMS 201–995). Ann Intern Med 1986;105(6):856–61.

[91] Freda PU. Somatostatin analogs in acromegaly. J Clin Endocrinol Metab 2002;87(7): 3013–8.

[92] Biermasz NR, Romijn JA, Pereira AM, et al. Current pharmacotherapy for acromegaly: a review. Expert Opin Pharmacother 2005;6(14):2393–405.

[93] Ben-Shlomo A, Melmed S. Somatostatin agonists for treatment of acromegaly. Molecular and Cellular Endocrinology, in press.

[94] Colao A, Attanasio R, Pivonello R, et al. Partial surgical removal of growth hormone-secreting pituitary tumors enhances the response to somatostatin analogs in acromegaly. J Clin Endocrinol Metab 2006;91(1):85–92.

[95] Bronstein M, Musolino N, Jallad R, et al. Pharmacokinetic profile of lanreotide autogel in patients with acromegaly after four deep subcutaneous injections of 60, 90 or 120 mg every 28 days. Clin Endocrinol (Oxf) 2005;63(5):514–9.

[96] Attanasio R, Baldelli R, Pivonello R, et al. Lanreotide 60 mg, a new long-acting formulation: effectiveness in the chronic treatment of acromegaly. J Clin Endocrinol Metab 2003; 88(11):5258–65.

[97] Ayuk J, Stewart SE, Stewart PM, et al. Long-term safety and efficacy of depot long-acting somatostatin analogs for the treatment of acromegaly. J Clin Endocrinol Metab 2002;87(9): 4142–6.

[98] Bevan JS, Atkin SL, Atkinson AB, et al. Primary medical therapy for acromegaly: an open, prospective, multicenter study of the effects of subcutaneous and intramuscular slow-release octreotide on growth hormone, insulin-like growth factor-I, and tumor size. J Clin Endocrinol Metab 2002;87(10):4554–63.

[99] Colao A, Ferone D, Marzullo P, et al. Long-term effects of depot long-acting somatostatin analog octreotide on hormone levels and tumor mass in acromegaly. J Clin Endocrinol Metab 2001;86(6):2779–86.

[100] Chanson P, Boerlin V, Ajzenberg C, et al. Comparison of octreotide acetate LAR and lanreotide SR in patients with acromegaly. Clin Endocrinol (Oxf) 2000;53(5):577–86.

[101] Cozzi R, Dallabonzana D, Attanasio R, et al. A comparison between octreotide-LAR and lanreotide-SR in the chronic treatment of acromegaly. Eur J Endocrinol 1999;141(3): 267–71.

[102] Turner HE, Vadivale A, Keenan J, et al. A comparison of lanreotide and octreotide LAR for treatment of acromegaly. Clin Endocrinol (Oxf) 1999;51(3):275–80.

[103] Lancranjan I, Atkinson AB. Results of a European multicentre study with Sandostatin LAR in acromegalic patients. Sandostatin LAR Group. Pituitary 1999;1(2):105–14.

[104] Davies PH, Stewart SE, Lancranjan L, et al. Long-term therapy with long-acting octreotide (Sandostatin-LAR) for the management of acromegaly. Clin Endocrinol (Oxf) 1998;48(3): 311–6.

[105] Flogstad AK, Halse J, Bakke S, et al. Sandostatin LAR in acromegalic patients: long-term treatment. J Clin Endocrinol Metab 1997;82(1):23–8.

[106] Lancranjan I, Bruns C, Grass P, et al. Sandostatin LAR: a promising therapeutic tool in the management of acromegalic patients. Metabolism 1996;45(8 Suppl 1):67–71.

[107] Amato G, Mazziotti G, Rotondi M, et al. Long-term effects of lanreotide SR and octreotide LAR on tumour shrinkage and GH hypersecretion in patients with previously untreated acromegaly. Clin Endocrinol (Oxf) 2002;56(1):65–71.

[108] Verhelst JA, Pedroncelli AM, Abs R, et al. Slow-release lanreotide in the treatment of acromegaly: a study in 66 patients. Eur J Endocrinol 2000;143(5):577–84.

[109] Baldelli R, Colao A, Razzore P, et al. Two-year follow-up of acromegalic patients treated with slow release lanreotide (30 mg). J Clin Endocrinol Metab 2000;85(11):4099–103.

[110] Caron P, Morange-Ramos I, Cogne M, et al. Three year follow-up of acromegalic patients treated with intramuscular slow-release lanreotide. J Clin Endocrinol Metab 1997;82(1): 18–22.

[111] al-Maskari M, Gebbie J, Kendall-Taylor P. The effect of a new slow-release, long-acting somatostatin analogue, lanreotide, in acromegaly. Clin Endocrinol (Oxf) 1996;45(4): 415–21.

[112] Ambrosio MR, Franceschetti P, Bondanelli M, et al. Efficacy and safety of the new 60-mg formulation of the long-acting somatostatin analog lanreotide in the treatment of acromegaly. Metabolism 2002;51(3):387–93.

[113] Caron P, Cogne M, Raingeard I, et al. Effectiveness and tolerability of 3-year lanreotide autogel treatment in patients with acromegaly. Clin Endocrinol (Oxf) 2006;64(2):209–14.

[114] Lucas T, Astorga R. Efficacy of lanreotide Autogel administered every 4–8 weeks in patients with acromegaly previously responsive to lanreotide microparticles 30 mg: a phase III trial. Clin Endocrinol (Oxf) 2006;65(3):320–6.

[115] Gutt B, Bidlingmaier M, Kretschmar K, et al. Four-year follow-up of acromegalic patients treated with the new long-acting formulation of Lanreotide (Lanreotide Autogel). Exp Clin Endocrinol Diabetes 2005;113(3):139–44.

[116] Caron P, Beckers A, Cullen DR, et al. Efficacy of the new long-acting formulation of lanreotide (lanreotide Autogel) in the management of acromegaly. J Clin Endocrinol Metab 2002;87(1):99–104.

[117] Ronchi CL, Varca V, Beck-Peccoz P, et al. Comparison between six-year therapy with long-acting somatostatin analogs and successful surgery in acromegaly: effects on cardiovascular risk factors. J Clin Endocrinol Metab 2006;91(1):121–8.

[118] Freda PU, Katznelson L, van der Lely AJ, et al. Long-acting somatostatin analog therapy of acromegaly: a meta-analysis. J Clin Endocrinol Metab 2005;90(8):4465–73.

[119] Ben-Shlomo A, Melmed S. Clinical review 154: the role of pharmacotherapy in perioperative management of patients with acromegaly. J Clin Endocrinol Metab 2003;88(3): 963–8.

[120] Colao A, Spinelli L, Cuocolo A, et al. Cardiovascular consequences of early-onset growth hormone excess. J Clin Endocrinol Metab 2002;87(7):3097–104.

[121] Baldelli R, Ferretti E, Jaffrain-Rea ML, et al. Cardiac effects of slow-release lanreotide, a slow-release somatostatin analog, in acromegalic patients. J Clin Endocrinol Metab 1999;84(2):527–32.

[122] Hradec J, Kral J, Janota T, et al. Regression of acromegalic left ventricular hypertrophy after lanreotide (a slow-release somatostatin analog). Am J Cardiol 1999;83(10):1506–9.

[123] Al-Khatib SM, LaPointe NM, Kramer JM, et al. What clinicians should know about the QT interval. JAMA 2003;289(16):2120–7.

[124] Ronchi C, Epaminonda P, Cappiello V, et al. Effects of two different somatostatin analogs on glucose tolerance in acromegaly. J Endocrinol Invest 2002;25(6):502–7.

[125] Newman CB, Melmed S, Snyder PJ, et al. Safety and efficacy of long-term octreotide therapy of acromegaly: results of a multicenter trial in 103 patients—a clinical research center study. J Clin Endocrinol Metab 1995;80(9):2768–75.

[126] Rx List, The Internet Drug Index. Sandostatin LAR. Available at: www.rxlist.com.

[127] Lucas T, Astorga R, Catala M. Preoperative lanreotide treatment for GH-secreting pituitary adenomas: effect on tumour volume and predictive factors of significant tumour shrinkage. Clin Endocrinol (Oxf) 2003;58(4):471–81.

[128] Giusti M, Gussoni G, Cuttica CM, et al. Effectiveness and tolerability of slow release lanreotide treatment in active acromegaly: six-month report on an Italian multicenter study. Italian multicenter slow release lanreotide Study Group. J Clin Endocrinol Metab 1996;81(6):2089–97.

[129] Marek J, Hana V, Krsek M, et al. Long-term treatment of acromegaly with the slow-release somatostatin analogue lanreotide. Eur J Endocrinol 1994;131(1):20–6.

[130] Morange I, De Boisvilliers F, Chanson P, et al. Slow release lanreotide treatment in acromegalic patients previously normalized by octreotide. J Clin Endocrinol Metab 1994;79(1):145–51.

[131] Bruttomesso D, Fongher C, Silvestri B, et al. Combination of continuous subcutaneous infusion of insulin and octreotide in Type 1 diabetic patients. Diabetes Res Clin Pract 2001;51(2):97–105.

[132] Schade R, Andersohn F, Suissa S, et al. Dopamine agonists and the risk of cardiac-valve regurgitation. N Engl J Med 2007;356(1):29–38.

[133] Chen WY, White ME, Wagner TE, et al. Functional antagonism between endogenous mouse growth hormone (GH) and a GH analog results in dwarf transgenic mice. Endocrinology 1991;129(3):1402–8.

[134] Chen WY, Wight DC, Wagner TE, et al. Expression of a mutated bovine growth hormone gene suppresses growth of transgenic mice. Proc Natl Acad Sci USA 1990;87(13):5061–5.

[135] Fuh G, Cunningham BC, Fukunaga R, et al. Rational design of potent antagonists to the human growth hormone receptor. Science 1992;256(5064):1677–80.

[136] Muller AF, Kopchick JJ, Flyvbjerg A, et al. Clinical review 166: growth hormone receptor antagonists. J Clin Endocrinol Metab 2004;89(4):1503–11.

[137] Kopchick JJ, Parkinson C, Stevens EC, et al. Growth hormone receptor antagonists: discovery, development, and use in patients with acromegaly. Endocr Rev 2002;23(5):623–46.

[138] Trainer PJ, Drake WM, Katznelson L, et al. Treatment of acromegaly with the growth hormone-receptor antagonist pegvisomant. N Engl J Med 2000;342(16):1171–7.

[139] van der Lely AJ, Hutson RK, Trainer PJ, et al. Long-term treatment of acromegaly with pegvisomant, a growth hormone receptor antagonist. Lancet 2001;358(9295):1754–9.

[140] Barkan AL, Burman P, Clemmons DR, et al. Glucose homeostasis and safety in patients with acromegaly converted from long-acting octreotide to pegvisomant. J Clin Endocrinol Metab 2005;90(10):5684–91.

[141] Colao A, Pivonello R, Auriemma RS, et al. Efficacy of 12-month treatment with the GH receptor antagonist pegvisomant in patients with acromegaly resistant to long-term, high-dose somatostatin analog treatment: effect on IGF-I levels, tumor mass, hypertension and glucose tolerance. Eur J Endocrinol 2006;154(3):467–77.

[142] Lindberg-Larsen R, Moller N, Schmitz O, et al. The impact of pegvisomant treatment on substrate metabolism and insulin sensitivity in patients with acromegaly. J Clin Endocrinol Metab 2007;92(5):1724–8.

[143] De Marinis L, Bianchi A, Fusco A, et al. Long-term effects of the combination of pegvisomant with somatostatin analogs (SSA) on glucose homeostasis in non-diabetic patients with active acromegaly partially resistant to SSA. Pituitary 2007;10(3):227–32.

[144] Frohman LA, Bonert V. Pituitary tumor enlargement in two patients with acromegaly during pegvisomant therapy. Pituitary 2007;10(3):283–9.

[145] Feenstra J, van Aken MO, de Herder WW, et al. Drug-induced hepatitis in an acromegalic patient during combined treatment with pegvisomant and octreotide long-acting repeatable attributed to the use of pegvisomant. Eur J Endocrinol 2006;154(6):805–6.

[146] Biering H, Saller B, Bauditz J, et al. Elevated transaminases during medical treatment of acromegaly: a review of the German pegvisomant surveillance experience and a report of a patient with histologically proven chronic mild active hepatitis. Eur J Endocrinol 2006; 154(2):213–20.

[147] Jorgensen JO, Feldt-Rasmussen U, Frystyk J, et al. Cotreatment of acromegaly with a somatostatin analog and a growth hormone receptor antagonist. J Clin Endocrinol Metab 2005;90(10):5627–31.

[148] Feenstra J, de Herder WW, ten Have SM, et al. Combined therapy with somatostatin analogues and weekly pegvisomant in active acromegaly. Lancet 2005;365(9471):1644–6.

[149] Maffei P, Martini C, Pagano C, et al. Lipohypertrophy in acromegaly induced by the new growth hormone receptor antagonist pegvisomant. Ann Intern Med 2006;145(4):310–2.

[150] Colao A, Ferone D, Marzullo P, et al. Effect of different dopaminergic agents in the treatment of acromegaly. J Clin Endocrinol Metab 1997;82(2):518–23.

[151] Abs R, Verhelst J, Maiter D, et al. Cabergoline in the treatment of acromegaly: a study in 64 patients. J Clin Endocrinol Metab 1998;83(2):374–8.

[152] Muratori M, Arosio M, Gambino G, et al. Use of cabergoline in the long-term treatment of hyperprolactinemic and acromegalic patients. J Endocrinol Invest 1997;20(9):537–46.

[153] Zanettini R, Antonini A, Gatto G, et al. Valvular heart disease and the use of dopamine agonists for Parkinson's disease. N Engl J Med 2007;356(1):39–46.

[154] Jenkins PJ, Bates P, Carson MN, et al. Conventional pituitary irradiation is effective in lowering serum growth hormone and insulin-like growth factor-I in patients with acromegaly. J Clin Endocrinol Metab 2006;91(4):1239–45.

[155] Eastman RC, Gorden P, Glatstein E, et al. Radiation therapy of acromegaly. Endocrinol Metab Clin North Am 1992;21(3):693–712.

[156] Jezkova J, Marek J, Hana V, et al. Gamma knife radiosurgery for acromegaly—long-term experience. Clin Endocrinol (Oxf) 2006;64(5):588–95.

[157] Jallad RS, Musolino NR, Kodaira S, et al. Does partial surgical tumour removal influence the response to octreotide-LAR in acromegalic patients previously resistant to the somatostatin analogue? Clin Endocrinol (Oxf) 2007;67(2):310–5.

ELSEVIER
SAUNDERS

Endocrinol Metab Clin N Am
37 (2008) 123–134

ENDOCRINOLOGY
AND METABOLISM
CLINICS
OF NORTH AMERICA

Thyrotropinomas

Paolo Beck-Peccoz, MD[a],*, Luca Persani, MD, PhD[b]

[a]Department of Medical Sciences, University of Milan, Fondazione Ospedale Maggiore
Policlinico IRCCS, Milan, Italy
[b]Department of Medical Sciences, University of Milan, Istituto Auxologico Italiano IRCCS,
Milan, Italy

Thyrotropinomas are infrequent pituitary adenomas but easily recognized, owing to their characteristic biochemical presentation (ie, high levels of circulating free thyroid hormones [FT4 and FT3] in the presence of normal/high serum thyrotropin concentrations). The diagnostic work-up of thyrotropinomas is facilitated by the routine use of ultrasensitive immunometric assays for thyrotropin measurement, which allows a clear distinction between patients who have suppressed and those who have nonsuppressed circulating thyropin concentrations (ie, between patients who have primary hyperthyroidism [Graves' disease or toxic nodular goiter] and those who have central hyperthyroidism [thyrotropinomas or pituitary resistance to thyroid hormones (PRTH)]). In approximately 25% of patients who have thyrotropinoma, a concomitant secretion of other pituitary hormones can be found [1–3]. Mixed thyrotropin/GH-secreting adenomas (hyperthyroidism and acromegaly) are the most common among them, followed by mixed thyrotropin/PRL-secreting and thyrotropin/gonadotropin–secreting adenomas. Mixed thyrotropin/ACTH adenomas never have been documented. Moreover, a high and unbalanced hypersecretion of glycoprotein hormone alpha-subunit (α-GSU) accompanies thyrotropin secretion from several thyrotropinomas; in particular cases, it may be found in cells not necessarily containing thyrotropin-b subunit, suggesting the presence of a mixed thyrotropin/α-GSU adenomas [4].

The majority of thyrotropinomas reported in the literature are macroadenomas that may be intrasellar, extrasellar, or invasive in 29%, 36%, and 35% of cases, respectively (Fig. 1). The occurrence of invasive macroadenomas is high, particularly in patients who have had previous thyroid ablation by surgery or radioiodine, a figure underlying the deleterious effects of

---

* Corresponding author.
E-mail address: paolo.beckpeccoz@unimi.it (P. Beck-Peccoz).

doi:10.1016/j.ecl.2007.10.001

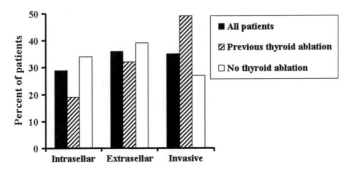

Fig. 1. Effect of mistaken thyroid ablation on the volume and invasiveness of thyrotropinomas. In patients who had previous thyroid ablation, invasive tumors are significantly higher, whereas in those who had intrasellar tumors, they are significantly lower compared with the results observed in patients who did not have thyroid ablation.

incorrect diagnosis and treatment of these rare adenomas (see Fig. 1). Such an aggressive tumor transformation resembles that occurring in Nelson's syndrome after adrenalectomy for Cushing's disease.

Because of the ultrasensitive and highly specific thyrotropin and free thyroid hormone measurement methods and more sensitive imaging procedures, thyrotropinomas today are diagnosed earlier, before the stage of large and invasive macroadenoma [2,5]. Because the characteristic biochemical features of thyrotropinomas are shared with patients who have resistance to thyroid hormones (RTH), in particular the "selective" PRTH, a correct differential diagnosis between the two disorders is mandatory [1,2,6]. Failure to recognize these different disorders may result in dramatic consequences, such as improper thyroid ablation in patients who have thyrotropinomas or unnecessary pituitary surgery in those who have RTH. Conversely, early diagnosis and correct treatment of thyrotropinomas may prevent the occurrence of neurologic and endocrine complications, such as headache, visual field defects, and hypopituitarism, and should improve the rate of cure.

Pathogenesis

As for the majority of pituitary adenomas, the pathogenesis of thyrotropinomas remains obscure. Analysis of X-chromosome inactivation demonstrates that thyrotropinomas derive from the clonal expansion of a single initially transformed cell [2]. Accordingly, the presence of a transforming event providing gain of proliferative function followed by secondary mutations or alterations favoring tumor progression presumably applies to thyrotropinomas as to other neoplastic lesions [7].

Mutations of proto-oncogenes, tumor suppressor genes, and pituitary-specific genes, able to confer growth advantage to pituitary cells, have been screened extensively. No mutations in oncogenes commonly activated in human cancer, particularly *Ras*, are reported in thyrotropinomas. In contrast to GH-secreting adenomas, in which the oncogene, *gsp*, frequently is found, none of the thyrotropinomas screened has been shown to express activating mutations of genes encoding for G protein subunits, such as αs, αq, α11, or αi2, or for thyrotopin-releasing hormone (TRH) receptor [8]. Because the transcription factor Pit-1 plays a crucial role in cell differentiation and in PRL, GH, and thyrotropin gene expression, Pit-1 gene has been screened for mutations in 14 thyrotropinomas and found to be wild type [2]. In contrast, as it occurs in GH-omas, Pit-1 also is overexpressed in thyrotropinomas, although the proliferative potential of this finding remains to be elucidated.

Possible alterations of antioncogenetic factors (p53, retinoblastoma gene, and others) also have been investigated and found normal. Another candidate gene investigated is the menin, the gene responsible for the multiple endocrine neoplasia type 1 (MEN1). Sporadic pituitary adenomas show loss of heterozygosity (LOH) on 11q13, where menin is located, and LOH on this chromosome seems to be associated with the transition from the noninvasive to the invasive phenotype. In a previous study performed on 13 thyrotropinomas using polymorphic markers on 11q13, the authors showed LOH in three, but menin mutations were absent in all [9]. Hyperthyroidism resulting from thyrotropinomas is reported in five cases within a familial setting of MEN1 syndrome [10].

Alterations in the feedback control mechanisms, as potential pathogenetic factors in the development of thyrotropinomas, recently have been investigated. The absence of expression of thyroid hormone receptors, such as TRa1, TRa2, and TRb1, was reported in one thyrotropinoma, but somatic mutations of TRb and aberrant alternative splicing of TRb2 mRNA encoding a TRb variant lacking T3-binding activity recently were shown as mechanisms for impaired T3-dependent negative regulation of thyrotropin-β and α-GSU in tumoral tissue [11,12].

Finally, LOH and particular polymorphisms at the somatostatin receptor type 5 gene locus seem to be associated with an aggressive phenotype and resistance to somatostatin analog treatment, possibly because of lack of somatostatin-induced inhibition of thyrotropin secretion [13]. Moreover, overexpression of basic fibroblast growth factor (bFGF) by some thyrotropinomas suggests the possibility that it may play a role in the development of fibrosis and tumor cell proliferation of this unusual type of pituitary neoplasm [14]. This overexpression of bFGF could be the cause of some tumor with the consistency of "stones" [15].

Diagnostic procedures

Patients who have thyrotropinoma present with signs and symptoms of hyperthyroidism that usually are milder than expected owing to the levels of circulating thyroid hormones, probably because of the long duration of the disease. In patients who have mixed thyrotropin/GH adenoma, clinical features of hyperthyroidism can be overshadowed by those of acromegaly, emphasizing the importance of systematic measurement of thyrotropin and FT4 in patients who have pituitary tumor. Goiter is present in almost all patients, even in those who have previous partial thyroidectomy, because thyroid residue may regrow as a consequence of the continuous thyrotropion hyperstimulation [1,2,5,16]. Approximately one third of patients who have thyrotropinoma were diagnosed as having primary hyperthyroidism (Graves' disease or toxic goiter) and, thus, mistakenly treated with thyroid ablation (thyroidectomy or radioiodine). Occurrence of uni- or multinodular goiter is frequent (approximately 72% of reported cases), but progression toward functional autonomy seems rare [1,5]. The presence of differentiated thyroid carcinomas also seems rare [2,17].

Hyperthyroid features frequently are associated with those related to tumor expansion, such as visual field defects (25% of patients), headache (20%), and hypopituitarism (50%) [1,5,16]. Alteration of hypothalamic-pituitary-gonadal axis is frequent, with menstrual disorders present in all patients who have mixed thyrotropin/PRL adenomas and in one third of those who have pure thyrotropinomas. Central hypogonadism, delayed puberty, and decreased libido also were found in several men who had thyrotropinomas or mixed thyrotropin/FSH adenomas. GH deficiency is reported in few cases.

From a biochemical viewpoint, along with the elevated levels of FT4 and FT3 in the presence of measurable thyrotropin concentrations, 80% of patients who have thyrotropinomas present an unbalanced hypersecretion of circulating free α-GSU levels and elevated α-GSU/thyrotropin molar ratio (Table 1) [1,4,5,16]. Recent data indicate that serum α-GSU levels almost always are normal in microadenomas, suggesting that the unbalanced α-GSU hypersecretion could be a phenomenon of progressive differentiation when the adenoma reaches a given volume. Moreover, measurements of several parameters of peripheral thyroid hormone action are proposed as quantifying the degree of tissue hyperthyroidism [2]. In particular, liver (sex hormone–binding globulin [SHBG]) and bone (carboxyterminal cross-linked telopeptide of type I collagen [ICTP]) parameters are used successfully to differentiate hyperthyroid patients who have thyrotropinoma from those who have PRTH [1,18]. As it occurs in the common forms of hyperthyroidism, patients who have thyrotropinoma have high serum SHBG and ICTP levels, whereas they are in the normal range in patients who have PRTH (see Table 1).

Stimulatory and inhibitory tests are useful for the diagnosis of thyrotropinoma. Classically, the T3 suppression test has been used to assess the presence of thyrotropinomas. A complete inhibition of thyrotropin secretion after T3 suppression test (80–100 mg per day per 8 to 10 days) never has been recorded (see Table 1). In patients who have had previous thyroid ablation, T3 suppression seems the most sensitive and specific test in assessing the presence of such a pituitary tumor [1,5,16]. This test is

Table 1
Differential diagnosis between thyrotropinomas and pituitary resistance to thyroid hormones

Parameter	Thyrotropinomas	Pituitary resistance to thyroid hormones	Significance (P)
Female/male ratio	1.3	1.4	NS
Familial cases (%)	0	85	<0.0001
Thyrotropin mU/L	2.7 ± 0.6	2.1 ± 0.3	NS
FT4 pmol/L	40.0 ± 4.2	30.5 ± 2.6	NS
FT3 pmol/L	14.5 ± 1.4	12.7 ± 1.2	NS
SHBG nmol/L[a]	113 ± 17	60 ± 5	<0.0001
Presence of lesion at CT scan or MRI (%)	98	5	<0.0001
High α-GSU levels (%)	65	3	<0.0001
High α-GSU/thyrotropin m.r. (%)	81	2	<0.0001
Abnormal thyrotropin response to T3 suppression test (%)[b]	100	100	NS
Blunted thyrotropin response to TRH test (%)	94	4	<0.0001

Only patients who had intact thyroid were taken into account. Data were obtained from patients followed at the authors' institute (38 thyrotropinomas and 58 PRTH) and are expressed as mean ± SE.

[a] SHBG measured as a parameter of thyroid hormone action at the peripheral tissue level.

[b] Werner's test (80–100 mg T3 for 8–10 days). Quantitatively normal responses to T3 (ie, complete inhibition of basal and TRH-stimulated thyrotropin levels) have never been recorded in either group of patients. Nonetheless, the majority of patients who have PRTH shows a qualitatively normal thyrotropin response to T3 suppression test.

contraindicated in elderly patients and in those who have coronary heart disease. Therefore, the stimulatory TRH test has been used widely in the work-up of thyrotropinomas. In the majority of patients, thyrotropin and α-GSU levels do not increase after TRH injection (see Table 1). The finding of a discrepant response to TRH between thyrotropin and α-GSU (or GH in the case of acromegaly), however, is pathognomonic of pituitary adenomas cosecreting thyrotropin and other hormones (Fig. 2) [4].

The administration of native somatostatin or its analogs (octreotide and lanreotide) induces a reduction of circulating thyrotropin levels in normal and in the majority of the tumoral thyrotropes [19–25]. In thyrotropinomas, the inhibitory response of thyrotropin to these agents may be predictive of the efficacy of long-term treatment. Recently, the authors have chronically treated a series of patients who had thyrotropinomas or PRTH with long-acting somatostatin analogs, documenting a marked decrease of FT3 and FT4 levels in all but one patient who had tumor; patients who had PRTH did not respond at all (Fig. 3). Thus, administration of long-acting somato-statin analogs for at least 2 to 3 months can be useful in the differential

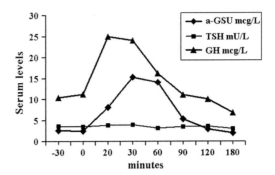

Fig. 2. Responses of serum pituitary α-GSU, thyrotropin (TSH), and GH to TRH injection in a patient who had a mixed thyrotropin/GH pitutary tumor. Note the lack of thyrotropin response to TRH that clearly is dissociated from those of α-GSU and GH. Such dissociation is pathognomonic of the presence of a pituitary adenoma secreting thyrotropin and other hormones.

diagnosis of problematic cases of central hyperthyroidism [26]. Nevertheless, because none of these tests is of clear-cut diagnostic value, the use of T3 suppression and TRH test is recommended whenever possible, because the combination of their results increases the specificity and sensitivity of the diagnostic work-up [1,5,16].

Finally, nuclear MRI currently is the preferable tool for the visualization of a thyrotropinoma. If MRI is contraindicated (eg, in the presence of a pacemaker), high-resolution CT is the alternative imaging investigation.

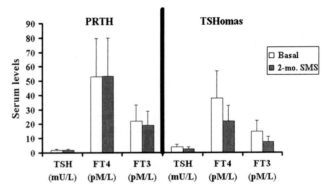

Fig. 3. Serum thyrotropin (TSH), FT4, and FT3 concentrations after 2 months' treatment with somatostatin analogs (octreotide 20–30 mg every 28 days) in 11 patients who had thyrotropinoma and in six patients who had PRTH. Note the lack of effects in patients who had PRTH and the significant reduction of FT4 and FT3 in patients who had thyrotropinomas. Only one patient who had thyrotropinoma did not have normalized serum FT4 and FT3 concentrations. These findings show that the administration of long-acting somatostatin analogs for at least 2 months can be useful in the differential diagnosis of problematic cases of central hyperthyroidism.

Recently, pituitary scintigraphy with radiolabeled octreotide (octreoscan) has been shown to successfully localize thyrotropinomas expressing somatostatin receptors [27]. The specificity of octreoscan is low, however, as positive scans can be seen in the case of a pituitary mass of different types, either secreting or nonsecreting. Such a procedure may be useful in the recognition of the possible ectopic localization of a thyrotropinoma, as two cases of thyrotropinomas recently were found in the nasopharyngeal region [28,29].

Differential diagnosis

In the differential work-up, the first step is to exclude the presence of methodologic interferences that may give falsely elevated serum levels of thyrotropin or free thyroid hormones (ie, rule out the presence of primary hyperthyroidism and the various forms of euthyroid hyperthyroxinemia) [1]. Once the existence of central hyperthyroidism is confirmed, additional diagnostic steps have to be performed to differentiate thyrotropinoma from RTH, in particular PRTH. The presence of neurologic signs and symptoms (eg, visual defects and headache) or clinical features of concomitant hypersecretion of other pituitary hormones, as in the case of acromegaly or amenorrhea/galactorrhea syndrome, points to the presence of a thyrotropinoma. Moreover, alterations of the pituitary gland on MRI or CT scan strongly support the diagnosis of a thyrotropinoma. Nonetheless, the differential diagnosis with PRTH may be difficult when the pituitary adenoma is small or in the case of confusing lesions, such as ectopic tumors, empty sella, or pituitary incidentalomas, the latter found frequently in the general population [30]. In these cases, elevated α-GSU concentrations or high α-GSU/thyrotropin molar ratio and thyrotropin unresponsiveness to TRH stimulation or to T3 suppression tests, or both, favor the presence of a thyrotropinoma. Moreover, the finding of similar biochemical data in family relatives definitely points to the presence of RTH, as familial cases of thyrotropinomas are not documented, apart from the setting of MEN1 syndrome. Finally, an apparent association between thyrotropinoma and RTH recently has been reported [31] and somatic mutations in the thyroid-hormone receptor are found in some tumors [11,12]; thus, the occurrence of thyrotropinoma in patients who have RTH should be considered carefully.

Treatment

The primary goals of the treatment of thyrotropinomas are the removal of pituitary tumor and restoration of euthyroidism. As a consequence, the first therapeutic approach should be the transsphenoidal or subfrontal adenomectomy, the route choice depending on the tumor volume and its suprasellar extension. This may be difficult particularly because of the marked fibrosis of these tumors, possibly related to high expression of bFGF [14,15]. Moreover, some adenomas are locally invasive involving the cavernous sinus, internal carotid artery, or optic chiasm, rendering the complete resection impossible or dangerous.

To restore euthyroidism before surgery, different drugs may be used, including antithyroid drugs (methimazole or propylthiouracil), propranolol, and somatostatin analogs (octreotide or lanreotide). They may overcast the postoperative course of thyrotropin secretion, however, which is expected to be inhibited totally if the tumor removal is achieved completely and, therefore, a useful criterion to assess definitive cure of the disease may be lost [32]. If surgery is contraindicated or declined, pituitary radiotherapy (no less than 45 Gy fractionated at 2 Gy per day or 10–25 Gy in a single dose if a stereotactic Gamma Unit is available) should be considered. A successful treatment of an invasive thyrotropinoma associated with an unruptured aneurysm by two-stage operation and gamma knife recently has been reported [33].

Fig. 4 shows the general outcome after surgery alone or combined with radiotherapy; data was collected from 211 patients reported in the literature. Normalization of thyroid hormone circulating levels and apparent complete removal of tumor mass was observed in 38% of patients who, therefore, may be considered apparently cured (follow-up ranged from 2 to 121 months). An additional 28% of patients were judged improved, as normalization of thyroid hormone circulating levels was achieved in all, although there was no complete removal of the adenoma. Together these findings indicate that approximately two thirds of thyrotropinomas are under control with surgery or irradiation. In the remaining patients, thyrotropin hypersecretion was unchanged, reflecting the surgical difficulties resulting from the large volume and invasiveness of the tumor. Because of the

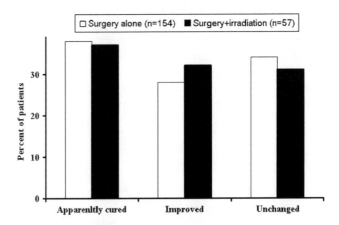

Fig. 4. Results of pituitary surgery alone and pituitary surgery plus irradiation in 211 patients who had thyrotropinomas (data collected from the literature as of June 2007). Apparently cured are the patients who became euthyroid and showed no residual tumor, whereas improved are the patients who became euthyroid but showed tumoral residues.

possible iatrogenic hypopituitarism, evaluation of other pituitary functions, in particular ACTH secretion, should be undertaken carefully soon after surgery and checked again every year, especially in patients treated with radiotherapy. In addition, in the case of surgical cure, postoperative thyrotropin is undetectable and may remain low for many weeks or even months, causing central hypothyroidism. A permanent central hypothyroidism may occur resulting from compression by the tumor on the pituitary stalk or surgical damage of the normal thyrotropes. Transient or permanent L-T4 replacement therapy may be necessary. Finally, in few patients, total thyroidectomy was performed after pituitary surgery failure, as the patients were at risk for thyroid storm [2,34].

Although the surgical cure rate of thyrotropinomas has improved in recent years, at least 30% of patients require medical therapy to control the hyperthyroidism. The physiologic inhibition of thyrotropin secretion by somatostatin and the expression of somatostatin receptors on the tumoral cells suggest trials with somatostatin analogs to block tumoral hypersecretion of thyrotropin [1,5,16,20–26]. There is a good correlation between somatostatin binding capacity and maximal biologic response, as quantified by inhibition of thyrotropin secretion and in vivo restoration of euthyroid state [19]. Moreover, the presence of dopamine receptors in thyrotropinomas was the rationale for therapeutic trials with dopaminergic agonists, such as bromocriptine and cabergoline. This treatment seems particularly effective in the mixed thyrotropin/PRL adenomas [1,2]. The combined use of somatostatin and dopaminergic drugs has never been tried in patients who have thyrotropinomas but should be re-evaluated in light of the demonstration of possible heterodimerization of somatostatin receptor type 5 and dopamine D2 receptor on cell surface [35]. Nevertheless, the medical treatment of thyrotropinomas rests on long-acting somatostatin analogs, such as octreotide LAR, lanreotide SR, or lanreotide Autogel [1,5,16,20–26]. Treatment with these analogs leads to a reduction of thyrotropin and α-GSU secretion in almost all cases, with restoration of the euthyroid state in the majority (Table 2). Circulating thyroid hormone levels normalized in 95% of patients who were not previously thyroidectomized. Pituitary tumor mass shrinkage occurred in approximately 42% of patients and vision improvement was documented in 66%. Goiter size was reduced significantly by somatostatin analog therapy in 20% of cases. Resistance to somatostatin analog treatment, true escape of thyrotropin secretion from the inhibitory effects of the drugs, or discontinuation of treatment because of side effects was documented in a minority of cases. Somatostatin analog treatment in pregnant women was effective in restoring euthyroidism in mothers and had no side effects on development and thyroid function of the fetuses [36]. Moreover, in almost all patients who had mixed thyrotropin/GH hypersecretion, signs and symptoms of acromegaly disappeared concomitantly. Patients on somatostatin analogs must be monitored carefully, as untoward side effects, such as cholelithiasis and carbohydrate

Table 2
Results of treatment with somatostatin analogs (octreotide LAR, lanreotide SR, or lanreotide Autogel) in 128 patients who had thyrotropinoma recorded in the literature as of June 2007

Thyrotopin reduction (> 50% versus basal)	88%
α-GSU reduction	93%
Thyrotopin and α-GSU normalization	72%
Thyroid hormone normalization (long-term studies)	95%
Tumor mass shrinkage	42%
Vision improvement	66%
Goiter size reduction	20%
True escape	9%
Resistance	4%
Discontinuation of therapy because of side effects	6%

intolerance, may become manifest. The administered dose should be tailored for each patient, depending on therapeutic response and tolerance (including gastrointestinal side effects). The tolerance usually is good, as gastrointestinal side effects are transient with long-acting analogs. The marked somatostatin-induced suppression of thyrotropin secretion and consequent biochemical hypothyroidism seen in some patients may require L-T4 substitution.

In conclusion, whether or not somatostatin analog treatment may be an alternative to surgery or irradiation in patients who have thyrotropinoma remains to be established. The therapeutic success of octreotide and lanreotide administration is high, however, approaching 95% of treated patients. Somatostatin analogs, therefore, may represent a useful tool for long-term treatment of such rare pituitary tumors.

References

[1] Beck-Peccoz P, Brucker-Davis F, Persani L, et al. Thyrotropin-secreting pituitary tumors. Endocr Rev 1996;17:610–38.
[2] Beck-Peccoz P, Persani L. Thyrotropin-secreting pituitary adenomas. In: Thyroid disease manager. Available at: http://www.thyroidmanager.org/.
[3] Greenman Y, Melemd S. Thyrotropin-secreting pituitary tumors. In: Melmed S, editor. The pituitary. 2nd edition. London: Blackwell Publishing; 2002. p. 561–74.
[4] Terzolo M, Orlandi F, Bassetti M, et al. Hyperthyroidism due to a pituitary adenoma composed of two different cell types, one secreting alpha-subunit alone and another cosecreting alpha-subunit and thyrotropin. J Clin Endocrinol Metab 1991;72:415–21.
[5] Socin HV, Chanson P, Delemer B, et al. The changing spectrum of TSH-secreting pituitary adenomas: diagnosis and management in 43 patients. Eur J Endocrinol 2003;148:433–42.
[6] Refetoff S, Weiss RE, Usala SJ. The syndromes of resistance to thyroid hormone. Endocr Rev 1993;14:348–99.
[7] Melmed S. Mechanisms for pituitary tumorigenesis: the plastic pituitary. J Clin Invest 2003; 112:1603–18.
[8] Dong Q, Brucker-Davis F, Weintraub BD, et al. Screening of candidate oncogenes in human thyrotroph tumors: absence of activating mutations of the Gaq, Ga11, Gas, or thyrotropin-releasing hormone receptor genes. J Clin Endocrinol Metab 1996;81:1134–40.

[9] Asteria C, Anagni M, Persani L, et al. Loss of heterozigosity of the MEN1 gene in a large series of TSH-secreting pituitary adenomas. J Endocrinol Invest 2001;24:796–801.

[10] Taylor TJ, Donlon SS, Bale AE, et al. Treatment of a thyrotropinoma with octreotide-LAR in a patient with multiple endocrine neoplasia-1. Thyroid 2000;10:1001–7.

[11] Ando S, Sarlis NJ, Oldfield EH, et al. Somatic mutation of TRbeta can cause a defect in negative regulation of TSH in a TSH-secreting pituitary tumor. J Clin Endocrinol Metab 2001;86:5572–6.

[12] Ando S, Sarlis NJ, Krishnan J, et al. Aberrant alternative splicing of thyroid hormone receptor in a TSH-secreting pituitary tumor is a mechanism for hormone resistance. Mol Endocrinol 2001;15:1529–38.

[13] Filopanti M, Ballare E, Lania AG, et al. Loss of heterozygosity at the SS receptor type 5 locus in human GH- and TSH-secreting pituitary adenomas. J Endocrinol Invest 2004;27:937–42.

[14] Ezzat S, Horvath E, Kovacs K, et al. Basic fibroblast growth factor expression by two prolactin and thyrotropin-producing pituitary adenomas. Endocr Pathol 1995;6:125–34.

[15] Webster J, Peters JR, Smith J, et al. Pituitary stone: two cases of densely calcified thyrotrophin-secreting pituitary adenomas. Clin Endocrinol (Oxf) 1994;40:137–43.

[16] Brucker-Davis F, Oldfield EH, Skarulis MC, et al. Thyrotropin-secreting pituitary tumors: diagnostic criteria, thyroid hormone sensitivity, and treatment outcome in 25 patients followed at the National Institutes of Health. J Clin Endocrinol Metab 1999;84:476–86.

[17] Brown RL, Muzzafar T, Wollman R, et al. A pituitary carcinoma secreting TSH and prolactin: a non-secreting adenoma gone awry. Eur J Endocrinol 2006;154:639–43.

[18] Persani L, Preziati D, Matthews CH, et al. Serum levels of carboxyterminal cross-linked telopeptide of type I collagen (ICTP) in the differential diagnosis of the syndromes of inappropriate secretion of TSH. Clin Endocrinol (Oxf) 1997;47:207–14.

[19] Bertherat J, Brue T, Enjalbert A, et al. Somatostatin receptors on thyrotropin-secreting pituitary adenomas: comparison with the inhibitory effects of octreotide upon in vivo and in vitro hormonal secretions. J Clin Endocrinol Metab 1992;75:540–6.

[20] Gancel A, Vuillermet P, Legrand A, et al. Effects of a slow-release formulation of the new somatostatin analogue lanreotide in TSH-secreting pituitary adenomas. Clin Endocrinol 1994;40:421–8.

[21] Chanson P, Weintraub BD, Harris AG. Octreotide therapy for thyroid stimulating-secreting pituitary adenomas. A follow-up of 52 patients. Ann Intern Med 1993;119:236–40.

[22] Kuhn JM, Arlot S, Lefebvre H, et al. Evaluation of the treatment of thyrotropin-secreting pituitary adenomas with a slow release formulation of the somatostatin analog lanreotide. J Clin Endocrinol Metab 2000;85:1487–91.

[23] Kienitz T, Quinkler M, Strasburger CJ, et al. Long-term management in five cases of TSH-secreting pituitary adenomas: a single center study and review of the literature. Eur J Endocrinol 2007;157:39–46.

[24] Horiguchi K, Yamada M, Umezawa R, et al. Somatostatin receptor subtypes mRNA in TSH-secreting pituitary adenomas: a case showing a dramatic reduction in tumor size during short octreotide treatment. Endocr J 2007;54:371–8.

[25] Yoshihara A, Isozaki O, Hizuka N, et al. Expression of type 5 somatostatin receptor in TSH-secreting pituitary adenomas: a possible marker for predicting long-term response to octreotide therapy. Endocr J 2007;54:133–8.

[26] Mannavola D, Persani L, Vannucchi G, et al. Different response to chronic somatostatin analogues in patients with central hyperthyroidism. Clin Endocrinol (Oxf) 2005;62:176–81.

[27] Losa M, Magnani P, Mortini P, et al. Indium-111 pentetreotide single-photon emission tomography in patients with TSH-secreting pituitary adenomas: correlation with the effect of a single administration of octreotide on serum TSH levels. Eur J Nucl Med 1997;24:728–31.

[28] Cooper DS, Wenig BM. Hyperthyroidism caused by an ectopic TSH-secreting pituitary tumor. Thyroid 1996;6:337–42.

[29] Pasquini E, Faustini-Fustini M, Sciarretta V, et al. Ectopic TSH-secreting pituitary adenoma of the vomerosphenoidal junction. Eur J Endocrinol 2003;148:253–7.

[30] Hall WA, Luciano MG, Doppman JL, et al. Pituitary magnetic resonance imaging in normal human volunteers: occult adenomas in the general population. Ann Intern Med 1994;120: 817–82.

[31] Watanabe K, Kameya T, Yamauchi A, et al. Thyrotropin-producing adenoma associated with pituitary resistance to thyroid hormone. J Clin Endocrinol Metab 1993;76:1025–31.

[32] Losa M, Giovanelli M, Persani L, et al. Criteria of cure and follow-up of central hyperthyroidism due to thyrotropin-secreting pituitary adenomas. J Clin Endocrinol Metab 1996;81: 3086–90.

[33] Ohki M, Sato K, Tuchiya D, et al. [A case of TSH-secreting pituitary adenoma associated with an unruptured aneurysm: successful treatment by two-stage operation and gamma knife]. No To Shinkei 1999;51:895–9 [in Japanese].

[34] Daousi C, Foy PM, MacFarlane IA. Ablative thyroid treatment for thyrotoxicosis due to thyrotropin-producing pituitary tumours. J Neurol Neurosurg Psychiatry 2007;78:93–5.

[35] Rocheville M, Lange DC, Kumar U, et al. Receptors for dopamine and somatostatin: formation of hetero-oligomers with enhanced functional activity. Science 2000;288:154–7.

[36] Blackhurst G, Strachan MW, Collie D, et al. The treatment of a thyrotropin-secreting pituitary macroadenoma with octreotide in twin pregnancy. Clin Endocrinol (Oxf) 2002; 57:401–4.

ELSEVIER
SAUNDERS

Endocrinol Metab Clin N Am
37 (2008) 135–149

ENDOCRINOLOGY
AND METABOLISM
CLINICS
OF NORTH AMERICA

Cushing's Syndrome

Rosario Pivonello, MD, PhD*,
Maria Cristina De Martino, MD, Monica De Leo, MD,
Gaetano Lombardi, MD, Annamaria Colao, MD, PhD

*Department of Molecular and Clinical Endocrinology and Oncology, Federico II University,
Via Sergio Pansini 5, 80131 Naples, Italy*

Cushing's syndrome results from chronic exposure to excessive concentrations of circulating glucocorticoids [1]. The most common cause of Cushing's syndrome, the "exogenous Cushing's syndrome," is usually caused by the use of supraphysiologic amounts of exogenous glucocorticoids. On the other hand, the "endogenous Cushing's syndrome" is caused by the endogenous oversecretion of glucocorticoids by the adrenal glands [1]. The incidence of the disorder, which is more common in women than in men, ranges from 0.7 to 2.4 per million population per year [2], although recent screening studies in patients with diabetes mellitus, especially those with obesity and hypertension, suggest that Cushing's syndrome is more common than previously thought (ie, the prevalence of the disease in these patients ranges from 2%–5%) [3]. Endogenous Cushing's syndrome is divided into two main forms: the corticotropin-dependent and the corticotropin-independent. The corticotropin-dependent Cushing's syndrome accounts for about 80% to 85% of cases, and of these, 80% are due to pituitary tumors, with the remaining 20% due to ectopic corticotropin secretion syndrome, which usually derives from carcinoid tumors or small-cell carcinoma of the lung. Corticotropin-independent Cushing's syndrome, accounting for about 15% to 20%, is due in most instances to an adrenal tumor or, more rarely, corticotropin-independent macronodular adrenal hyperplasia, primary pigmented nodular adrenal disease (either as isolated disease or as part of Carney complex), or McCune-Albright syndrome [1]. This article focuses on endogenous Cushing's syndrome; mainly, the pituitary-dependent disease (ie, Cushing's disease).

* Corresponding author.
E-mail address: rpivone@tin.it (R. Pivonello).

0889-8529/08/$ - see front matter © 2008 Elsevier Inc. All rights reserved.
doi:10.1016/j.ecl.2007.10.010

Clinical picture

The clinical picture of Cushing's syndrome is significantly variable, depending on the sex and age of the patient as well as the severity and the duration of the disease [4]. The most common feature of Cushing's syndrome is central obesity, which is due to excessive deposits of visceral fat at the abdominal level, associated with thinning of the limbs as a result of muscle atrophy. Typical features of the disease are represented by rounded face with facial plethora; "buffalo hump" formed by the fat deposit in the posterior region of the neck; purple striae, located mainly in the lateral region of the abdomen, in the axillary region, and in the internal region of the thighs; and body bruising. Gonadal dysfunction is a common feature of the disease, being present in more than 75% of patients. It is differently manifested in men and women; indeed, men have sexual disturbances mainly owing to decreased libido and erectile dysfunction, whereas women have menstrual irregularity. Hirsutism and alopecia occur in a certain percentage of women, owing to the concomitant increase of circulating androgens, directly secreted by the adrenal glands, or as consequence of a polycystic ovary syndrome. Infertility is common in men and women. The most important systemic complication of Cushing's syndrome is represented by the metabolic syndrome, occurring in around 75% of patients, owing to visceral obesity, hypertension, glucose intolerance, and dyslipidemia, which commonly complicate the disease [5]. The metabolic syndrome, together with the thrombosis diathesis, and the presence of increased homocysteine and decreased taurine levels determine the association of the disease with an increased cardiovascular risk, partially persisting also after the disease cure [6–8]. Nephrolithiasis is present in 50% of patients, although they are usually not apparent clinically [9]. Osteoporosis is also present in 50% of patients and often induces skeletal fractures [10,11], which usually recover after disease cure, although it often requires specific treatments [12].

Neurologic or psychiatric syndrome complicate a greater part of patients with Cushing's syndrome. The former includes impairment of cognition and memory and is associated with a reduction in apparent brain volume, whereas the latter ranges from anxiety to psychosis, manifested mainly as depression. Neurologic syndromes slowly recover, whereas psychiatric syndromes often persist after disease cure [13,14]. An impaired quality of life is consistently documented in patients with Cushing's syndrome even after resolution of cortisol excess [15]. It is noteworthy that central obesity and delayed growth and puberty are the most important features in children and adolescent patients with Cushing's syndrome. Table 1 summarizes the clinical picture of Cushing's syndrome.

Diagnosis

The diagnosis and differential diagnosis of Cushing's syndrome are complicated procedures that require a combination of several laboratory tests

Table 1
List of the main symptoms and signs associated with Cushing's syndrome

Symptoms and signs	Prevalence (%)
	90–100
Central obesity	
Rounded face ("moon face")	
Facial plethora	
Decreased libido	
	70–90
Purple striae	
Menstrual disturbances	
Hirsutism	
Erectile dysfunction	
Hypertension	
	50–70
Muscle weakness	
Posterior neck fat deposit ("buffalo hump")	
Body bruising	
Glucose intolerance/diabetes	
Osteopenia/osteoporosis	
Emotional lability/depression	
	20–50
Headache	
Backache	
Limb edema	
Recurrent infections	
Hypokaliemic alkalosis	
Nephrolithiasis	
	0–20
Acne	
Alopecia	

and radiologic examinations [16]. The first step in the diagnostic procedure of chronic endogenous hypercortisolism is the diagnosis of Cushing's syndrome, which means distinguishing Cushing's syndrome from normal individuals and patients with pseudo-Cushing's states, including primarily obesity but also depression, alcoholism, and polycystic ovary syndrome, where hypercortisolism is a common feature. None of the commonly used first-line screening tests has proven a 100% diagnostic accuracy. These tests mainly include 24-hour urinary-free cortisol (UFC) and overnight low-dose dexamethasone suppression test (LD-DST). The 24-hour UFC gives an integrated index of the unbound cortisol that circulated in the blood during this period of time. In contrast to plasma cortisol levels, which measure total cortisol, unbound and bound, it is not affected by factors that influence corticosteroid-binding globulin levels [17,18]. However, urine collection modality and renal function may affect this test. Therefore, urinary creatinine should be measured to verify the adequacy of the urine collection. Moreover, a glomerular filtration rate less than 30 mL/min should induce to consider whether UFC may be falsely normal [16–18]. UFC values can be extremely variable in Cushing's syndrome. Nonetheless, if cortisol excretion results are normal in three collections, Cushing's syndrome is highly unlikely, whereas UFC values fourfold greater than the upper limit of normal can be considered diagnostic for Cushing's syndrome. UFC values between normal values and this cutoff value do not permit any conclusion to be drawn on the diagnosis of the syndrome. The overnight 1-mg LD-DST consists of the oral intake of 1-mg dexamethasone between 11 PM and midnight, followed by measurement of fasting plasma cortisol between 8 and 9 AM the following morning. The original criterion for normal level of suppression was a plasma cortisol level below 5 µg/dL (138 nmol/L), although more recently this cutoff level has been reduced to less than 1.8 µg/dL (50 nmol/L) [10,11], greatly enhancing the sensitivity of the test. A serum cortisol level below 1.8 µg/dL excludes Cushing's syndrome. The specificity of the test is, however, limited, owing to potential misclassification of patients with pseudo-Cushing states and, occasionally, healthy individuals [16–18]. A recent screening test is represented by the late-night salivary cortisol, a simple and potentially useful test, whose accuracy still needs to be validated [19]. The second-line screening tests consist of plasma cortisol circadian rhythm/midnight plasma cortisol and 2 days' LD-DST. Patients with Cushing's syndrome often have early-morning serum cortisol concentrations within or slightly above the normal range but lack a normal circadian rhythm. Plasma cortisol levels are above a cutoff value of 1.8 µg/dL when measured at midnight in hospitalized patients with Cushing's syndrome. This cutoff value has a high degree of sensitivity, but its specificity is sensibly lower than sensitivity. A higher cutoff value (7.5 µg/dL) has been proposed to achieve the best specificity. The classic 2 days' LD-DST consists of taking 0.5-mg dexamethasone orally every 6 hours and collecting urine for UFC at baseline and on the second day of dexamethasone administration, or, alternatively, measuring serum cortisol at baseline and 48 hours after the starting of dexamethasone administration. A normal response consists of a decrease of UFC to less than 10 µg (27 nmol) every 24 hours on the second day of dexamethasone administration or of plasma cortisol to less than 1.8 µg/dL on the morning after the last dose of dexamethasone. Use of the plasma cortisol end point results in a sensitivity and specificity of more than 95%. Adequate urine collections and normal bioavailability and metabolism of dexamethasone are required for the procedure to be valid [16–18]. The combined LD-DST+CRH (corticotrophin-releasing hormone) test has been proposed as a possible useful test, but it has shown controversial results and its accuracy still needs to be validated [20,21].

The second step in the diagnostic procedure of chronic endogenous hypercortisolim is represented by the differentiation between the three forms of Cushing's syndrome. This step is initially based on the measurement of plasma adrenocorticotropic hormone (ACTH) levels. If ACTH is suppressed (<5 pg/mL), adrenal-dependent Cushing's syndrome is suspected, and an adrenal CT/MRI scanning will identify the type of adrenal lesion responsible for the disease. An ACTH between 5 and 20 pg/mL is doubtful and may require a stimulation test to be clearly interpreted. Conversely, if ACTH is not suppressed (>20 pg/mL), ACTH-dependent causes should be investigated. ACTH levels tend to be higher in ectopic ACTH-secreting than in pituitary ACTH-secreting Cushing's syndrome. However, the overlap in ACTH values is such that ACTH values alone rarely distinguish between the two conditions; dynamic tests are therefore needed [16–18]. On the other hand, an occult ectopic source of ACTH may mimic pituitary-dependent disease because such tumors may express glucocorticoid and/or CRH and/or vasopressin (AVP) receptors, and thus behave as a misplaced pituitary in the course of all standard dynamic tests. The most important dynamic test is the high-dose DST (HD-DST). High doses of glucocorticoids partially suppress ACTH secretion from most corticotroph pituitary tumors, whereas ectopic tumors are generally resistant to feedback inhibition. There are several versions of the HD-DST, including the standard 2 days' oral high dose (2 mg every 6 h for eight doses), the 8-mg overnight oral, and the intravenous (IV) 4- to 7-mg tests. Plasma and/or urinary cortisol levels are evaluated before, during, and/or after dexamethasone administration. These tests distinguish pituitary from ectopic sources of ACTH with a sensitivity varying from 60% to 80% and with high specificity when it is used as cutoff of plasma cortisol suppression above 50%. The specificity can be improved using a cutoff of cortisol suppression greater than 80%, although a specificity of 100% can never be attained. Two further useful dynamic tests are represented by CRH and desmopressin (DD-AVP) tests. Most pituitary tumors respond to CRH administration with an increase in plasma ACTH and cortisol levels. The test is performed by injecting IV 100-μg synthetic ovine or human CRH. Variability in the interpretation depends on the type of CRH used (human versus ovine), biochemical parameters considered (increase above baseline in ACTH, 35%–50%; cortisol, 14%–20%), and evaluated time points (ACTH, 15–30 min; cortisol, 15–45 min). However, because ectopic ACTH-producing tumors can also respond to CRH, increasing the cutoff level of the response will not produce 100% specificity, thus preventing complete reliance on this test alone. Most pituitary tumors also respond to DD-AVP administration with an increase of ACTH and cortisol levels. However, the evidence that a certain percentage of ectopic ACTH-secreting tumors also respond to DD-AVP limits its usefulness in distinguishing the source of ACTH excess [16–18]. A pituitary MRI with gadolinium enhancement should be performed in all patients with ACTH-dependent Cushing's syndrome. This procedure will reveal a discrete pituitary adenoma in around 60% of patients. In the patient with a classic clinical presentation and dynamic biochemical studies compatible with pituitary Cushing's syndrome, the presence of a focal lesion (>5 mm) disclosed on pituitary MRI may provide a definitive diagnosis, and no further evaluation may be required. However, it is important to realize that 10% of the general population harbor incidental pituitary tumors disclosed on MRI, although the majority of these lesions are less than 5 mm in diameter [22]. Bilateral inferior petrosal sinus sampling (BIPSS) for ACTH determination should be recommended for patients with ACTH-dependent Cushing's syndrome whose clinical, biochemical, or radiologic studies are discordant or equivocal. After the radiologist catheterizes both inferior petrosal sinuses (IPSs), blood samples for ACTH are obtained in the basal state and at 3, 5, and 10 minutes after IV ovine or human CRH (100 µg IV) simultaneously from both IPSs and a peripheral vein. An IPS-to-peripheral ACTH ratio (IPS/P) greater than 2.0 in the basal state and/or greater than 3.0 after CRH is consistent with Cushing's disease. BIPSS in experienced centers has a very high sensitivity (95%–99%). However, technical factors as well as anomalous venous drainage may produce false-negative results in patients with a pituitary source of ACTH. Lower IPS/P ratios suggest an ectopic ACTH-secreting tumor with a specificity of 95% to 99% [23,24]. In recent years, different sites of venous sampling (cavernous and jugular veins) have been used, but BIPPS remains the best test for the identification of Cushing's disease. If BIPSS confirms the lack of a pituitary ACTH gradient, CT and/or MRI of the neck, thorax, and abdomen should be performed to search for the ectopic ACTH-secreting tumors [16–18]. Despite the entire series of laboratory tests and radiologic examinations commonly used for the diagnosis and the differential diagnosis of Cushing's syndrome, the clear definition of the syndrome and the identification of its cause usually require a long period of time, which consequently delays the starting of the correct definitive treatment and worsens the prognosis of the disease. Fig. 1 presents a flow chart of the procedures used to diagnose Cushing's syndrome.

Treatment

The treatment of Cushing's syndrome is strongly dependent on the etiologic form of the syndrome. Indeed, surgery is the first-line treatment for all causes of Cushing's syndrome. In the majority of cases, however, surgical removal of the cortisol-secreting adrenal lesion or the ACTH-secreting neuroendocrine tumor represents the definitive treatment for the adrenal-dependent and the ectopic Cushing's syndrome, respectively, and requires additional therapies only in selected cases in which malignancy surgery failure is documented. The treatment of Cushing's disease, in general, requires different approaches (eg, pituitary and adrenal surgery, pituitary-targeted and adrenal-targeted pharmacotherapy, and radiotherapy) [1]. The following section focuses on the treatment of Cushing's disease.

Pituitary surgery

The first-line treatment of Cushing's disease is the surgical removal of the pituitary tumor by transphenoidal approach [25,26]. Transphenoidal

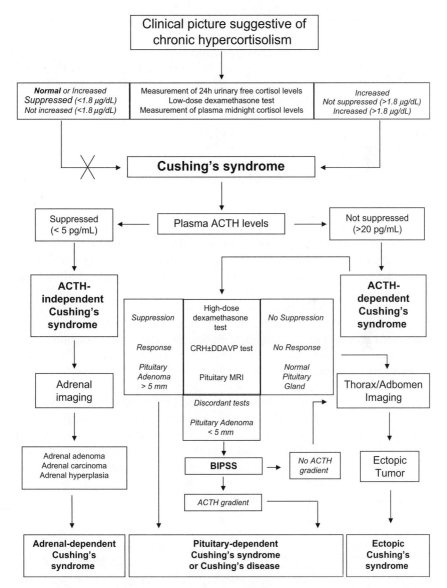

Fig. 1. Schematic procedure for the diagnosis and differential diagnosis of Cushing's syndrome.

surgery is associated with an initial remission rate between 60% and 80% (<15% for macroadenomas), but with a relapse rate of up to 20% during the first 10 years after surgery. It is probable that these variations result from different surgical skill, and controversy persists about the characterization of remission or persistence of Cushing's disease after surgery. Patients with hypocortisolism in the immediate postoperative period need glucocorticoid treatment until the recovery of the hypothalamo-pituitary-adrenal axis. On long-term follow-up, the overall remission rate is about 50% to 60% and pituitary deficiencies occur in up to 50% of patients. Although long-term remission is most probable when postoperative concentration of cortisol in serum is low (<1.8 μg/dL, <50 nmol/L), there is no threshold value that fully excludes possible recurrence [27,28]. The frequent failure of pituitary surgery in inducing disease cure is probably related to the small size of ACTH-secreting pituitary tumors and the documented presence of corticotroph cell hyperplasia instead of defined corticotroph tumors, which makes visualization of the tumors by standard imaging techniques difficult and, consequently, their surgical removal. These data emphasize the ongoing need for alternative therapies directed against the pituitary gland.

Adrenal surgery

The second-line treatment of Cushing's disease is the surgical removal of the adrenal glands [29]. Total bilateral adrenalectomy is indicated, especially in patients who are not candidates for a re-operation after the failure of the first pituitary surgery and have a severe disease not easy controlled by medical treatment. Total bilateral adrenalectomy induces rapid suppression of cortisol secretion and, consequently, a rapid resolution of the clinical picture, although lifelong treatment with glucocorticoids and mineralocorticoids are needed after surgery. As laparoscopic surgery has demonstrated lower morbidity than has classic laparotomic adrenal surgery, the former is becoming the main approach for this type of treatment, which is being considered more frequently than before, especially in cases of patient preference. A major concern after bilateral adrenalectomy in patients with Cushing's disease is the development of Nelson's syndrome, a locally aggressive pituitary tumor associated with severely increased secreting ACTH levels and consequent skin pigmentation that therefore needs specific treatment with surgery and/or radiotherapy. Whether a preventive radiotherapy at the time of total bilateral adrenalectomy is useful to reduce the risk of development of Nelson's syndrome is controversial [30].

Medical therapy

Medical therapy has a minor role in the management of Cushing's disease. Two different categories of drugs are used in the management of the disease: adrenal-blocking drugs, which act directly at the adrenal level, and neuromodulatory drugs, which act at the pituitary level [31].

Adrenal-blocking drugs mainly include metyrapone, ketoconazole, aminoglutethimide, and mitotane, all of which are capable of lowering cortisol by directly inhibiting synthesis and secretion in the adrenal gland. The first three agents have the capacity to inhibit the function of the adrenal enzymes; the last agent, an adrenolytic effect. In clinical practice, the most commonly used agent is the antifungal drug ketoconazole, which has a rapid onset of action but is frequently associated with loss of control of hypercortisolism, a phenomenon known as "escape," owing to ACTH oversecretion.

Ketoconazole is affected by gastrointestinal side effects, including a liver dysfunction, which rarely induces a severe hepatitis with acute liver failure. Metyrapone and aminoglutethimide have similar characteristics of ketoconazole. These drugs are not usually effective as the sole long-term treatment of the disorder, and are used mainly either in preparation for surgery or as adjunctive treatment after surgery and/or radiotherapy while the definitive effectiveness of these procedures is pending. These medical treatments can also be used in patients who are unwilling or unfit to undergo surgery. The anesthetic drug etomidate is sporadically used to induce an acute inhibition of cortisol secretion. Mitotane is a potent drug with delayed onset but long-lasting action, and it is not associated with escape occurrence. However, mitotane is associated with severe neurologic side effects, and induces a medical adrenalectomy, therefore limiting its use only in cases of severe disease or malignancy [32].

The neuromodulatory drugs include a long series of drugs that, during several past decades, have been tested as potential inhibitors of ACTH secretion from the corticotroph pituitary tumor. However, no single agent has ever demonstrated a great effectiveness for routine use in the management of Cushing's disease. In the past, cyproheptadine and valproate, respectively, acting at the level of serotonin and γ-Amino butyric acid receptors, have episodically demonstrated effectiveness in control of ACTH and cortisol secretion. The use of the somatostatin analog octreotide produced disappointing results, being effective only in a minority of cases tested for a short period of time. The only neuromodulatory agent that demonstrated such an effectiveness to be suggested as a possible agent for treatment of Cushing's disease was the dopamine agonist bromocriptine. Yet, although bromocriptine demonstrated an effectiveness in more than one third of patients with Cushing's disease after short-term treatment, the long-term results were also disappointing [33–35].

Recently, there has been renewed interest in the use of neuromodulatory drugs. The peroxisome proliferator-activated receptor γ (PPARγ) agonist rosiglitazone has been demonstrated to reduce ACTH and cortisol concentrations and prevent tumor growth in an animal model of Cushing's disease [36]. Despite the documented expression of PPARγ in human pituitary corticotroph tumors [37], studies in patients with Cushing's disease have, unfortunately, been almost uniformly disappointing. Rosiglitazone achieved only short-term control of cortisol, with later escape [38,39]. The PPARγ agonist pioglitazone has shown similar results [40]; moreover, it failed to demonstrate an inhibitory effect on ACTH levels in Nelson's syndrome [41]. Although the results of PPARγ agonists have been disappointing, it might be that higher doses or more potent agonists are needed to obtain a significant effectiveness. At present, the use of PPARγ ligands cannot be recommended in the treatment of Cushing's disease. In recent years, the possible role of dopamine agonists in the treatment of Cushing's disease has been reconsidered owing to the demonstration of disease remission in different cases with silent or active corticotroph tumors following the administration of the potent dopamine agonist cabergoline [42,43] and the demonstration of the expression of dopamine receptors in corticotroph tumors [44]. Indeed, short-term treatment with cabergoline at a dose of 1 to 3 mg each week was demonstrated to decrease cortisol secretion in 60% and to normalize cortisol secretion in 40% of patients with Cushing's disease [44]. Fig. 2 shows the effect of 3 months of cabergoline treatment on 10 patients with persistent Cushing's disease following surgery. Preliminary data on long-term (24 months) treatment suggested that more than one third of patients are controlled by cabergoline administration at doses ranging from 1 to 7 mg each week [45]. Cabergoline has also been found to be effective in controlling ACTH secretion in Nelson's syndrome [46–48]. Therefore, although this evidence needs to be confirmed on a large population of patients, cabergoline seems to be the most promising agent for the medical treatment of Cushing's disease.

The possible role of somatostatin analogs has also been reevaluated in the treatment of Cushing's disease as a newer somatostatin analog; namely pasireotide has been demonstrated to reduce ACTH secretion in cell culture of corticotroph tumor [49]. However, no definitive data are available on clinical trials; a preliminary experience on very short-term treatment, however, looks encouraging [50]. These data on the effectiveness of specific dopamine agonists and somatostatin analogs suggest that their combination may also be a possible therapeutic approach, considering that the combined use of cabergoline and lanreotide was demonstrated to be of benefit in ectopic Cushing's syndrome [51], especially when an escape from treatment with the only cabergoline occurs [52]. Finally, preliminary data in an animal model suggest that retinoic acid might cause direct inhibition of ACTH secretion from corticotroph tumors and should be considered as a possible therapeutic agent in the future [53].

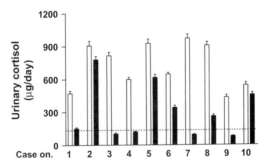

Fig. 2. Response of urinary cortisol levels to cabergoline treatment in 10 patients with Cushing's disease. White columns indicate the baseline values; black columns indicate the 3-month follow-up values. Broken line indicates the upper limit of normal of urinary cortisol levels. (*Reprinted from* Pivonello R, Ferone D, de Herder WW, et al. Dopamine receptor expression and function in corticotroph pituitary tumors. J Clin Endocrinol Metab 2004;89:2452–62; with permission. Copyright © 2004, The Endocrine Society.)

Fig. 3 represents a schematic treatment algorithm, outlining the possible role of medical therapy during the entire period of disease management.

Radiotherapy

Radiotherapy directed at residual pituitary tumor is a treatment option in patients with persistent hypercortisolaemia after surgery. Conventional fractionated radiotherapy is a very effective means of treatment, although its effectiveness is delayed—up to 10 years—and it is associated with long-term

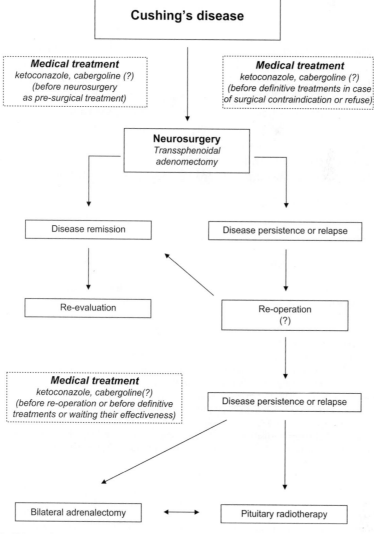

Fig. 3. Schematic algorithm for treatment of Cushing's disease with emphasis on the possible role of medical therapy during the entire period of disease management.

hypopituitarism [54]. Stereotactic radiosurgery has been demonstrated to be more rapidly effective, but a relapse rate of up to 20% after treatment has been shown, and it does not compare favorably with conventional radiotherapy. Radiotherapy is being used today less than in the past, and it is mostly reserved for patients with severe disease. This is especially the case when repeated pituitary surgery has failed to cure the disease and total bilateral adrenalectomy is not indicated, is refused by the patient, and/or medical therapy does not easily control hypercortisolism, as well as in the event of particularly aggressive tumors [55].

Summary

Cushing's syndrome is a rare and severe disease, associated with severe morbidities and an increased mortality. The major systemic complications and the main cause of death are represented by cardiovascular disease. The prognosis of the disease is mainly affected by the difficulties in the diagnosis and treatment of the disease, which remain a considerable challenge. Therefore, research efforts to develop new methods for the disclosure of Cushing's syndrome and the rapid identification of the causing tumor, as well as to develop new strategies for its treatment—especially for Cushing's disease and ecopic Cushing's syndrome—are needed and should be emphasized in the future.

References

[1] Newell-Price J, Bertagna X, Grossman AB, et al. Cushing's syndrome. Lancet 2006;367: 1605–17.
[2] Lindholm J, Juul SJ, Jorgensen JO, et al. Incidence and late prognosis of Cushing's syndrome: a population-based study. Clin Endocrinol Metab 2001;86:117–23.
[3] Catargi B, Rigalleau V, Poussin A, et al. Occult Cushing's syndrome in type-2 diabetes. J Clin Endocrinol Metab 2003;88:5808–13.
[4] Pecori Giraldi F, Moro M, Cavagnini F. Gender-related differences in the presentation and course of Cushing's disease. J Clin Endocrinol Metab 2003;88:1554–8.
[5] Pivonello R, Faggiano A, Lombardi G, et al. The metabolic syndrome and cardiovascular risk in Cushing's syndrome. Endocrinol Metab Clin North Am 2005;34:327–39.
[6] Faggiano A, Pivonello R, Spiezia S, et al. Cardiovascular risk factors and common carotid artery caliber and stiffness in patients with Cushing's disease during active disease and 1 year after disease remission. J Clin Endocrinol Metab 2003;88:2527–33.
[7] Faggiano A, Melis D, Alfieri R, et al. Sulfur amino acids in Cushing's disease: insight in homocysteine and taurine levels in patients with active and cured disease. J Clin Endocrinol Metab 2005;90:6616–22.
[8] Colao A, Pivonello R, Spiezia S, et al. Persistence of increased cardiovascular risk in patients with Cushing's disease after five years of successful cure. J Clin Endocrinol Metab 1999;84: 2664–72.
[9] Faggiano A, Pivonello R, Melis D, et al. Nephrolithiasis in Cushing's disease: prevalence, etiopathogenesis, and modification after disease cure. J Clin Endocrinol Metab 2003;88: 2076–80.

[10] Di Somma C, Pivonello R, Loche S, et al. Severe impairment of bone mass and turnover in Cushing's disease: comparison between childhood-onset and adulthood-onset disease. Clin Endocrinol (Oxf) 2002;56:153–8.

[11] Tauchmanovà L, Pivonello R, Di Somma C, et al. Bone demineralization and vertebral fractures in endogenous cortisol excess: role of disease etiology and gonadal status. J Clin Endocrinol Metab 2006;91:1779–84.

[12] Di Somma C, Colao A, Pivonello R, et al. Effectiveness of chronic treatment with alendronate in the osteoporosis of Cushing's disease. Clin Endocrinol (Oxf) 1998;48:655–62.

[13] Forget H, Lacroix A, Cohen H. Persistent cognitive impairment following surgical treatment of Cushing's syndrome. Psychoneuroendocrinology 2002;27:367–83.

[14] Bourdeau I, Bard C, Noel B, et al. Loss of brain volume in endogenous Cushing's syndrome and its reversibility after correction of hypercortisolism. J Clin Endocrinol Metab 2002;87:1949–54.

[15] Lindsay JR, Nansel T, Baid S, et al. Long-term impaired quality of life in Cushing's syndrome despite initial improvement after surgical remission. J Clin Endocrinol Metab 2006;91:447–53.

[16] Arnaldi G, Angeli A, Atkinson AB, et al. Diagnosis and complications of Cushing's syndrome: a consensus statement. J Clin Endocrinol Metab 2003;88:5593–602.

[17] Newell-Price J, Trainer P, Besser GM, et al. The diagnosis and differential diagnosis of Cushing's syndrome and pseudo-Cushing's states. Endocr Rev 1998;19:647–72.

[18] Boscaro M, Barzon L, Sonino N. The diagnosis of Cushing's syndrome: atypical presentations and laboratory shortcomings. Arch Intern Med 2000;160:3045–53.

[19] Papanicolaou DA, Mullen N, Kyrou I, et al. Nighttime salivary cortisol: a useful test for the diagnosis of Cushing's syndrome. J Clin Endocrinol Metab 2002;87:4515–21.

[20] Yanovski JA, Cutler GB Jr, Chrousos GP, et al. Corticotropin-releasing hormone stimulation following low-dose dexamethasone administration. A new test to distinguish Cushing's syndrome from pseudo-Cushing's states. JAMA 1993;269:2232–8.

[21] Pecori Giraldi F, Pivonello R, Ambrogio AG, et al. The dexamethasone-suppressed corticotropin-releasing hormone stimulation test and the desmopressin test to distinguish Cushing's syndrome from pseudo-Cushing's states. Clin Endocrinol (Oxf) 2007;66:251–7.

[22] Invitti C, Pecori Giraldi F, de Martin M, et al. Diagnosis and management of Cushing's syndrome: results of an Italian multicentre study. Study Group of the Italian Society of Endocrinology on the Pathophysiology of the Hypothalamic-Pituitary-Adrenal Axis. J Clin Endocrinol Metab 1999;84:440–8.

[23] Oldfield EH, Doppman JL, Nieman LK, et al. Petrosal sinus sampling with and without corticotropin-releasing hormone for the differential diagnosis of Cushing's syndrome. N Engl J Med 1991;325:897–905.

[24] Colao A, Faggiano A, Pivonello R, et al. Study Group of the Italian Endocrinology Society on the Pathophsiology of the Hypothalamic-Pituitary-Adrenal Axis. Inferior petrosal sinus sampling in the differential diagnosis of Cushing's syndrome: results of an Italian multicenter study. Eur J Endocrinol 2001;144:499–507.

[25] Rees DA, Hanna FW, Davies JS, et al. Long-term follow-up results of transsphenoidal surgery for Cushing's disease in a single centre using strict criteria for remission. Clin Endocrinol (Oxf) 2002;56:541–51.

[26] Atkinson AB, Kennedy A, Wiggamvan MI, et al. Long-term remission rates after pituitary surgery for Cushing's disease: the need for long-term surveillance. Clinical Endocrinol (Oxf) 2005;63:549–59.

[27] Pereira AM, van Aken MO, van Dulken H, et al. Long-term predictive value of postsurgical cortisol concentrations for cure and risk of recurrence in Cushing's disease. J Clin Endocrinol Metab 2003;88:5858–64.

[28] Yap LB, Turner HE, Adams CB, et al. Undetectable postoperative cortisol does not always predict long-term remission in Cushing's disease: a single centre audit. Clin Endocrinol (Oxf) 2002;56:25–31.

[29] Porpiglia F, Fiori C, Bovio S, et al. Bilateral adrenalectomy for Cushing's syndrome: a comparison between laparoscopy and open surgery. J Endocrinol Invest 2004;27:654–8.

[30] Assie G, Bahurel H, Bertherat J, et al. The Nelson's syndrome revisited. Pituitary 2004;7: 209–15.

[31] Miller JW, Crapo L. The medical treatment of Cushing's syndrome. Endocr Rev 1993;14: 443–58.

[32] Nieman LK. Medical therapy of Cushing's disease. Pituitary 2002;5:77–82.

[33] Lamberts SW, Birkenhäger JC. Bromocriptine in Nelson's syndrome and Cushing's disease. Lancet 1976;2:811.

[34] Lamberts SW, Klijn JG, de Quijada M, et al. The mechanism of the suppressive action of bromocriptine on adrenocorticotropin secretion in patients with Cushing's disease and Nelson's syndrome. J Clin Endocrinol Metab 1980;51:307–11.

[35] Invitti C, De Martin M, Danesi L, et al. Effect of injectable bromocriptine in patients with Cushing's disease. Exp Clin Endocrinol Diabetes 1995;103:266–71.

[36] Heaney AP, Fernando M, Yong WH, et al. Functional PPARgamma receptor is a novel therapeutic target for ACTH-secreting pituitary adenomas. Nat Med 2002;8:1281–7.

[37] Heaney AP, Fernando M, Melmed S. PPAR-gamma receptor ligands: novel therapy for pituitary adenomas. J Clin Invest 2003;111:1381–8.

[38] Ambrosi B, Dall'Asta C, Cannavo S, et al. Effects of chronic administration of PPAR-gamma ligand rosiglitazone in Cushing's disease. Eur J Endocrinol 2004;151:173–8.

[39] Pecori Giraldi F, Scaroni C, Arvat E, et al. Effect of protracted treatment with rosiglitazone, a PPARgamma agonist, in patients with Cushing's disease. Clin Endocrinol (Oxf) 2006;64: 219–24.

[40] Suri D, Weiss RE. Effect of pioglitazone on adrenocorticotropic hormone and cortisol secretion in Cushing's disease. J Clin Endocrinol Metab 2005;90:1340–6.

[41] Munir A, Song F, Ince P, et al. Ineffectiveness of rosiglitazone therapy in Nelson's syndrome. J Clin Endocrinol Metab 2007;92:1758–63.

[42] Petrossians P, Ronci N, Valdés Socin H, et al. ACTH silent adenoma shrinking under cabergoline. Eur J Endocrinol 2001;144:51–7.

[43] T'Sjoen G, Defeyter I, van de Saffele J, et al. Macroprolactinoma associated with Cushing's disease, successfully treated with cabergoline. J Endocrinol Invest 2002;25:172–5.

[44] Pivonello R, Ferone D, de Herder WW, et al. Dopamine receptor expression and function in corticotroph pituitary tumors. J Clin Endocrinol Metab 2004;89:2452–62.

[45] Pivonello R, De Martino MC, Faggiano A, et al. Cabergoline treatment in Cushing's disease: effect on hypertension, glucose metabolism and dyslipidemia. Presented at the 9th European Congress of Endocrinology, Budapest, Hungary, April 29–May 2, 2007.

[46] Pivonello R, Faggiano A, Di Salle F, et al. Complete remission of Nelson's syndrome after 1-year treatment with cabergoline. J Endocrinol Invest 1999;22:860–5.

[47] Casulari LA, Naves LA, Mello PA, et al. Nelson's syndrome: complete remission with cabergoline but not with bromocriptine or cyproheptadine treatment. Horm Res 2004;62:300–5.

[48] Shraga-Slutzky I, Shimon I, Weinshtein R. Clinical and biochemical stabilization of Nelson's syndrome with long-term low-dose cabergoline treatment. Clinical and biochemical stabilization of Nelson's syndrome with long-term low-dose cabergoline treatment. Pituitary 2006;9:151–4.

[49] Hofland LJ, van der Hoek J, Feelders R, et al. The multi-ligand somatostatin analogue SOM230 inhibits ACTH secretion by cultured human corticotroph adenomas via somatostatin receptor type 5. Eur J Endocrinol 2005;152:645–54.

[50] Boscaro M, Atkinson A, Bertherat J, et al. SOM230 Cushing's disease study group. Early data on the efficacy and safety of the novel multi-ligand somatostatin analog, SOM230, in patients with Cushing's disease. Presented at the 87th Annual Meeting of the Endocrine Society. San Diego (CA), June 4–7, 2005.

[51] Pivonello R, Ferone D, Lamberts SW, et al. Cabergoline plus lanreotide for ectopic Cushing's syndrome. N Engl J Med 2005;352:2457–8.

[52] Pivonello R, Ferone D, de Herder WW, et al. Dopamine receptor expression and function in corticotroph ectopic tumors. J Clin Endocrinol Metab 2007;92:66–9.

[53] Paez-Pereda M, Kovalovsky D, Hopfner U, et al. Retinoic acid prevents experimental Cushing syndrome. J Clin Invest 2001;108:1123–31.

[54] Estrada J, Boronat M, Mielgo M, et al. The long-term outcome of pituitary irradiation after unsuccessful transsphenoidal surgery in Cushing's disease. N Engl J Med 1997;336:172–7.

[55] Sheehan JM, Vance ML, Sheehan JP, et al. Radiosurgery for Cushing's disease after failed transsphenoidal surgery. J Neurosurg 2000;93:738–42.

ELSEVIER
SAUNDERS

Endocrinol Metab Clin N Am
37 (2008) 151–171

ENDOCRINOLOGY
AND METABOLISM
CLINICS
OF NORTH AMERICA

Nonfunctioning Pituitary Tumors and Pituitary Incidentalomas

Mark E. Molitch, MD

Division of Endocrinology, Metabolism, and Molecular Medicine, Northwestern University Feinberg School of Medicine, 645 North Michigan Avenue, Suite 530, Chicago, IL 60611, USA

Clinically nonfunctioning adenomas (CNFAs) range from being completely asymptomatic, and therefore detected at autopsy or as incidental findings on head MRI or CT scans performed for other reasons, to causing significant hypothalamic/pituitary dysfunction and visual symptoms because of their large size. Approximately three quarters of CNFAs are actually gonadotroph adenomas, based on the finding that patients who have such tumors produce intact gonadotropins or their glycoprotein subunits (α or β) in vivo or in vitro, as shown by measurement of these products in the blood, staining on immunohistochemistry, or measurement of the mRNA for these products in the tumors [1]. Rarely, clinically nonfunctioning tumors are found to stain positively for adrenocorticotropin (ACTH), growth hormone (GH), prolactin (PRL), or thyrotropin (TSH) but do not secrete these hormones in sufficient quantities so as to cause clinical syndromes; such tumors are referred to as "silent" corticotroph, somatotroph, lactotroph, or thyrotroph adenomas [2]. In this discussion, asymptomatic and symptomatic tumors are reviewed.

Several other lesions may be found in the sellar area that may mimic a pituitary adenoma, including aneurysms of the internal carotid artery, craniopharyngiomas, Rathke's cleft cysts, meningiomas of the tuberculum sellae, gliomas of the hypothalamus and optic nerves, dysgerminomas, cysts, hamartomas, metastases, sarcoidosis, eosinophilic granulomas, sphenoid sinus mucoceles, and focal areas of infarction [3–6]. Lymphocytic infiltration of the pituitary can also masquerade as a pituitary adenoma [7]. Some normal individuals statistically must have pituitaries that exceed the normal size boundary of 9 mm (+3 SDs in healthy subjects) [8–10], and Chanson and colleagues [11] have reported several such patients. These individuals with

E-mail address: molitch@northwestern.edu

"normal pituitary hypertrophy" had pituitaries that had homogeneous iso-intense signals and enhanced homogeneously with contrast on MRI [11]. Furthermore, surgical specimens showed normal pituitary tissue in two cases [11]. Artifacts mimicking pituitary lesions include beam-hardening effects with CT and susceptibility distortions with MRI [4,6] (for more details regarding the radiologic characteristics of adenomas versus other lesions, see the article by Chandler and Barkan elsewhere in this issue).

Asymptomatic, incidental, clinically nonfunctioning adenoma (pituitary incidentaloma)

Autopsy findings

Pituitary adenomas have been found at autopsy in 1.5% to 27% of subjects not suspected of having pituitary disease while alive (Table 1) [3,12–40]. The average frequency of finding an adenoma for these studies, which examined a total of 18,631 pituitaries, was 10.6%. The tumors were distributed equally throughout the age groups (range: 16–86 years old) and between the genders. In the studies in which PRL immunohistochemistry was performed, 22% to 66% stained positively for PRL [18,20,21,26,29–31,33–36,38,39]. Buurman and Saeger [39] provide a detailed breakdown of the 334 pituitary adenomas found in 316 pituitaries of the 3048 autopsy cases they examined, finding 39.5% staining for PRL, 13.8% staining for ACTH, 7.2% staining for gonadotropins or α-subunits, 1.8% staining for GH, 0.6% staining for TSH, and 3.0% staining for multiple hormones.

In these postmortem studies, all but seven of the tumors were less than 10 mm in diameter. The relative lack of macroadenomas in these studies suggests that growth from micro- to macroadenomas must be an exceedingly uncommon event or that virtually all macroadenomas come to clinical attention, and thus are not included in autopsy findings. There is a separate report of an additional three macroadenomas being found at autopsy [41].

CT and MRI scans in normal individuals

Three series have evaluated CT scans of the sellar area in normal subjects who were having such scans for reasons unrelated to possible pituitary disease. Chambers and colleagues [3] found discrete areas of low density greater than 3 mm in diameter in 10 of 50 such subjects. In the author's study of 107 normal women, 7 women were found who had focal hypodense areas and 5 were found who had focal high-density regions greater than 3 mm in diameter [42]. In a third study, Peyster and colleagues [43] found focal hypodense areas greater than 3 mm in diameter in only 8 of 216 subjects.

Two similar studies have been performed using MRI. Chong and colleagues [44] found focal pituitary gland hypodensities 2 to 5 mm (mean of 3.9 mm) in 20 of 52 normal subjects with nonenhanced images using a 1.5-T scanner and 3-mm-thick sections. With similar scans but with

Table 1
Frequency of pituitary adenomas found at autopsy

Series	No. pituitaries examined	No. adenomas found	Frequency (%)	No. macroadenomas found	Stain PRL-positive (%)
Susman [12]	260	23	8.8	—	—
Close [13]	250	23	9.2	—	—
Costello [14]	1000	225	22.5	0	—
Sommers [15]	400	26	6.5	0	—
McCormick and Halmi [16]	1600	140	8.8	0	—
Haugen [17]	170	33	19.4		
Kovacs et al [18]	152	20	13.2	2	53
Landolt [19]	100	13	13.0	0	—
Mosca et al [20]	100	24	24.0	0	—
Burrows et al [21]	120	32	26.7	0	41
Parent [22]	500	42	8.4	1	—
Muhr et al [23]	205	3	1.5	0	—
Max [24]	500	9	1.8	—	—
Schwezinger and Warzok [25]	5100	485	9.5	0	—
Chambers et al [3]	100	14	14.0	0	—
Coulon et al [26]	100	10	10.0	0	60
Siqueira and Guembarovski [27]	450	39	8.7	0	—
Char and Persaud [28]	350	35	10.0	0	—
Gorczyca and Hardy [29]	100	27	27.0	0	30
El-Hamid et al [30]	486	97	20.0	0	48
Scheithauer et al [31]	251	41	16.3	0	66
Kontogeorgos et al [32]	470	49	10.4	0	—
Marin et al [33]	210	35	16.7	0	32
Sano et al [34]	166	15	9.0	0	47
Teramoto et al [35]	1000	51	5.1	0	30
Camaris et al [36]	423	14	3.2	0	44
Tomita and Gates [37]	100	24	24.0		
Kurosaki [38]	692	79	11.4	1	24
Buurman and Saeger [39]	3048	334	11.0	3	40
Rittierodt and Hori [40]	228	7	3.0	0	
Total	18,631	1,969	10.6%	7	

Each series is identified by the authors and by the reference number.

PRL-positive indicates the percentage of tumors that had positive immunostaining for PRL, indicating that they were prolactinomas.

gadolinium–diethylenetriamine penta-acetic acid (DTPA) enhancement, Hall and colleagues [45] found that focal areas of decreased intensity greater than 3 mm in diameter compatible with the diagnosis of adenoma were found in 34, 10, and 2 of 100 normal volunteers, depending on whether there was agreement on the diagnosis between one, two, or three independent reviewing neuroradiologists.

Sellar lesions greater than 10 mm in diameter have not been found in these studies of consecutive normal individuals, similar to the limited number found at autopsy. Nammour and colleagues [46] found that of 3550 consecutive CT scans done in men with a mean age of 57 years for the symptoms of change in mental status, headache, or possible metastases, 7 (0.2%) demonstrated pituitary macroadenomas ranging from 1.0 to 2.5 cm in size; all were thought to be CNFAs after hormonal evaluation. Similarly, Yue and colleagues [47] found that when 3672 nonenhanced MRI scans were performed without specific views of the sellar area, 0.16% of subjects were found to have adenomas, with all being macroadenomas. Furthermore, macroadenomas have been reported as incidental findings [48].

In the eight series of patients reported to have pituitary incidentalomas [49–56], 301 (68%) of the 445 patients had macroadenomas (Table 2). Several of these patients had tumors 2 cm or more in maximum diameter. This proportion of patients who have macroadenomas found clinically is much greater than would be expected based on the autopsy findings, suggesting that the mass effects of such tumors may have resulted in some of the symptomatology causing the patients to have the scans in the first place.

Endocrinologic evaluation of the asymptomatic incidental mass

Because the most common lesion in the sella is a pituitary adenoma, it is reasonable to evaluate patients for hormone oversecretion, regardless of the

Table 2
Changes in pituitary incidentaloma size

| Series followed | Microadenomas | | | | Macroadenomas | | | | Years |
	Total	Increased	Decreased	No change	Total	Enlarged	Decreased	No change	
Donovan and Corenblum [49]	15	0	0	15	16	4[a]	0	12	6 – 7
Reincke et al [50]	7	1	1	5	7	2	0	5	8
Nishizawa et al [51]					28	2[a]	0	26	5.6
Feldkamp et al [52]	31	1	1	29	19	5	1	13	2.7
Igarashi et al [53]	1	0	0	1	22	6	10	6	5.1
Sanno et al [54]	74	10	7	57	165	20[a]	22	123	2.3
Fainstein Day et al [55]	11	1	0	10	7	1	0	6	3.2
Arita et al [56]	5	2	0	3	37	19[a]	0	18	5.2
Total	144	15 (10%)	9 (6%)	120 (84%)	301	59 (20%)	33 (11%)	209 (69%)	

Each series is identified by the authors and by the reference number.

[a] Total of seven cases in these series had tumor enlargement attributable to apoplexy.

size of the lesion seen. Many of the changes occurring with hormone over-secretion syndromes may be quite subtle and only slowly progressive; there-fore, screening for hormonal oversecretion is warranted even in patients with no clinical evidence of hormone oversecretion. Silent somatotroph and corticotroph adenomas have been reported many times, but it is not clear whether such patients with minimal clinical evidence of hormone over-secretion are free from the increased risk for the more subtle cardiovascular, bone, oncologic, and possibly other adverse effects that we usually associate with such tumors. Indeed, there is emerging evidence that subclinical Cush-ing's syndrome attributable to adrenal incidentalomas is associated with significantly increased prevalences of diabetes, hypertension, obesity, osteo-porosis, and cardiovascular risk [57]. Whether there is a similar increased risk for these comorbidities with silent corticotroph adenomas is unknown. Furthermore, there is some evidence that silent corticotroph adenomas have a worse prognosis than those with overt disease with respect to aggressive-ness after initial surgery [58]. It is not clear how many of these patients have nonsuppressible serum cortisol levels or elevated urinary free cortisol levels, but Lopez and colleagues [59] have found suppressed ACTH secretion and hypocortisolism in 2 of 12 patients after resection of silent ACTH-secreting adenomas.

Screening for hormone oversecretion in such patients has been ques-tioned as to its cost-effectiveness [60,61]. Evidence from the series of Fain-stein Day and colleagues [55] cited previously suggests that such screening is worthwhile, because 7 of their 46 patients turned out to have prolactino-mas and of the 13 patients who ended up going to surgery and having immunohistochemistry performed, 2 adenomas (15%) were GH-positive, 3 adenomas (23%) were gonadotropin-positive, and 4 (31%) were plurihor-monal adenomas.

A serum PRL level should be obtained, but it may be difficult to distin-guish between PRL production by a tumor versus hyperprolactinemia from stalk dysfunction in the case of macroadenomas, especially those with suprasellar extension. For such tumors, PRL levels are usually greater than 200 ng/mL with hormone-secreting tumors and lower numbers suggest stalk dysfunction [62,63]. For extremely large tumors, the sample should be diluted to a 1:100 ratio to avoid the "hook effect" [64,65]. An insulin-like growth factor-1 (IGF-1) level is probably sufficient to screen for acromegaly, but if this test cannot be performed, it may be necessary to demonstrate nonsuppression of GH levels during an oral glucose tolerance test [66]. The best screening tests for Cushing's syndrome have traditionally been the overnight dexamethasone suppression test, the 24-hour urinary free cor-tisol test, and, more recently, the assessment of a midnight salivary cortisol level [67,68]. Any abnormality found on such screening would then need to be pursued with more definitive testing (see the article by Pivonello and col-leagues elsewhere in this issue). Most CNFAs are gonadotroph adenomas, as shown by immunohistochemistry [1]. Because gonadotropin oversecretion rarely causes clinical symptoms, however, and the finding of such hormone oversecretion would not influence therapy, there is no reason to screen for this.

Microadenomas do not generally cause disruption of normal pituitary function. Of the 22 patients who had suspected microadenomas evaluated in the series of Reincke and colleagues [50] and Donovan and Corenblum [49], all had normal pituitary function. Larger lesions may cause varying degrees of hypopituitarism because of compression of the hypothalamus, the hypothalamic-pituitary stalk, or the pituitary itself. Of the various series reported, between 0% and 41% of patients who had macroadenomas were found to have hypopituitarism, depending on whether the patients were reported from an endocrinology or neurosurgery service [49,50,55,56]. Thus, all patients who have macroadenomas should be screened for hypopituitarism (see the article by Toogood and Stewart elsewhere in this issue for details regarding the evaluation of hypopituitarism).

Natural history and follow-up of incidental clinically nonfunctioning adenomas

Eight separate series have been reported on the follow-up of patients who had pituitary incidentalomas (see Table 2). Of the 144 patients who had microadenomas reported in these series, 15 (10%) experienced tumor growth, 9 (6%) showed evidence of a decrease in tumor size, and 84% had tumors that remained unchanged in size on follow-up MRI scans over periods of up to 8 years [49–56]. Of the 301 patients who had macroadenomas, 59 (20%) showed evidence of tumor enlargement, 33 (11%) showed evidence of a decrease in tumor size, and 69% had tumors that remained unchanged in size on follow-up MRI scans over periods of up to 8 years [49–56]. It should be mentioned that of the 59 macroadenomas with an increase in tumor size, this was attributable to hemorrhage into the tumor in 7 macroadenomas (see Table 2).

Management of incidental clinically nonfunctioning adenomas

Therapy is indicated for tumors that are hypersecreting. Therefore, prolactinomas would generally be treated with dopamine agonists and those producing GH or ACTH would be treated with surgery (see the articles by Chandler and Barkan elsewhere in this issue). For tumors not oversecreting these hormones, the indications for surgery are based primarily on size, size change, and mass effects of the tumors.

For patients who have microadenomas, the data presented previously suggest that significant tumor enlargement occurs in only 10%. Therefore, surgical resection is generally not indicated, and repeat scanning for 1 to 2 years is indicated to detect tumor enlargement; subsequently, this can be done at less frequent intervals (Fig. 1). Surgery is performed only for significant tumor enlargement.

Tumors greater than 1 cm in diameter have already indicated a propensity for growth. A careful evaluation of the mass effects of these tumors is indicated,

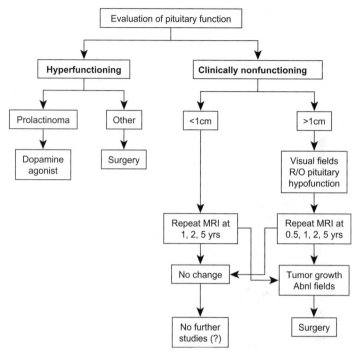

Fig. 1. Flow diagram indicates the approach to the patient found to have a pituitary inciden-taloma. The first step is to evaluate patients for pituitary hyperfunction and then to treat those found to be hyperfunctioning. Of patients who have tumors that are clinically nonfunctioning, those with macroadenomas are evaluated further for evidence of chiasmal compression and hypopituitarism. Scans are then repeated at progressively longer intervals to assess for enlarge-ment of the tumors.

including evaluation of pituitary function and visual field examination if the tumor abuts the chiasm. If there are visual field defects, surgery is indicated. Because hypopituitarism is potentially correctable with tumor resection, this is also an indication for surgery. In the author's opinion, tumors larger than 2 cm should also be considered for surgery simply because of their already dem-onstrated propensity for growth. If a completely asymptomatic lesion is thought to be a pituitary adenoma on the basis of radiologic and clinical findings, a de-cision could be made simply to repeat scans on a yearly basis, with surgery being deferred until there is evidence of tumor growth. As indicated previously, signif-icant tumor growth can be expected in approximately 20% of such patients. Hemorrhage into such tumors is uncommon, but anticoagulation may predis-pose to this complication. When there is no evidence of visual field defects or hypopituitarism and the patient is asymptomatic, an attempt at medical therapy with a dopamine agonist or octreotide is reasonable, realizing that only approx-imately 10% to 20% of such patients respond with a decrease in tumor size. Sur-gery is indicated if surveillance scans show evidence of tumor enlargement, especially when such growth is accompanied by compression of the optic chiasm or the development of pituitary hormone deficiencies (see Fig. 1).

Symptomatic clinically nonfunctioning adenomas

Presenting symptoms

CNFAs usually present because of symptoms attributable to the mass effects of the tumor. Data from eight representative series are shown in Table 3. Clearly, the most common symptoms and signs are visual field disturbance, headache, and hypopituitarism, although the last was often only found with detailed testing. Testing of pituitary function in nine series [69–80] showed that the loss of hormones was on the order of loss of GH greater than loss of luteinizing hormone (LH)/follicle-stimulating hormone (FSH), greater than loss of ACTH, greater than loss of TSH (Table 4). In many older series, testing for GH deficiency in adults was not performed because it was believed that the finding of GH deficiency would not change therapy. The multitude of studies performed in recent years showing the potential benefit of GH therapy in GH-deficient adults suggest that GH testing should be done in all such patients, however, if such therapy would be appropriate for the given patient [81]. When it is done, more than 90% of patients are found to be GH deficient (see Table 4).

Diagnostic evaluation

MRI with gadolinium is preferred to CT because it can reveal far more anatomic detail of the lesion itself and its relation to surrounding structures

Table 3
Signs and symptoms in patients who have clinically nonfunctioning adenomas

Series	Toronto	Rochester	Montreal	Cardiff	Naples	Tel Aviv	Erlangen	Milan
Reference no.	69	70	71	72	73	74	75	76
No. patients	153	100	126	35	84	122	721	378
Symptoms/signs (%)								
Visual field defects	66	68	78	71	39	18	31	60
Hypopituitarism	58	61	75	89	74	34	48	71
Headaches	44	36	56	17	75	29	19	—
Visual acuity reduction	—	—	—	54	26	32	—	—
Ophthalmoplegia	—	5	12	11	16	14	—	4
Apoplexy	—	5	8	—	—	4	10	—

Each series is identified by the city of the first hospital mentioned of the authors and by the reference number. In the series from Rochester [70], although all were CNAFs, on immunohistochemistry, 82 were null-cell adenomas, 9 were prolactinomas, 2 were silent corticotroph adenomas, 4 were gonadotroph adenomas, 1 was a plurihormonal adenoma, and 2 were not assessed.

Table 4
Frequency of endocrine deficiencies and hyperprolactinemia at presentation in patients who have clinically nonfunctioning adenomas

Series	Rochester	Cleveland	Montreal	Hiroshima	Naples	Tel Aviv	Erlangen	Milan	Leiden
Reference no.	70	77	71	78	73	74	75	76	79
No. patients	100	26	126	33	84	122	721	378	109
Hormone lost									
LH/FSH	36	96	75	52	56	69	78	71	75
ACTH	17	62	36	48	23	27	32	21	53
TSH	32	81	18	19	8	29	20	23	43
GH	NT	100	NT	97	93	NT	0	NT	77
Hyperprolactinemia	NT	46	65	42	42	43	28	43	NT

Each series is identified by the city of the first hospital mentioned of the authors and by the reference number.
Abbreviation: NT, not tested.

and can provide characteristics distinguishing an adenoma from other mass lesions, such as craniopharyngiomas or Rathke's cleft cysts [4,6]. MRI can demonstrate the decreased signal of flowing blood, and therefore can better determine the presence of aneurysms. Aneurysms and adenomas may coexist, however, and, rarely, magnetic resonance arteriography may be necessary (see the article by Chandler and Barkan elsewhere in this issue for more detail regarding the radiologic characteristics of adenomas). Somatostatin receptor imaging shows that most CNFAs have somatostatin receptors [82], and dopamine receptor imaging shows that many CNFAs have dopamine receptors [83]; however, the imaging with these compounds is considerably less sensitive than MRI or CT for showing anatomic detail, and, as yet, they do not accurately predict those tumors that might respond to somatostatin analogues or dopamine agonists with size reduction [82,83]. Positron emission tomography is another technique that is in the development stage for the diagnosis and assessment of tumor bioactivity, but it remains a research tool to date [84].

The endocrinologic evaluation for hormonal over- and undersecretion has been discussed previously.

Treatment

Treatment options for CNFAs include no treatment with careful observation, surgery with or without postoperative radiotherapy, radiotherapy alone, and medical therapy. Transsphenoidal resection usually is recommended for patients who have enlarging tumors or tumors with mass effects. Rarely, craniotomy with subfrontal resection is required for extremely large tumors, but this technique is associated with higher morbidity. The effectiveness of each treatment modality can be assessed clinically with assessment of resolution or amelioration of symptoms (eg, headache) and signs (eg, visual field defects), biochemically with assessment of reversal of pituitary hormonal deficits, and structurally with assessment of tumor size by MRI. Postoperative MRI scans ideally should be done at least 3 to 4 months after surgery [85,86] to assess completeness of resection, because the appearance can be deceiving in the immediate postoperative period because of surgical packing, edema, and debris. Once this postoperative baseline has been established, MRI scans should be repeated yearly for 3 to 5 years to detect regrowth and then less frequently if stable. Tumors should be followed by MRI in a similar fashion after radiotherapy or with medical treatment.

Surgery

Outcome data from series in which transsphenoidal surgery was performed are often difficult to analyze, because many series mix results from patients who may or may not have received postoperative radiotherapy, often without an early postoperative scan to determine the presence of residual tumor. Whether patients were cured or not, resection of the bulk of the tumor mass often resulted in improvement of pituitary function with resolution of hyperprolactinemia that was attributable to stalk dysfunction (Table 5). In general, surgical success highly depends on the skill and experience of the neurosurgeon [87,88] and on specific tumor characteristics, such as size, invasiveness, and parasellar extension. The best way to assess completeness of resection is to obtain an MRI scan 3 to 4 months after surgery and then to follow with serial MRI scans as noted previously.

Resolution of one or more hormonal deficits by surgery can be expected in 15% to 50% of patients, with resolution of hyperprolactinemia in more than two thirds of patients (see Table 5). Conversely, surgery may induce an additional loss of one or more pituitary hormones when they were normal before surgery in 2% to 15% of patients [71,75,76]. Transient diabetes insipidus (DI) can be expected in approximately one third of patients [74], but permanent DI occurs in 0.5% to 5% [71,75,76,89]. Other complications of surgery occurring in less than 1% of patients each include postoperative cerebrospinal fluid (CSF) leak, meningitis, rebleeding, cranial nerve injury, and visual function deterioration (for more details, see the article by Chandler and Barkan elsewhere in this issue). Mortality remains approximately 0.3% to 0.5% and is seen more often in patients who have extremely large tumors and require craniotomy. Patients who have giant tumors, defined as being greater than 4 cm in diameter, do particularly poorly, with low cure rates and relatively high morbidity and mortality rates [90–93].

Radiotherapy

Radiotherapy as primary therapy is rarely done and is mainly restricted to those patients who would not be able to tolerate surgery. More commonly, radiotherapy is given as adjunctive therapy after surgery. Before the institution of policies of routine surveillance with MRI scans, many series reported postoperative recurrence rates in patients who did or did not have routine postoperative irradiation. In many of those series, the criteria for choosing which patients received postoperative irradiation were not

Table 5
Results of transsphenoidal surgery for clinically nonfunctioning pituitary adenomas on pituitary function

Series	Cleveland	Montreal	Madrid	Hiroshima	Naples	Erlangen
Reference no.	77	71	80	78	73	75
Hormone axis normalized						
LH/FSH	32	11	29	13	34	15
ACTH	38	41	57	73	10	35
TSH	57	14	13	67	57	33
Hyperprolactinemia	58	NT	NT	85	68	95

Each series is identified by the city of the first hospital mentioned of the authors and by the reference number.

Abbreviation: NT, not tested.

specified. Reports from nine series of patients showed that the recurrence rates for tumors after surgery were 10.3% of 224 patients who received routine postoperative radiotherapy and 25.5% of 428 patients who did not receive such routine radiotherapy (Table 6) [70–72,93–98]. More recent series have reported similar data stratified by the presence or absence of tumor on the initial postoperative MRI scan [73,75,78,99–103]. For those patients who had no visible tumor on postoperative MRI, none of 11 who received routine radiotherapy had recurrences and only 13.1% of 359 patients who did not receive routine radiotherapy experienced recurrences (see Table 6). For those patients who had visible tumor on postoperative MRI, 22.9% of 83 patients who received routine radiotherapy had growth of tumor remnants, whereas 41.0% of 200 patients who did not receive routine radiotherapy experienced growth of tumor remnants (see Table 6). Thus, the risk for tumor recurrence/growth is low when no tumor is visible after surgery, but such a risk is considerably higher when a tumor remnant is visible, and this risk can be approximately halved with postoperative irradiation. In addition to postoperative irradiation, the age of the patient significantly affects tumor growth, with those older than of 61 years of age having a more than twofold slower doubling time compared with those younger than 61 years of age [104].

Conventional radiotherapy has substantial complications, including a risk for hypopituitarism in more than 50% of patients, a twofold increase in stroke, and a three- to fourfold increase in the development of brain tumors [105,106]. The last of these is unclear, however, because there is a clear ascertainment bias attributable to the routine surveillance MRI scans done in patients who have had pituitary irradiation compared with none in the general population [106]. Cognitive dysfunction is rare when conventional radiotherapy doses are used [105,106].

Over the past decade, the mode of radiotherapy has changed in most institutions around the world from conventional to stereotactic. With conventional radiotherapy, radiation is given through two or three ports 5 days per week for 5 weeks, thereby giving a total dose of approximately 45 Gy over 25 sessions. With stereotactic radiotherapy (often referred to as "radiosurgery"), after tumor anatomy is defined by MRI, radiation is given in a single fraction by means of linear accelerator (LINAC) beams that are shaped or through multiple cobalt sources (gamma knife) in higher doses to the tumor with lower doses to the surrounding brain tissue (for a review of these techniques, see the article by Brada and Jankowska elsewhere in this issue). In a recent review summarizing 17 series in which 452 patients who had CNFAs were treated with these newer stereotactic techniques, only 1% of patients experienced tumor growth, but this was only over a 2- to 4-year period [107]. Because of the short period of follow-up, the true long-term tumor size control rate is as yet unknown.

The complications rates of stereotactic radiotherapy are also only beginning to be appreciated after this short follow-up period. In one detailed

Table 6
Regrowth of pituitary adenomas after transsphenoidal surgery with and without postoperative radiotherapy and with and without residual tumor visible after surgery

Series	Postoperative MRI status unknown				No visible tumor on postoperative MRI				Visible tumor on postoperative MRI			
	RT		No RT		RT		No RT		RT		No RT	
	Total	Regrowth	Total	Regrowth	Total	Regrowth	Total	Regrowth	Total	Regrowth	Total	Regrowth
Ebersold et al [70]	50	9	42	5								
Comtois et al [71]			71	15								
Colao et al [73]	10	0	22	5								
Bradley et al [94]			73	8								
Greenman et al [74]	57	9	25	4								
Gittoes et al [95]	63	4	63	27								
Park et al [96]	44	1	132	45								
Brada et al [97]	208	6										
Breen et al [98]	120	15										
Lillihei et al [99]							32	2				
Turner et al [100]							57	13				
Woollons et al [101]							11	2	41	13	11	8
Soto-Ares et al [102]							17	0			34	13
Nomikos et al [75]					11	0	30	6	14	5	78	41
Alameda et al [103]							11	1	22	1	5	3
Arafah [77]							174	23				
Marzuela et al [80]							27	0	6	0	64	9
Total	552	44 (8.0%)	428	109 (25.5%)	11	0 (0%)	359	47 (13.1%)	83	19 (22.9%)	200	82 (41.0%)

Each series is identified by the authors and by the reference number. The numbers shown are numbers of cases. For each category, the total number of cases evaluated and the number in which there was recurrence/regrowth of the tumors are shown.

Abbreviation: RT, radiotherapy.

report, it was found that after a mean of 4.6 years after gamma knife radiotherapy, new pituitary hormone deficiencies requiring replacement therapy were 21.7% for FSH/LH, 23.9% for TSH, 8.7% for ACTH, and 13% for GH [108]. Thus, the ultimate rate for hypopituitarism is likely to be quite similar to that for conventional radiotherapy. The optic nerves and optic chiasm are radiosensitive; thus, stereotactic radiotherapy is not given to tumors less than 5 mm from the optic chiasm [109,110]. The cranial nerves coursing through the cavernous sinus (III, IV, V_1, V_2, and VI) are much more radioresistant [109,110]; therefore, stereotactic radiotherapy is quite good for treating residual tumor in the cavernous sinus. Acute symptoms of headache, fatigue, nausea, and vomiting usually developing within 2 days but up to 10 days after irradiation may also occur in up to 50% of patients [111]. An MRI scan should be done to exclude apoplexy in such circumstances. Dexamethasone at a dose of approximately 8 mg/d has been used for these acute complications, but results have been variable.

Surgery for tumor regrowth has had variable success. In a series of 42 such patients, Benveniste and colleagues [112] reported that visual loss improved in only 57%, residual tumor was still present in 75%, and late relapse after this second operation occurred in 15%. Stereotactic radiotherapy has also been given to a limited number of patients who have had prior surgery and prior conventional radiotherapy but have had continued tumor growth or hypersecretion, with some success and no increase in adverse events [113].

Medical therapy

CNFAs have been shown to have high-affinity dopaminergic binding sites using [^{3}H]spiperone as a radioligand with affinities similar to those seen for normal pituitary tissue and prolactinomas; however, the number of binding sites was only 18.8% of that seen in prolactinomas but similar to that seen in normal pituitaries [114]. In a more recent study, Pivonello and colleagues [115] showed that the dopamine D_2 receptor was expressed in 67% of 18 cases. Clinically, however, bromocriptine has been shown to be effective in shrinking CNFAs in less than 20% of cases [114,116,117]. Conversely, Greenman and colleagues [118] recently reported giving bromocriptine to patients who had CNFAs and residual tumor on MRI after surgery, finding that the tumor mass decreased or remained stable in 18 of 20 patients. In this same study, bromocriptine was started in 13 subjects when tumor remnant growth became evident during the course of routine follow-up, and this growth stabilized or decreased in 8 (62%) [118]. In contrast, tumor size increased in 29 (62%) of 47 subjects who had neither bromocriptine nor radiotherapy [118]. Cabergoline, a long-acting dopamine agonist with greater activity on prolactinomas than bromocriptine, has also been found to have somewhat better in vivo activity on CNFAs. Lohmann and colleagues [119] found greater than 10% (range: 10%–18%) tumor shrinkage in 7 of 13 patients treated with cabergoline at a dosage of 1 mg/wk for

1 year and Pivonello and colleagues [115] found a more significant tumor size reduction (range: 28.6%–62.4%) in 5 of 9 patients treated with cabergoline at a dosage of 3 mg/wk for 1 year. Caution is needed when using high doses of cabergoline, however, in that patients using extremely high doses (>3 mg/d) for Parkinson's disease have been found to be at increased risk for fibrotic cardiac valvular lesions [120,121].

Somatostatin receptors are also present in most CNFAs [122]. Octreotide, a somatostatin analogue, has been shown to reduce tumor size modestly, with improvement in visual field defects in 25% to 30% of patients in several small series [122–126]. Interestingly, Andersen and colleagues [127] found a 60% response rate with the combination of octreotide at a dose of 200 µg administered subcutaneously three times daily and cabergoline at a dose of 0.5 mg/d, with the six responders being those who had elevated blood levels of gonadotropin subunits and the four nonresponders having no elevation of gonadotropin subunits. New chimeric drugs that act on the dopamine and somatostatin receptors are currently being developed, but their utility in patients who have CNFAs has not yet been determined.

Management of the symptomatic patient

Transsphenoidal resection usually is recommended for patients who havev enlarging tumors, tumors that cause hypopituitarism, or tumors that press on the optic chiasm. Because of its generally limited success, medical therapy would be an option only in those patients with comorbidities so severe as to preclude surgery. Postoperative MRI scans should be done 3 to 4 months after surgery to assess completeness of resection and then repeated yearly for 3 to 5 years and subsequently less frequently if stable. If tumor resection is shown to be complete by postoperative MRI scans, routine radiotherapy may well not be needed, because the tumor recurrence rate for such patients is only 10% to 15% and patients can be followed with periodic MRI scans as stated previously. Radiotherapy, repeat surgery, or even medical therapy can be given at the time tumor size increase is documented. If tumor resection is incomplete, postoperative radiotherapy may be indicated, because radiotherapy can reduce the recurrence rate from 26% to 50% to approximately 20%. The recent demonstration by Greenman and colleagues [118] regarding the control of postoperative growth suggests that a trial of a dopamine agonist is perhaps reasonable in the patient who has residual tumor; irradiation (stereotactic) would then only be given to those not responding to the dopamine agonist.

References

[1] Young WF, Scheithauer BW, Kovacs KT, et al. Gonadotroph adenoma of the pituitary gland: a clinicopathologic analysis of 100 cases. Mayo Clin Proc 1996;71:649–56.

[2] Yamada S, Kovacs K, Horvath E, et al. Morphological study of clinically nonsecreting pituitary adenomas in patients under 40 years of age. J Neurosurg 1991;75:902–5.

[3] Chambers EF, Turski PA, LaMasters D, et al. Regions of low density in the contrast-enhanced pituitary gland: normal and pathologic processes. Radiology 1982;144:109–13.

[4] Elster AD. Modern imaging of the pituitary. Radiology 1993;187:1–14.

[5] Freda PU, Wardlaw SL, Post KD. Unusual causes of sellar/parasellar masses in a large transsphenoidal surgical series. J Clin Endocrinol Metab 1996;81:3455–9.

[6] Naidich MJ, Russell EJ. Current approaches to imaging of the sellar region and pituitary. Endocrinol Metab Clin North Am 1999;28:45–79.

[7] Powrie JK, Powell M, Ayers AB, et al. Lymphocytic adenohypophysitis: magnetic resonance imaging features of two new cases and a review of the literature. Clin Endocrinol 1995;42:315–22.

[8] Doraiswamy PM, Potts JM, Axelson DA, et al. MR assessment of pituitary gland morphology in healthy volunteers: age- and gender-related differences. Am J Neuroradiol 1992;13:1295–9.

[9] Elster AD, Chen MY, Williams DWD, et al. Pituitary gland: MR imaging of physiologic hypertrophy in adolescence. Radiology 1999;174:681–5.

[10] Tsunoda A, Okuda O, Sato K. MR height of the pituitary gland as a function of age and sex: especially physiological hypertrophy in adolescence and in climacterium. Am J Neuroradiol 1997;18:551–4.

[11] Chanson P, Daujat F, Young J, et al. Normal pituitary hypertrophy as a frequent cause of pituitary incidentalomas: a follow-up study. J Clin Endocrinol Metab 2001;86:3009–15.

[12] Susman W. Pituitary adenoma. Br Med J 1933;2:1215.

[13] Close HG. The incidence of adenoma of the pituitary body in some types of new growth. Lancet 1934;1:732–4.

[14] Costello RT. Subclinical adenoma of the pituitary gland. Am J Pathol 1936;12:205–15.

[15] Sommers SC. Pituitary cell relations to body states. Lab Invest 1959;8:588–621.

[16] McCormick WF, Halmi NS. Absence of chromophobe adenomas from a large series of pituitary tumors. Arch Pathol 1971;92:231–8.

[17] Haugen OA. Pituitary adenomas and the histology of the prostate in elderly men. Acta Path Microbiol Scand Section A 1973;81:425–34.

[18] Kovacs K, Ryan N, Horvath E. Pituitary adenomas in old age. J Gerontol 1980;35:16–22.

[19] Landolt AM. Biology of pituitary microadenomas. In: Faglia G, Giovanelli MA, MacLeod RM, editors. Pituitary microadenomas. New York: Academic Press; 1980. p. 107–22.

[20] Mosca L, Solcia E, Capella C, et al. Pituitary adenomas: surgical versus post-mortem findings today. In: Faglia G, Giovanelli MA, MacLeod RM, editors. Pituitary microadenomas. New York: Academic Press; 1980. p. 137–42.

[21] Burrows GN, Wortzman G, Rewcastle NB, et al. Microadenomas of the pituitary and abnormal sellar tomograms in an unselected autopsy series. N Engl J Med 1981;304:156–8.

[22] Parent AD, Bebin J, Smith RR. Incidental pituitary adenomas. J Neurosurg 1981;54:228–31.

[23] Muhr C, Bergstrom K, Grimelius L, et al. A parallel study of the roentgen anatomy of the sella turcica and the histopathology of the pituitary gland in 205 autopsy specimens. Neuroradiology 1981;21:55–65.

[24] Max MB, Deck MDF, Rottenberg DA. Pituitary metastasis: incidence in cancer patients and clinical differentiation from pituitary adenoma. Neurology 1981;31:998–1002.

[25] Schwezinger G, Warzok R. Hyperplasien und adenome der hypophyse im unselektierten sektionsgut. Zentralbi Allg Pathol 1982;126:495–8.

[26] Coulon G, Fellmann D, Arbez-Gindre F, et al. Les adenome hypophysaires latents. Etude autopsique. Sem Hop Paris 1983;59:2747–50.

[27] Siqueira MG, Guembarovski AL. Subclinical pituitary microadenomas. Surg Neurol 1984;22:134–40.

[28] Char G, Persaud V. Asymptomatic microadenomas of the pituitary gland in an unselected autopsy series. West Indian Med J 1986;35:275–9.

[29] Gorczyca W, Hardy J. Microadenomas of the human pituitary and their vascularization. Neurosurgery 1988;22:1–6.

[30] El-Hamid MWA, Joplin GF, Lewis PD. Incidentally found small pituitary adenomas may have no effect on fertility. Acta Endocrinol 1988;117:361–4.

[31] Scheithauer BW, Kovacs KT, Randall RV, et al. Effects of estrogen on the human pituitary: a clinicopathologic study. Mayo Clin Proc 1989;64:1077–84.

[32] Kontogeorgos G, Kovacs K, Horvath E, et al. Multiple adenomas of the human pituitary. A retrospective autopsy study with clinical implications. J Neurosurg 1991;74:243–7.

[33] Marin F, Kovacs KT, Scheithauer BW, et al. The pituitary gland in patients with breast carcinoma: a histologic and immunocytochemical study of 125 cases. Mayo Clin Proc 1992;67: 949–56.

[34] Sano T, Kovacs KT, Scheithauer BW, et al. Aging and the human pituitary gland. Mayo Clin Proc 1993;68:971–7.

[35] Teramoto A, Hirakawa K, Sanno N, et al. Incidental pituitary lesions in 1,000 unselected autopsy specimens. Radiology 1994;193:161–4.

[36] Camaris C, Balleine R, Little D. Microadenomas of the human pituitary. Pathology 1995; 27:8–11.

[37] Tomita T, Gates E. Pituitary adenomas and granular cell tumors. Incidence, cell type, and location of tumor in 100 pituitary glands at autopsy. Am J Clin Pathol 1999;111: 817–25.

[38] Kurosaki M, Saeger W, Lüdecke DK. Pituitary tumors in the elderly. Pathol Res Pract 2001;197:493–7.

[39] Buurman H, Saeger W. Subclinical adenomas in postmortem pituitaries: classification and correlations to clinical data. Eur J Endocrinol 2006;154:753–8.

[40] Rittierodt M, Hori A. Pre-morbid morphological conditions of the human pituitary. Neuropathology 2007;27:43–8.

[41] Auer RN, Alakija P, Sutherland GR. Asymptomatic large pituitary adenomas discovered at autopsy. Surg Neurol 1996;46:28–31.

[42] Wolpert SM, Molitch ME, Goldman JA, et al. Size, shape and appearance of the normal female pituitary gland. Am J Neuroradiol 1984;5:263–7.

[43] Peyster RG, Adler LP, Viscarello RR, et al. CT of the normal pituitary gland. Neuroradiology 1986;28:161–5.

[44] Chong BW, Kucharczyk AW, Singer W, et al. Pituitary gland MR: a comparative study of healthy volunteers and patients with microadenomas. Am J Neuroradiol 1994;15:675–9.

[45] Hall WA, Luciano MG, Doppman JL, et al. Pituitary magnetic resonance imaging in normal volunteers: occult adenomas in the general population. Ann Intern Med 1994; 120:817–20.

[46] Nammour GM, Ybarra J, Naheedy MH, et al. Incidental pituitary macroadenoma: a population-based study. Am J Med Sci 1997;314:287–91.

[47] Yue NC, Longsteth WT Jr, Elster AD, et al. Clinically serious abnormalities found incidentally at MR imaging of the brain: data from the Cardiovascular Health Study. Radiology 1997;202:41–6.

[48] Chacko AG, Chandy MJ. Incidental pituitary macroadenomas. Br J Neurosurg 1992;6: 233–6.

[49] Donovan LE, Corenblum B. The natural history of the pituitary incidentaloma. Arch Intern Med 1995;153:181–3.

[50] Reincke M, Allolio B, Saeger W, et al. The 'incidentaloma' of the pituitary gland. Is neurosurgery required? JAMA 1990;263:2772–6.

[51] Nishizawa S, Ohta S, Yokoyama T, et al. Therapeutic strategy for incidentally found pituitary tumors ("pituitary incidentalomas"). Neurosurgery 1998;43:1344–8.

[52] Feldkamp J, Santen R, Harms E, et al. Incidentally discovered pituitary lesions: high frequency of macroadenomas and hormone-secreting adenomas—results of a prospective study. Clin Endocrinol 1999;51:109–13.

[53] Igarashi T, Saeki N, Yamaura A. Long-term magnetic resonance imaging follow-up of asymptomatic sellar tumors. Their natural history and surgical indications. Neurol Med Chir (Tokyo) 1999;39:592–9.

[54] Sanno N, Oyama K, Tahara S, et al. A survey of pituitary incidentaloma in Japan. Eur J Endocrinol 2003;149:123–7.

[55] Fainstein Day P, Guitelman M, Artese R, et al. Retrospective multicentric study of pituitary incidentalomas. Pituitary 2004;7:145–8.

[56] Arita K, Tominaga A, Sugiyama K, et al. Natural course of incidentally found nonfunctioning pituitary adenoma, with special reference to pituitary apoplexy during follow-up examination. J Neurosurg 2006;104:884–91.

[57] Angeli A, Terzolo M. Adrenal incidentaloma—a modern disease with old complications. J Clin Endocrinol Metab 2002;87:4869–71.

[58] Bradley KJ, Wass JAH, Turner HE. Non-functioning pituitary adenomas with positive immunoreactivity for ACTH behave more aggressively than ACTH immunonegative tumours but do not recur more frequently. Clin Endocrinol 2003;58:59–64.

[59] Lopez JA, Kleinschmidt-DeMasters BK, Sze C-I, et al. Silent corticotroph adenomas: further clinical and pathological observations. Hum Pathol 2004;35:1137–47.

[60] King JT Jr, Justice AC, Aron DC. Management of incidental pituitary microadenomas: a cost-effectiveness analysis. J Clin Endocrinol Metab 1997;82:3625–32.

[61] Krikorian A, Aron D. Evaluation and management of pituitary incidentalomas—revisiting an acquaintance. Nat Clin Pract Endocrinol Metab 2006;2:138–45.

[62] Molitch ME, Reichlin S. Hypothalamic hyperprolactinemia: neuroendocrine regulation of prolactin secretion in patients with lesions of the hypothalamus and pituitary stalk. In: MacLeod RM, Thorner MO, Scapagnini U, editors. Prolactin. Basic and clinical correlates. Padova (Italy): Liviana Press; 1985. p. 709–19.

[63] Arafah MB, Neki KE, Gold RS, et al. Dynamics of prolactin secretion in patients with hypopituitarism and pituitary macroadenomas. J Clin Endocrinol Metab 1995;80: 3507–12.

[64] St-Jean E, Blain F, Comtois R. High prolactin levels may be missed by immunoradiometric assay in patients with macroprolactinomas. Clin Endocrinol 1996;44:305–9.

[65] Barkan AL, Chandler WF. Giant pituitary prolactinoma with falsely low serum prolactin: the pitfall of the "high-dose hook effect": case report. Neurosurgery 1998;42:913–5.

[66] The Growth Hormone Research Society and Pituitary Society Consensus Conference. Biochemical assessment and long-term monitoring in patients with acromegaly. J Clin Endocrinol Metab 2004;89:3099–102.

[67] Arnaldi G, Angeli A, Atkinson AB, et al. Diagnosis and complications of Cushing's syndrome: a consensus statement. J Clin Endocrinol Metab 2003;88:5593–602.

[68] Findling JW, Raff H. Cushing's syndrome: important issues in diagnosis and management. J Clin Endocrinol Metab 2006;91:3746–53.

[69] Erlichman C, Meakin JW, Simpson WJ. Review of 154 patients with non-functioning pituitary tumors. Int J Radiat Oncol Biol Phys 1979;5:1981–6.

[70] Ebersold MJ, Quast LM, Laws ER, et al. Long-term results in transsphenoidal removal of nonfunctioning pituitary adenomas. J Neurosurg 1986;64:713–9.

[71] Comtois R, Beauregard H, Somma M, et al. The clinical and endocrine outcome to transsphenoidal microsurgery of nonsecreting pituitary adenomas. Cancer 1991;68:860–6.

[72] Shone GR, Richards SH, Hourihan MD, et al. Non-secretory adenomas of the pituitary treated by trans-ethmoidal sellotomy. J R Soc Med 1991;84:140–3.

[73] Colao A, Cerbone G, Cappabianca P, et al. Effect of surgery and radiotherapy on visual and endocrine function in nonfunctioning pituitary adenomas. J Endocrinol Invest 1998;21: 284–90.

[74] Greenman Y, Ouaknine G, Veshchev I, et al. Postoperative surveillance of clinically nonfunctioning pituitary macroadenomas: markers of tumour quiescence and regrowth. Clin Endocrinol 2003;58:763–9.

[75] Nomikos P, Ladar C, Fahlbusch R, et al. Impact of primary surgery on pituitary function in patients with non-functioning pituitary adenomas—a study on 721 patients. Acta Neurochir (Wien) 2004;146:27–35.

[76] Mortini P, Losa M, Barzaghi R, et al. Results of transsphenoidal surgery in a large series of patients with pituitary adenoma. Neurosurgery 2005;56:1222–33.

[77] Arafah AM. Reversible hypopituitarism in patients with large nonfunctioning pituitary adenomas. J Clin Endocrinol Metab 1986;62:1173–9.

[78] Tominaga A, Uozumi T, Arita K, et al. Anterior pituitary function in patients with nonfunctioning pituitary adenoma: results of longitudinal follow-up. Endocr J 1995;42: 421–7.

[79] Dekkers OM, Pereira AM, Roelfsema F, et al. Observation alone after transsphenoidal surgery for nonfunctioning pituitary macroadenoma. J Clin Endocrinol Metab 2006;91: 1796–801.

[80] Marzuela M, Astigarraga B, Vicente A, et al. Recovery of visual and endocrine function following transsphenoidal surgery of large nonfunctioning pituitary adenomas. J Endocrinol Invest 1994;17:703–7.

[81] Molitch ME, Clemmons DR, Malozowski S, et al. Evaluation and treatment of adult growth hormone deficiency: an Endocrine Society Clinical Practice Guideline. J Clin Endocrinol Metab 2006;91:1621–34.

[82] De Herder WW, Kwekkeboom DJ, Feelders RA, et al. Somatostatin receptor imaging for neuroendocrine tumors. Pituitary 2006;9:243–8.

[83] De Herder WW, Reijs AE, Feelders RA, et al. Diagnostic imaging of dopamine receptors in pituitary adenomas. Eur J Endocrinol 2007;156(Suppl 1):S53–6.

[84] Lucignani G, Losa M, Moresco RM, et al. Differentiation of clinically non-functioning pituitary adenomas from meningiomas and craniopharyngiomas by positron emission tomography with [^{18}F]fluoro-ethyl-spiperone. Eur J Nucl Med 1997;24:1149–55.

[85] Steiner E, Knosp E, Herold CJ, et al. Pituitary adenomas: findings of postoperative MR imaging. Radiology 1992;185:521–7.

[86] Dina TS, Feaster SH, Laws ER. MR of the pituitary gland postsurgery: serial MR studies following transsphenoidal resection. Am J Neuroradiol 1993;14:763–9.

[87] Ciric I, Ragin A, Baumgartner C, et al. Complications of transsphenoidal surgery: results of a national survey, review of the literature, and personal experience. Neurosurgery 1997;40: 225–36.

[88] Barker FG II, Klibanski A, Swearingen B. Transsphenoidal surgery for pituitary tumors in the United States, 1996–2000; mortality, morbidity, and the effects of hospital and surgeon volume. J Clin Endocrinol Metab 2003;88:4709–19.

[89] Nemergut EC, Zuo Z, Jane JA, et al. Predictors of diabetes insipidus after transsphenoidal surgery: a review of 881 patients. J Neurosurg 2005;103:448–54.

[90] Ciric I, Mikhael M, Stafford T, et al. Transsphenoidal microsurgery of pituitary macroadenomas with long-term follow-up results. J Neurosurg 1983;59:395–401.

[91] Pia HW, Grote E, Hildebrandt G. Giant pituitary adenomas. Neurosurg Rev 1985;8: 207–20.

[92] Mohr G, Hardy J, Comtois R, et al. Surgical management of giant pituitary adenomas. Can J Neurol Sci 1990;17:62–6.

[93] Alleyne CH Jr, Barrow DL, Oyesiku NM. Combined transsphenoidal and pterional craniotomy approach to giant pituitary tumors. Surg Neurol 2002;57:380–90.

[94] Bradley KM, Adams CBT, Potter CPS, et al. An audit of selected patients with non-functioning pituitary adenoma treated by transsphenoidal surgery without irradiation. Clin Endocrinol 1994;41:655–9.

[95] Gittoes NJL, Bates AS, Tse W, et al. Radiotherapy for non-functioning pituitary tumours. Clin Endocrinol 1998;48:331–7.

[96] Park P, Chandler WF, Barkan AL, et al. The role of radiation therapy after surgical resection of nonfunctional pituitary macroadenomas. Neurosurgery 2004;55:100–7.

[97] Brada M, Rajan B, Traish D, et al. The long-term efficacy of conservative surgery and radiotherapy in the control of pituitary adenomas. Clin Endocrinol 1993;38:571–8.

[98] Breen P, Flickinger JC, Kondziolka D, et al. Radiotherapy for nonfunctional pituitary adenoma: analysis of long-term tumor control. J Neurosurg 1998;89:933–8.

[99] Lillehei KO, Kirschman DL, Kleinschmidt-DeMasters BK, et al. Reassessment of the role of radiation therapy in the treatment of endocrine-inactive pituitary macroadenomas. Neurosurgery 1998;43:432–9.

[100] Turner HE, Stratton IM, Byrne JV, et al. Audit of selected patients with nonfunctioning pituitary adenomas treated without irradiation—a follow-up study. Clin Endocrinol 1999;51:281–4.

[101] Woollons AC, Hunn MK, Rajapakse YR, et al. Non-functioning pituitary adenomas: indications for postoperative radiotherapy. Clin Endocrinol 2000;53:713–7.

[102] Soto-Ares G, Cortet-Rudelli C, Assaker R, et al. MRI protocol technique in the optimal therapeutic strategy of non-functioning pituitary adenomas. Eur J Endocrinol 2002;146: 179–86.

[103] Alameda C, Lucas T, Peneda E, et al. Experience in the management of 51 non-functioning pituitary adenomas: indications for post-operative radiotherapy. J Endocrinol Invest 2005; 23:18–22.

[104] Tanaka Y, Hongo K, Tada T, et al. Growth pattern and rate in residual nonfunctioning pituitary adenomas: correlations among tumor volume doubling time, patient age, and MIB-1 index. J Neurosurg 2003;98:359–65.

[105] Hansen LK, Molitch ME. Postoperative radiotherapy for clinically nonfunctioning pituitary adenomas. Endocrinologist 1998;8:71–8.

[106] Gittoes NJL. Radiotherapy for non-functioning pituitary tumors—when and under what circumstances. Pituitary 2003;6:103–8.

[107] Sheehan JP, Niranjan A, Sheehan JM, et al. Stereotactic radiosurgery for pituitary adenomas: an intermediate review of its safety, efficacy, and role in the neurosurgical treatment armamentarium. J Neurosurg 2005;102:678–91.

[108] Feigl GC, Bonelli CM, Berghold A, et al. Effects of gamma knife radiosurgery of pituitary adenomas on pituitary function. J Neurosurg 2002;97(Suppl 5):415–21.

[109] Tishler RB, Loeffler JS, Lunsford LD, et al. Tolerance of cranial nerves of the cavernous sinus to radiosurgery. Int J Radiat Oncol Biol Phys 1993;27:215–21.

[110] Leber KA, Berglöff J, Pendl G. Dose-response tolerance of the visual pathways and cranial nerves of the cavernous sinus to stereotactic radiosurgery. J Neurosurg 1998;88:43–50.

[111] St. George EJ, Kudhail J, Perks J, et al. Acute symptoms after gamma knife radiosurgery. J Neurosurg 2002;97(Suppl 5):631–4.

[112] Benveniste RJ, King WA, Walsh J, et al. Repeated transsphenoidal surgery to treat recurrent or residual pituitary adenoma. J Neurosurg 2005;102:1004–12.

[113] Swords FM, Allan CA, Plowman PN, et al. Stereotactic radiosurgery SVI: a treatment for previously irradiated pituitary adenomas. J Clin Endocrinol Metab 2003;88:6334–40.

[114] Bevan JS, Burke CW. Non-functioning pituitary adenomas do not regress during bromocriptine therapy but possess membrane-bound dopamine receptors which bind bromocriptine. Clin Endocrinol 1986;25:561–72.

[115] Pivonello R, Matrone C, Filippella M, et al. Dopamine receptor expression and function in clinically nonfunctioning pituitary tumors: comparison with the effectiveness of cabergoline treatment. J Clin Endocrinol Metab 2004;89:1674–83.

[116] Grossman A, Ross R, Charlesworth M, et al. The effect of dopamine agonist therapy on large functionless pituitary tumours. Clin Endocrinol 1985;22:679–86.

[117] Van Schaardenburg D, Roelfsema F, Van Seters AP, et al. Bromocriptine therapy for non-functioning pituitary adenoma. Clin Endocrinol 1989;30:475–84.

[118] Greenman Y, Tordjman K, Osher E, et al. Postoperative treatment of clinically nonfunctioning pituitary adenomas with dopamine agonists decreases tumor remnant growth. Clin Endocrinol 2005;63:39–44.

[119] Lohmann T, Trantakis C, Biesold M, et al. Minor tumour shrinkage in nonfunctioning pituitary adenomas by long-term treatment with the dopamine agonist cabergoline. Pituitary 2001;4:173–8.

[120] Schade R, Andersohn F, Suissa S, et al. Dopamine agonists and the risk of cardiac-valve regurgitation. N Engl J Med 2007;356:29–38.

[121] Zanettini R, Antonini A, Gatto G, et al. Valvular heart disease and the use of dopamine agonists for Parkinson's disease. N Engl J Med 2007;356:39–46.

[122] De Bruin TWA, Kwekkeboom DJ, Van't Verlaat JW, et al. Clinically nonfunctioning pituitary adenoma and octreotide response to long term high dose treatment, and studies in vitro. J Clin Endocrinol Metab 1992;75:1310–7.

[123] Katznelson L, Oppenheim DS, Coughlin JF, et al. Chronic somatostatin analog administration in patients with α-subunit-secreting pituitary tumors. J Clin Endocrinol Metab 1992;75:1318–25.

[124] Duet M, Mundler O, Ajzenberg C, et al. Somatostatin receptor imaging in non-functioning pituitary adenomas: value of an uptake index. Eur J Nucl Med 1994;21:647–50.

[125] Plockinger U, Reichel M, Fett U, et al. Preoperative octreotide treatment of growth hormone-secreting and clinically nonfunctioning pituitary macroadenomas: effect on tumor volume and lack of correlation with immunohistochemistry and somatostatin receptor scintigraphy. J Clin Endocrinol Metab 1994;79:1416–23.

[126] Warnet A, Harris AG, Renard E, et al. A prospective multicenter trial of octreotide in 24 patients with visual defects caused by nonfunctioning and gonadotropin-secreting pituitary adenomas. Neurosurgery 1997;41:786–96.

[127] Andersen M, Bjerre P, Schrøder HD, et al. *In vivo* secretory potential and the effect of combination therapy with octreotide and cabergoline in patients with clinically non-functioning pituitary adenomas. Clin Endocrinol 2001;56:23–30.

ELSEVIER
SAUNDERS

Endocrinol Metab Clin N Am
37 (2008) 173–193

ENDOCRINOLOGY
AND METABOLISM
CLINICS
OF NORTH AMERICA

Craniopharyngiomas

Niki Karavitaki, MBBS, MSc, PhD,
John A.H. Wass, MA, MD, FRCP*

*Department of Endocrinology, Oxford Centre for Diabetes, Endocrinology, and Metabolism,
Old Road, Headington, Oxford, OX3 7LJ, United Kingdom*

Craniopharyngiomas are rare epithelial tumors arising along the path of the craniopharyngeal duct. Masses of cells resembling squamous epithelium along the pars distalis and pars tuberalis of the pituitary were first identified by Zenker [1] in 1857. In 1902, Saxer [2] described a tumor consisting of these cells. The first attempt for surgical removal of such a lesion ("from a patient presenting the symptoms associated with hypophyseal growths but without acromegaly") by Halstead [3] at St. Luke's Hospital (Chicago) was reported in 1910. Notably, the term *craniopharyngioma* was introduced by Cushing [4] in 1932.

Their incidence is reported as 0.13 cases per 100,000 person-years [5]. They account for 2% to 5% of all primary intracranial neoplasms [6] and 5.6% to 15% of intracranial tumors in children (the most common lesion of the hypothalamopituitary region in childhood populations) [7–10]. They show a bimodal age distribution (peak incidence rates in children from 5–14 years old and in adults from 50–74 years old), the reason for which has not been clarified [6]. Population-based studies from the United States and Finland suggest no gender differences [6,11].

Pathogenesis and pathologic findings

Craniopharyngiomas arise along the path of the craniopharyngeal duct, the canal connecting the stomodeal ectoderm with the evaginated Rathke's pouch. Two pathogenetic hypotheses have been proposed: neoplastic transformation of embryonic squamous cell rests of the involuted craniopharyngeal duct [12] or metaplasia of adenohypophyseal cells in the pituitary stalk or gland [13,14]. A subset of these tumors is monoclonal in origin [15].

---

* Corresponding author.
E-mail address: john.wass@noc.anglox.nhs.uk (J.A.H. Wass).

0889-8529/08/$ - see front matter
doi:10.1016/j.ecl.2007.10.012

Chromosomal abnormalities, including translocation, deletion, and increase in DNA copies, have been recognized [16–18]. β-Catenin gene mutations affecting exon 3 (which encodes the degradation targeting box of β-catenin) have been identified only in the adamantinomatous subtype [10,19], suggesting accumulation of nuclear β-catenin protein (a transcriptional activator of the Wnt signaling pathway) [20]. Furthermore, strong β-catenin expression has been demonstrated in the adamantinomatous subtype [20,21], indicating reactivation of the Wnt signaling pathway (which is implicated in the development of several neoplasms) [22]. In contrast, mutations in the p53 tumor suppressor gene [23] and the gsp or gip oncogene have not been demonstrated [15].

Craniopharyngiomas are histologically benign grade I tumors (World Health Organization [WHO] classification) [24]. Rare cases of malignant transformation (possibly triggered by previous irradiation) [25,26] have been reported. Two main histologic subtypes have been recognized, the adamantinomatous and papillary subtypes, but transitional or mixed forms have also been reported [27–30].

The adamantinomatous type (Fig. 1) may be diagnosed at all ages and predominantly affects young subjects during their first 2 decades of life [30–32]. It bears similarity to the adamantinoma of the jaw [33] and the calcifying odontogenic cyst [34], suggesting that it may develop from embryonic rests with enamel organ potential. Macroscopically, this type may show cystic or solid components, necrotic debris, fibrous tissue, and calcification [27,28,31,35,36]. Notably, bone [27,35] or teeth formation within the tumor has been reported [27,37,38]. The liquid within the cyst(s) ranges from "machinery oil" to shimmering cholesterol-laden fluid, and it is mostly

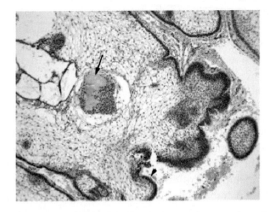

Fig. 1. Adamantinomatous craniopharyngioma. The epithelium consists of a palisaded basal layer of cells (*arrowhead*), the intermediate stellate reticulum, and a layer of flattened keratinized squamous cells. Nodules of "wet" keratin are characteristic (*arrow*) (hematoxylin-eosin, original magnification × 20). (*From* Karavitaki N, Cudlip S, Adams CBT, et al. Craniopharyngiomas. Endocr Rev 2006;27:373; with permission. Copyright © 2006, The Endocrine Society.)

composed of desquamated squamous epithelial cells, rich in membrane lipids and cytoskeleton keratin [6]. The borders of the tumor often merge into a peripheral zone of dense reactive gliosis, which may lead to the misdiagnosis of a glioma [6,39–41]. Furthermore, the margins are frequently sharp and irregular, posing significant difficulties in the manipulation of the surgical planes and the preservation of critical structures [6,35,39–41]. The epithelium is composed of a palisaded basal layer of small cells; an intermediate one with loose aggregates of stellate cells (stellate reticulum); and a top layer of abruptly enlarged, flattened, and keratinized to flat plate-like squamous cells [41]. The flat squames are desquamated singly or in distinctive stacked clusters forming nodules of "wet" keratin, which are often heavily calcified [28,30,40,41]. The keratinous debris may elicit an inflammatory and foreign body giant cell reaction [27]. The demonstration of adamantinomatous epithelium or of wet keratin alone is diagnostic; in contrast, a fibrohistiocytic reaction, necrotic debris, calcification, or cholesterol clefts cannot confirm the presence of an adamantinomatous craniopharyngioma [40].

The papillary variety (Fig. 2) has been almost exclusively described in adults [30,31]. Its cellular structure resembles the oropharyngeal mucosa [27]. Macroscopically, it tends to be solid or mixed with cystic and solid components [28,31,42,43]. Calcification is rarely seen [28,30,31,41,42], and the cyst content is usually viscous and yellow [28]. Infiltration of adjacent brain tissue is less frequent than in the adamantinomatous type [30]. Microscopically, it is composed of mature squamous epithelium forming pseudopapillae and of an anastomosing fibrovascular stroma, which includes

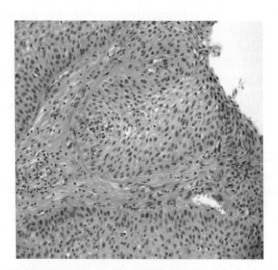

Fig. 2. Papillary craniopharyngioma. The epithelium is mature squamous-forming pseudopapillae (hematoxylin-eosin, original magnification × 10). (*From* Karavitaki N, Cudlip S, Adams CBT, et al. Craniopharyngiomas. Endocr Rev 2006;27:373; with permission. Copyright © 2006, The Endocrine Society.)

a small number of chronic inflammatory cells [28,30,31,42]. Discrete nodules of wet keratin are not present, but small aggregates of keratinized cells may be seen in some tumors [28,42]. The differential diagnosis between a papillary craniopharyngioma and a Rathke's cleft cyst may occasionally be perplexing because of the squamous differentiation that the epithelial lining of the Rathke's cysts may undergo [28]. In such cases, the lack of a solid component and the presence of extensive ciliation or mucin production are suggestive of a Rathke's cyst [40]. It has also been suggested that cytokeratins 8 and 20 are expressed only in Rathke's cysts [44].

Craniopharyngiomas express estrogen [45] and progesterone receptor mRNA [46] and protein [47]. It has been reported that treatment of craniopharyngioma cell cultures by progesterone results in decreased [^{3}H]thymidine uptake [46]. Strong insulin-like growth factor-I (IGF-I) receptor expression has been shown in cell lines and paraffin-embedded material in a subset of craniopharyngiomas; notably, in this group of tumors, treatment with an IGF-I receptor inhibitor caused growth arrest [48].

Clinical, hormonal, and imaging features at presentation

Craniopharyngiomas may exert pressure effects to various brain structures (visual pathways, brain parenchyma, ventricular system, major blood vessels, and hypothalamopituitary system), resulting in multiple clinical features (neurologic, visual, and hypothalamopituitary); headaches, nausea/vomiting, visual disturbances, growth failure (in children), and hypogonadism (in adults) are the most frequently described [49]. The duration of the symptoms until diagnosis ranges between 1 week and 372 months [49].

A substantial number of patients present with compromised pituitary function; reported rates for pituitary hormone deficits include 35% to 95% for growth hormone (GH), 38% to 82% for follicle-stimulating hormone (FSH)/luteinizing hormone (LH), 21% to 62% for corticotropin (ACTH), 21% to 42% for thyroid-stimulating hormone (TSH), and 6% to 38% for antidiuretic hormone (ADH) [49].

Most of the craniopharyngiomas are detected in the sellar/parasellar region; rare ectopic locations have also been described, including the pineal gland, the cerebellopontine angle, the temporal lobe, or completely within the third ventricle [49]. A suprasellar component has been reported in 94% to 95% of the cases (purely suprasellar in 20%–41%, both supra- and intrasellar in 53%–75%, and purely intrasellar in 5%–6%), and extension into the anterior or middle or posterior fossa has been reported in nearly 30% of them [49].

Useful imaging tools for the detection of craniopharyngiomas include plain skull radiographs, CT, MRI, and, occasionally, cerebral angiography. Plain skull radiographs may show calcification and abnormal sella [7,50–53]. CT is helpful for evaluation of the bony anatomy and for identification of calcifications and of the solid and cystic components (the cystic fluid appears hypodense and the solid portions and the cyst capsule show enhancement after contrast administration) (Fig. 3) [49]. MRI is particularly useful for the topographic and structural analysis of the tumor. The appearance depends on the proportion of the solid and cystic components, the content of the cyst(s) (eg, cholesterol, keratin, hemorrhage), and the amount of calcification present. A solid lesion appears as isointense or hypointense relative to the brain on precontrast T_1-weighted images, shows enhancement after gadolinium administration, and is usually of mixed hypointensity or hyperintensity on T_2-weighted sequences (Fig. 4). Large amounts of calcification may be visualized as areas of low signal on T_1-weighted and T_2-weighted images. A cystic element is usually hypointense on T_1-weighted sequences and hyperintense on T_2-weighted sequences. On T_1-weighted images, a thin, peripheral, contrast-enhancing rim of the cyst is demonstrated (see Fig. 4). Protein, cholesterol, and methemoglobin may cause high signal on T_1-weighted images, whereas concentrated protein and various blood products may be associated with low T_2-weighted signal [49]. Finally, cerebral angiography may clarify the anatomic relation of the tumor to the blood vessels [49].

The size of craniopharyngiomas, as evaluated by CT or MRI, has been reported as greater than 4 cm in 14% to 20% of the cases, 2 to 4 cm in 58% to 76%, and less than 2 cm in 4% to 28% [30,53]. Rare cases of "giant" tumors with a diameter up to 12 cm have also been described [54]. Their consistency is purely or predominantly cystic in 46% to 64% of cases, purely

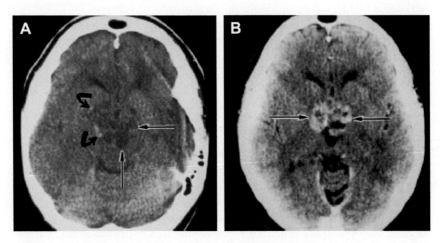

Fig. 3. Axial unenhanced (A) and contrast-enhanced (B) CT images demonstrating an inhomogeneously enhancing soft-tissue mass (straight arrows) in the suprasellar cistern extending into the third ventricle. Specks of calcium (curved arrows) and small cysts are also shown. (From Eldevik OP, Blaivas M, Gabrielsen TO, et al. Craniopharyngioma: radiologic and histologic findings and recurrence. AJNR Am J Neuroradiol 1996;17:1433; with permission. Copyright © 1996, American Society of Neuroradiology.)

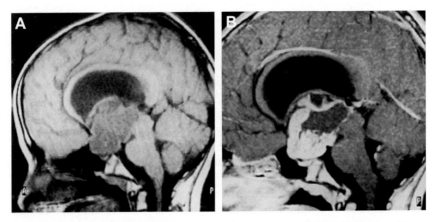

Fig. 4. Sagittal noncontrast (*A*) and contrast-enhanced (*B*) T$_1$-weighted MRI scans demonstrating a hypointense suprasellar tumor with peripherally enhancing cystic areas and an inhomogeneously enhancing solid tumor part. (*From* Sartoretti-Schefer S, Wichmann W, Aguzzi A, et al. MRI differentiation of adamantinous and squamous-papillary craniopharyngiomas. AJNR Am J Neuroradiol 1997;18:80; with permission. Copyright © 1997, American Society of Neuroradiology.)

or predominantly solid in 18% to 39%, and mixed in 8% to 36% [49]. Calcification has been shown in 45% to 57% of cases, and it is probably more common in children (78%–100% of cases) [49]. Hydrocephalus has been reported in 20% to 38% of cases and is probably more frequent in childhood populations (41%–54% of cases) [49]. There is no general agreement on the radiologic features discriminating the two histologic subtypes [49].

The differential diagnosis includes several sellar or parasellar lesions, primarily Rathke's cleft cyst, dermoid and epidermoid cyst, and cystic pituitary adenoma.

Treatment

Surgical removal combined or not with external beam irradiation

Surgery combined or not combined with adjuvant external beam irradiation is currently the most widely used first therapeutic approach. Craniopharyngiomas remain challenging tumors, even in the era of modern neurosurgery. This is mainly attributed to their sharp irregular margins and to their tendency to adhere to vital neurovascular structures, making surgical manipulations potentially hazardous to vital brain areas. Consequently, the attempted degree of excision has been a subject of long-standing debate. The extent of resection depends on the size (achieved in 0% of lesions >4 cm) and location (particularly difficult for retrochiasmatic or within the third ventricle) of the tumor, the presence of hydrocephalus, the presence of greater than 10% calcification and brain invasion, and the experience and individual judgment of a neurosurgeon [49]. Notably, in large series, radical surgery has been accomplished in 18% to 84% of the cases [49]. The perioperative mortality rate currently ranges between 1.7% and 5.4% for primary operations [49]. Radical excision may [55–60] or may not [53,61] associated with substantial perioperative morbidity and mortality [55–60].

The irradiation of cystic craniopharyngiomas carries the risk for enlargement, which may later regress [62] or necessitate further intervention [61,63]. In a series of 188 patients [63], 14% of them developed acute visual deterioration, hydrocephalus, or global deficit leading to loss of consciousness around the time of radiotherapy. These complications could not be predicted by patient or disease characteristics, and they did not seem to be influenced by the dose, fractionation, or technique of irradiation. Urgent surgical intervention significantly improved survival (mortality was 0% for the patients who had intervention and 86% for those who did not) [63].

Recurrence may arise even from small islets of craniopharyngioma cells in the gliotic brain adjacent to the tumor. The mean interval for their diagnosis after various primary treatment modalities ranges between 1 and 4.3 years [49]. Remote recurrences have also been described with possible mechanisms, including transplantation during the surgical procedures and dissemination by meningeal seeding or cerebrospinal fluid (CSF) spreading [64–67]. The 10-year recurrence rate after gross total removal ranges between 0% and 62% and between 25% and 100% after partial or subtotal resection. In cases of limited surgery, adjuvant radiotherapy significantly improves the local control (recurrence rates of 10%–63% at 10 years of follow-up). Finally, radiotherapy alone provides 10-year recurrence rates ranging between 0% and 23% [49,53,55,58,61,68,69]. Interestingly, Rajan and colleagues [68] found that the extent of surgery in patients who subsequently received irradiation was not an independent predictor of recurrence. In cases of predominantly cystic tumors, fluid aspiration provides relief of the obstructive manifestations and facilitates the subsequent removal of the solid tumor portion; the latter should not be delayed for more than a few weeks because of the significant risk for cyst refilling (reported in up to 81% of the cases at a median length of 10 months) [53,61]. It should be pointed out that interpretation of the data on the effectiveness of each therapeutic modality has to be done with caution, because the published studies are retrospective, nonrandomized, and often specialty biased. Although not widely accepted [70,71], it has been proposed that tumor control is affected by the irradiation dose [72–74]; relapse rates were around 50% with a tumor dose less than 5000 rads and around 15% with a dose of 5500 to 5700 rads [72].

The growth rate of craniopharyngiomas varies considerably and cannot be predicted from clinical, radiologic, and pathologic criteria [49]. Differences in the local control rates between tumors diagnosed during childhood or adult life [29,30,55,61,68,75,76] and between male and female patients [61,68,77] have not been confirmed. Notably, Eldevik and colleagues [29] did not find any imaging characteristics predictive of recurrence, and Duff and colleagues [55] and Weiner and colleagues [30] did not confirm the effect of tumor size on the prognosis. A number of reports suggest that the location (intrasellar, extrasellar, or both) [61]; the consistency of the tumor [61,70]; and the presence of calcification [70], hydrocephalus [61,77], or third ventricular wall/floor invasion [61] are not associated with an unfavorable outcome. A few series suggest that the papillary type may have a better outcome [31,32,78], although others do not support this view [28,30,55]. The prognostic value of MIB-1 immunoreactivity and of microvascular density is not consistent [79–84]. The recurrent tumors show lower levels of galectin-3 and macrophage migration inhibiting factor [85], lower levels of retinoic acid receptor-β, and higher levels of retinoic acid receptor-γ [86].

The management of recurrent tumors remains difficult, because scarring/adhesions from previous operations or irradiation decreases the chances of successful excision. In such cases, total removal is achieved at a substantially lower rate when compared with primary surgery (0%–25%) and is associated with increased perioperative morbidity and mortality (10.5%–24%) [49,53,61]. The beneficial effect of radiotherapy in recurrent lesions has been shown in several studies [49]. Kalapurakal and colleagues [87] found a 5-year second relapse-free survival of 100% in patients offered radiotherapy and 0% in those treated by surgery alone. Karavitaki and colleagues [61] showed a significant difference in the 2.5-year local control rates after partial removal (50%), radiotherapy alone (83%), or partial removal followed by radiotherapy (100%).

Recurrent lesions with a significant cystic component, in which total removal is not possible, may be treated by repetitive aspirations through an indwelling Ommaya reservoir apparatus [88].

Other treatment options

Intracavitary irradiation (brachytherapy) is a minimally invasive treatment modality involving stereotactically guided instillation of β-emitting isotopes into cystic craniopharyngiomas. It delivers a higher radiation dose to the cyst lining than that offered by external beam radiotherapy and leads to destruction of the secretory epithelial lining, elimination of fluid production, and cyst shrinkage. The efficacy of various β-emitting and γ-emitting isotopes (mainly [32]phosphate, [90]yttrium, [186]rhenium, and [198]gold) [89–94] has been assessed in several studies; because none of them has the ideal physical and biologic profile (ie, pure β-emitter with a short half-life and with tissue penetrance limited to cover only the cyst wall [95]), there is no consensus on which is the most suitable therapeutic agent. In several studies [90,91,93,94] with a mean or median follow-up ranging between 3.1 and 11.9 years and intracavitary irradiation (mainly with [90]yttrium or [32]phosphorus) providing a radiation dose of 200 to 267 Gy, complete or partial cyst resolution was seen in 71% to 88% of the cases, stabilization was seen in 3% to 19%, and an increase in size was seen in 5% to 10%. New cyst formation or an increase in the solid component of the tumor was observed in 6.5% to 20% of the cases. The published control rates, combined with its reported low surgical morbidity and mortality rates [49], render brachytherapy an attractive option for predominantly cystic tumors, particularly the monocystic ones. The most beneficial isotope and the impact on the quality of survival and long-term morbidity remain to be assessed [49].

The intracystic installation of the antineoplasmatic agent bleomycin results in at least a 50% decrease of the cystic tumor size in 64% to 86% of children during follow-up ranging from 3 to 12 years [96,97]. Less optimal results have been described by Frank and colleagues [98] in a series of six patients; all the cysts regrew within 1 year, with five of them requiring reoperation. Headache, nausea, and vomiting, along with transient fever, have been described as common minor adverse effects during bleomycin administration [99]. Direct leakage of the drug to surrounding tissues during the installation procedure, diffusion though the cyst wall, or high drug dose has been associated with more serious toxic (eg, hypothalamic damage, blindness, hearing loss, ischemic attacks, peritumoral edema) or even fatal effects. The value of this treatment option remains to be established in large series with appropriate follow-up [49].

Stereotactic radiosurgery delivers a single fraction of high-dose ionizing radiation on precisely mapped targets, keeping the exposure of adjacent structures to a minimum. Tumor volume and close attachment to critical structures are limiting factors for its application; 10 Gy and 15 Gy have been reported as the maximum tolerated doses to the optic apparatus and the other cranial nerves, respectively [100]. Mokry [101] treated 23 patients (15 adults and 8 children) with a mean prescription dose of 10.8 Gy (range: 8–15 Gy). In 10 subjects with cystic tumors, intracystic bleomycin preceded radiosurgery. Sixty-one percent (14 of 23) of the patients showed a decrease in their mean treated tumor volume from 3.8 cm^3 to 1.9 cm^3 during a mean follow-up of 22.6 months, and 13% (3 of 23 patients) required a second radiosurgical intervention, resulting in a reduction of the mean treated tumor volume from 2.8 cm^3 to 0.9 cm^3 at a mean interval of 18 months after the second therapy. The remaining 26% (6 of 23 patients) had further tumor growth during a mean follow-up of 26.7 months. The initial tumor volume was a significant prognostic factor for the response. In the group of good responders, monocystic lesions amenable to bleomycin instillation predominated, pointing out the importance of a multimodality approach. Chung and colleagues [102] treated 31 patients (22 adults and 9 children [in 6 as primary therapy and in 25 for recurrent disease]) with a mean margin dose of 12.2 Gy (range: 9.5–16 Gy). During a mean follow-up of 33 months, the overall response rate was complete (residual tumor volume <20% of the original volume) in 32.3% of the cases and partial (residual tumor volume 20%–50% of the original volume) in 32.3%. No change was observed in

22.6%, and uncontrolled tumor progression was observed in 12.8%. A total of 10.3% of the subjects experienced enlargement of the cystic component 5 to 17 months after radiosurgery. Smaller volume (<4.2 cm^3 or diameter <2 cm) or single-component tumors (solid or cystic) had a better control rate. Chiou and colleagues [103] performed 12 stereotactic radiosurgical procedures in 10 consecutive patients (aged 9–64 years) who had small (≤2.5 cm) residual or recurrent tumors previously treated by surgery with or without radiotherapy. The mean marginal dose was 16.4 Gy (range: 12.5–20 Gy). During a median follow-up of 63 months, 58.3% (7 of 12) of the lesions showed shrinkage or complete regression (within a median interval of 8.5 months). Kobayashi and colleagues [104] treated 100 patients (38 children and 62 adults) with a tumor margin dose of 11.5 Gy. During a mean follow-up period of 65.5 months (range: 6–148 months), the craniopharyngioma disappeared or decreased in size greater than 25% in 67.4% of the cases, remained stable or decreased in size less than 25% in 12.2%, and increased in size in 20%. Based on the published data, stereotactic radiosurgery achieves tumor control in a substantial number of patients who have small-volume lesions and it may be particularly useful for well-defined residual tissue after surgery or for the treatment of small solid recurrent tumors, especially after failure of conventional radiotherapy. In cases of large cystic portions, multimodality approaches with instillation of radioisotopes or bleomycin may provide further benefits [101,105].

Fractionated stereotactic radiotherapy combines the accurate focal dose delivery of stereotactic radiosurgery with the radiobiologic advantages of fractionation. The data on its usefulness for the management of craniopharyngiomas are limited. In a study comprising 26 patients, the 10-year local control rate was 100% [106], and in a second study that included 39 subjects, the 5-year progression-free survival rate was 92% [107]. Early enlargement of the cystic component was observed in 8% to 30% of the cases.

Systemic chemotherapy has been offered in a limited number of patients, mainly with aggressive tumors, with relative success [49]. Its application remains rather experimental, and its value, particularly in the treatment of aggressive tumors, remains to be established.

Long-term morbidity and mortality

Craniopharyngiomas are associated with significant long-term morbidity, which compromises normal psychosocial integration and the quality of living. These complications are attributed to the damage of critical structures by the primary or recurrent tumor or to the adverse effects of the therapeutic interventions. Notably, the severity of radiation-induced late toxicity is associated with the total and per-fraction doses, the volume of exposed normal tissue, and the young age in childhood populations [49].

The rates of individual hormone deficits range between 88% and 100% for GH, between 80% and 95% for FSH/LH, between 55% and 88% for

ACTH, between 39% and 95% for TSH, and between 25% and 86% for ADH [49]. In contrast to anterior pituitary tumors [108], restoration of pre-existing hormone deficits after surgical removal is absent [62,109–111] or uncommon [112]. Rare cases of precocious puberty after surgical intervention have been described [113,114]. Apart from symptomatic diabetes insipidus (DI), which is probably more common in surgically treated patients, the long-term endocrine morbidity is not influenced by the type of tumor therapy [49,61]. The phenomenon of growth without GH has been reported in some children with craniopharyngioma (having normal or even accelerated linear growth, despite their untreated GH deficiency), but its pathophysiologic mechanism has not been clarified [115]. Based on data of 183 adults with craniopharyngioma and 209 adults with nonfunctioning pituitary adenoma from the Pharmacia and Upjohn International Metabolic (KIMS) database (Pfizer International Metabolic Database) treated for 2 years with GH, the subjects with craniopharyngiomas responded equally well as those with nonfunctioning pituitary adenoma in the free-fat mass, lipid levels, and quality of life, but they were less likely to lose body fat [116]. Several reports suggest that GH replacement in children and adults does not increase the risk for tumor recurrence [117–120].

Compromised vision has been reported in up to 62.5% of the patients treated by surgery combined or not with radiotherapy during an observation period of 10 years [55]. The visual outcome is adversely affected by the presence of visual symptoms at diagnosis [121,122] and by daily irradiation doses greater than 2 Gy [123]. An adverse visual outcome is more common in those treated by partial removal, probably as a consequence of their significantly increased recurrence rates [61].

Hypothalamic damage may result in hyperphagia and uncontrollable obesity, disorders of thirst and water/electrolyte balance, behavioral and cognitive impairment, loss of temperature control, and disorders in the sleep pattern [49]. Among those, obesity is the most frequent, reported in 26% to 61% of the patients treated by surgery combined or not combined with radiotherapy. It is a consequence of the disruption of the mechanisms controlling satiety, hunger, and energy balance, and it often results in devastating metabolic and psychosocial complications [49]. DI with an absent or impaired sense of thirst has been reported in approximately 14% of patients treated by surgery combined or not combined with radiotherapy. It confers a significant risk for serious electrolyte imbalance and is one of the most difficult complications to manage [124,125]. Factors proposed to be associated with significant hypothalamic morbidity are young age at presentation, hypothalamic disturbance at diagnosis, hypothalamic invasion, attempts to remove adherent tumor from the region of the hypothalamus, multiple operations for recurrence, and hypothalamic radiation doses greater than 51 Gy [49].

The compromised neuropsychologic and cognitive function in patients who have craniopharyngioma after surgery and radiation therapy contributes significantly to poor academic and work performance, disrupted family and social relationships, and impaired quality of life [1]. In a series of 121 patients followed up for a mean period of 10 years, Duff and colleagues [55] found that 40% of them had a poor functional neuropsychiatric outcome. In a series of 75 children followed up for a mean period of 6.4 years, De Vile and colleagues [58] demonstrated that 40% of them had an IQ less than 80. Finally, in a series of 121 patients, Karavitaki and colleagues [61] found cumulative probabilities for permanent motor deficits, epilepsy, psychologic disorders necessitating treatment, and complete dependency for basal daily activities at 10 years of follow-up of 11%, 12%, 15%, and 9%, respectively. During the same period, almost one quarter of the adults or children were unable to work in their previous occupation or were behind their expected school status. De Vile and colleagues [58] found that the mean morbidity scores (based on endocrine deficiencies, vision, motor disorders and epilepsy, learning difficulties, behavioral problems, IQ, and hypothalamic dysfunction) were not different between children who received radiotherapy after subtotal removal and those who had complete removal. The scores of children with additional surgery for recurrence were higher than those after their initial surgery and higher than those of children without recurrence, however. In this study, severe hydrocephalus, occurrence of intraoperative complications (vascular or frontal lobe trauma), and young age at presentation were predictors of poor long-term outcome. Duff and colleagues [55] proposed that gross total removal is associated with better clinical outcome, whereas factors associated with poor outcome were lethargy; visual deterioration, papilledema, or hydrocephalus at presentation; tumor calcification; and adhesiveness to surrounding neurovascular structures. There is no consensus on the therapeutic option with the least unfavorable impact on the neurobehavioral outcome, necessitating prospective studies with formal neuropsychologic testing and specific behavioral assessment before and after any intervention [49]. Such data are particularly important for young children, in whom the uncertainties of whether delaying irradiation is a reasonable policy and the relative contributions of the recurrent disease, subsequent surgery, and irradiation need to be clarified.

Craniopharyngiomas are associated with decreased survival; overall mortality rates three to six times higher than that of the general population have been reported [126,127]. In studies published during the past decade, the 10-year mortality rates range between 83% and 92.7% [53,61,126,128,129]. Apart from those deaths directly attributed to the tumor (pressure effects to critical structures) and those related to the surgical interventions [53,61,69,127], the risk for cardiovascular or cerebrovascular [127,130] and respiratory [130] mortality is enhanced. It has also been suggested that in childhood populations, the hypoadrenalism and associated hypoglycemia and the metabolic consequences of ADH deficiency and absent thirst may contribute to the excessive mortality [124,129,131]. The unfavorable effect of tumor recurrence on mortality is widely accepted [61,72,127,132], with

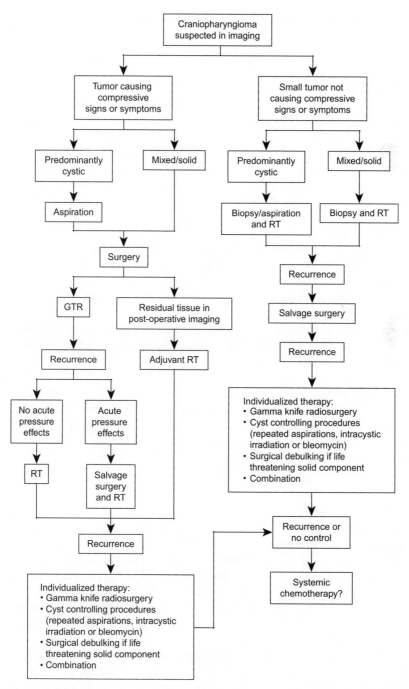

Fig. 5. Treatment algorithm for craniopharyngiomas. GTR, gross total removal; RT, radiotherapy. (*From* Karavitaki N, Cudlip S, Adams CBT, et al. Craniopharyngiomas. Endocr Rev 2006;27:391; with permission. Copyright © 2006, The Endocrine Society.)

10-year survival rates ranging between 29% and 70% depending on the subsequent treatment modalities [49].

Treatment algorithm

Based on the significant literature available, the proposed treatment algorithm is shown in Fig. 5 [49]. Surgical removal is suggested for all tumors resulting in compressive signs or symptoms (if a predominantly cystic lesion, the resection may be facilitated by previous aspiration of the cyst fluid). Gross total removal is a reasonable target, provided that it is performed by an experienced neurosurgeon and hazardous manipulations to vital brain structures are avoided. In cases of residual tumor after primary surgery, postoperative irradiation is recommended; this is because of the high risk for relapse and its negative impact on morbidity and mortality. Although this strategy may be debated for young children, the radiation toxicity to the developing brain needs to be balanced with the consequences of a recurrent mass and subsequent possible multiple surgical procedures. In small tumors not causing pressure effects, primary radiotherapy (preceded by biopsy for confirmation of the diagnosis) is an attractive option, avoiding the risks of surgery. The treatment of recurrent disease depends on the previous interventions and the severity of the clinical picture. In recurrent lesions not previously irradiated, radiotherapy provides satisfactory local control rates. Taking into account the high morbidity and mortality of a second operation, such an intervention is advocated only in cases of acute pressure effects. The treatment of further recurrence should be individualized, and options include gamma knife radiosurgery, cyst-controlling procedures, surgical debulking (for a significant solid life-threatening component), and systemic chemotherapy [49].

Summary

Craniopharyngiomas are rare epithelial tumors diagnosed during childhood or adult life. Two primary histologic subtypes have been recognized (adamantinomatous and papillary), with an as yet unclarified pathogenesis. Most of them are detected in the sellar or parasellar region. They may exert pressure effects to various brain structures (visual pathways, brain parenchyma, ventricular system, major blood vessels, and hypothalamopituitary system), resulting in multiple manifestations at presentation. Given the lack of randomized studies, their optimal treatment remains a subject of debate. Surgery combined or not combined with adjuvant external beam irradiation is currently the most widely used first therapeutic approach. In cases of limited surgery, adjuvant radiotherapy significantly improves local control. Intracystic irradiation or bleomycin, stereotactic radiosurgery or radiotherapy, and systemic chemotherapy are alternative approaches; their place in the management plan remains to be assessed in adequately powered long-term trials. The long-term morbidity of patients who have craniopharyngioma is considerable, and it is attributed to the damage of critical structures by the primary or recurrent tumor or to the adverse effects of the therapeutic interventions. It mainly involves endocrine, visual, hypothalamic, neurobehavioral, and cognitive sequelae, compromising normal psychosocial integration and the quality of life.

References

[1] Raimondi AJ, Rougerie J. A critical review of personal experiences with craniopharyngioma: clinical history, surgical technique and operative results. Pediatr Neurosurg 1994; 21:134–50.

[2] Saxer F. Ependymepithel, Gliome und epithelische Geschwuelste des Zentralenervensystems. Ziegler's Beitraege 1902;32:276.

[3] Lewis DD. A contribution to the subject of tumours of the hypophysis. JAMA 1910;55: 1002–8.

[4] Cushing H. The craniopharyngioma. In: Intracranial tumours. London: Bailliere, Tindall and Cox; 1932. p. 93–8.

[5] Bunin GR, Surawicz TS, Witman PA, et al. The descriptive epidemiology of craniopharyngioma. J Neurosurg 1998;89:547–51.

[6] Parisi JE, Mena H. Nonglial tumours. In: Nelson JS, Parisi JE, Schochet SS Jr, editors. Principles and practice of neuropathology. 1st edition. St. Louis (MO): Mosby; 1993. p. 203–66.

[7] Matson DD, Crigler JF Jr. Management of craniopharyngioma in childhood. J Neurosurg 1969;30:377–90.

[8] Schoenberg BC, Schoenberg DG, Christine BW, et al. The epidemiology of primary intracranial neoplasms of childhood. A population study. Mayo Clin Proc 1976;51: 51–6.

[9] Kuratsu J, Ushio Y. Epidemiological study of primary intracranial tumours in childhood. A population-based survey in Kumamoto Prefecture, Japan. Pediatr Neurosurg 1996; 25(5):240–6.

[10] DeVile CJ. Craniopharyngioma. In: Wass JAH, Shalet SM, editors. Oxford textbook of endocrinology and diabetes. 1st edition. Oxford (UK): Oxford University Press; 2002. p. 218–25.

[11] Sorva R, Heiskanen O. Craniopharyngioma in Finland. A study of 123 cases. Acta Neurochir (Wien) 1986;81(3–4):85–9.

[12] Goldberg GM, Eshbaught DE. Squamous cell nests of the pituitary gland as related to the origin of craniopharyngiomas: a study of their presence in the newborn and infants up to age four. Arch Pathol 1960;70:293–9.

[13] Hunter IJ. Squamous metaplasia of cells of the anterior pituitary gland. J Pathol Bacteriol 1955;69:141–5.

[14] Asa SL, Kovacs K, Bilbao JM. The pars tuberalis of the human pituitary: a histologic, immunohistochemical, ultrastructural and immunoelectron microscopic analysis. Virchows Arch A Pathol Anat Histopathol 1983;399:49–59.

[15] Sarubi JC, Bei H, Adams FF, et al. Clonal composition of human adamantinomatous craniopharyngiomas and somatic mutation analyses of the patched (PTCH), Gsalpha and Gi2alpha genes. Neurosci Lett 2001;310(1):5–8.

[16] Gorski GK, Morro LE, Donaldson MH, et al. Multiple chromosomal abnormalities in a case of craniopharyngioma. Cancer Genet Cytogenet 1992;60(2):212–3.

[17] Karnes PS, Tran TN, Cui MY, et al. Cytogenetic analysis of 39 pediatric central nervous system tumors. Cancer Genet Cytogenet 1992;59(1):12–9.

[18] Rienstein S, Adams EF, Pilzer D, et al. Comparative genomic hybridization analysis of craniopharyngiomas. J Neurosurg 2003;98:162–4.

[19] Sekine S, Shibata T, Kokubu A, et al. Craniopharyngioma of adamantinomatous type harbor β-catenin gene mutations. Am J Pathol 2002;161(6):1997–2001.

[20] Buslei R, Nolde M, Hofman B, et al. Common mutations of beta-catenin in adamantinomatous but not in other tumours originating from the sellar region. Acta Neuropathol (Berl) 2005;109:589–97.

[21] Hassanein AM, Glanz SM, Kessler HP, et al. Beta-catenin is expressed aberrantly in tumours expressing shadow cells. Pilomatricoma, craniopharyngioma, and calcifying odontogenic cyst. Am J Clin Pathol 2003;120(5):732–6.

[22] Kato K, Nakataki Y, Kanno H, et al. Possible linkage between specific histological structures and aberrant reactivation of the Wnt pathway in adamantinomatous craniopharyngioma. J Pathol 2004;203:814–21.

[23] Nozaki M, Tada M, Matsuko R. Rare occurrence of inactivating p53 gene mutations in primary non-astrocytic tumours of the central nervous system: reappraisal by yeast functional assay. Acta Neuropathol (Berl) 1998;95:291–6.

[24] Kleihnes P, Burger P, Scheithauer B. Histological typing of tumours of the central nervous system. In: WHO international histological classification of tumours. Heidelberg (Germany): Springer-Verlang; 1993.

[25] Nelson GA, Bastian FO, Schlitt M, et al. Malignant transformation of craniopharyngioma. Neurosurgery 1988;22:427–9.

[26] Kristopaitis T, Thomas C, Petruzzelli GJ, et al. Malignant craniopharyngioma. Arch Pathol Lab Med 2000;124:1356–60.

[27] Petito CK, De Girolami U, Earle K. Craniopharyngiomas. A clinical and pathological review. Cancer 1976;37:1944–52.

[28] Crotty TB, Scheithauer BW, Young WF, et al. Papillary craniopharyngioma: a clinicopathological study of 48 cases. J Neurosurg 1995;83:206–14.

[29] Eldevik OP, Blaivas M, Gabrielsen TO, et al. Craniopharyngioma: radiologic and histologic findings and recurrence. AJNR Am J Neuroradiol 1996;17:1427–39.

[30] Weiner HL, Wisoff JH, Rosenberg ME, et al. Craniopharyngiomas: a clinicopathological analysis of factors predictive of recurrence and functional outcome. Neurosurgery 1994;35(6):1001–11.

[31] Adamson TE, Wiestler OD, Kleihues P, et al. Correlation of clinical and pathological features in surgically treated craniopharyngiomas. J Neurosurg 1990;73:12–7.

[32] Kahn EA, Gosch HH, Seeger JF, et al. Forty-five years experience with the craniopharyngiomas. Surg Neurol 1973;1:5–12.

[33] Gorlin RJ, Chaudhry AP. The ameloblastoma and the craniopharyngioma; the similarities and differences. Oral Surg Oral Med Oral Pathol 1959;12:199–205.

[34] Bernstein ML, Buchino JJ. The histologic similarity between craniopharyngioma and odontogenic lesions: a reappraisal. Oral Surg Oral Med Oral Pathol 1983;56:502–11.

[35] Banna M. Craniopharyngioma: based on 160 cases. Br J Radiol 1976;49:206–23.

[36] Zhang YQ, Wang CC, Ma ZY. Pediatric craniopharyngiomas: clinicomorphological study of 189 cases. Pediatr Neurosurg 2002;36(2):80–4.

[37] Alvarez-Garijo JA, Froufe A, Taboada D, et al. Successful treatment of an odontogenic ossified craniopharyngioma: case report. J Neurosurg 1981;55:832–5.

[38] Seemayer TA, Blundell JS, Wiglesworth FW. Pituitary craniopharyngioma with tooth formation. Cancer 1972;29:423–30.

[39] Ghatak NR, Hirano A, Zimmerman HM. Ultrastructure of a craniopharyngioma. Cancer 1971;27(6):1465–75.

[40] Scheithauer BW. Region of the sella turcica. In: Burger PC, Scheithauer BW, Vogel FS, editors. Surgical pathology of the nervous system and its coverings. 4th edition. New York: Churchill Livingstone; 2002. p. 475–96.

[41] Miller DC. Pathology of craniopharyngiomas: clinical import of pathological findings. Pediatr Neurosurg 1994;21(Suppl 1):11–7.

[42] Giangaspero F, Burger PC, Osborne DR, et al. Suprasellar papillary squamous epithelioma ("papillary craniopharyngioma"). Am J Surg Pathol 1984;8(1):57–64.

[43] Sartoretti-Schefer S, Wichmann W, Aguzzi A, et al. MRI differentiation of adamantinous and squamous-papillary craniopharyngiomas. AJNR Am J Neuroradiol 1997;18(1):77–87.

[44] Xin W, Rubin MA, McKeever PE. Differential expression of cytokeratins 8 and 20 distinguishes craniopharyngioma from Rathke's cleft cyst. Arch Pathol Lab Med 2002;126:174–8.

[45] Thapar K, Stefaneanu K, Kovacs K, et al. Estrogen receptor gene expression in craniopharyngiomas: an in situ hybridization study. Neurosurgery 1994;35(6):1012–7.

[46] Honegger J, Renner C, Fahlbush R, et al. Progesterone expression in craniopharyngiomas and evidence for biological activity. Neurosurgery 1997;41:1359–64.

[47] Izumoto S, Suzuki T, Kinoshita M, et al. Immunohistochemical detection of female sex hormone receptors in craniopharyngiomas: correlation with clinical and histologic features. Surg Neurol 2005;63:520–5.

[48] Ulfarsson E, Karstrom A, Yin S, et al. Expression and growth dependency of the insulin-like growth factor I receptor in craniopharyngioma cells: a novel therapeutic approach. Clin Cancer Res 2005;11:4674–80.

[49] Karavitaki N, Cudlip S, Adams CB, et al. Craniopharyngiomas. Endocr Rev 2006;27: 371–97.

[50] Love JG, Marshall TM. Craniopharyngiomas (pituitary adamantinomas). Surg Gynec Obset 1950;90:591–601.

[51] Banna M, Hoare RD, Stanley P, et al. Craniopharyngioma in children. J Pediatr 1973; 83(5):781–5.

[52] Svolos DG. Craniopharyngiomas. A study based on 108 verified cases. Acta Chir Scand Suppl 1969;403:1–44.

[53] Fahlbush R, Honegger J, Paulus W, et al. Surgical treatment of craniopharyngiomas: experience with 168 patients. J Neurosurg 1999;90(2):237–50.

[54] Kurosaki M, Saeger W, Ludecke DK. Immunohistochemical localisation of cytokeratins in craniopharyngioma. Acta Neurochir (Wien) 2001;143(2):147–51.

[55] Duff JM, Meyer FB, Ilstrup DM, et al. Long-term outcomes for surgically resected craniopharyngiomas. Neurosurgery 2000;46(2):291–305.

[56] Hoffman HJ, DeSilva M, Humphreys RP, et al. Aggressive surgical management of craniopharyngiomas in children. J Neurosurg 1992;76:47–52.

[57] Shapiro K, Till K, Grant DN. Craniopharyngiomas in childhood. A rational approach to treatment. J Neurosurg 1979;50:617–23.

[58] De Vile CJ, Grant DB, Kendall BE, et al. Management of childhood craniopharyngioma: can the morbidity of radical surgery be predicted? J Neurosurg 1996;85:73–81.

[59] Yasargil GM, Curcic M, Kis M, et al. Total removal of craniopharyngiomas. Approaches and long-term results in 144 patients. J Neurosurg 1990;73:3–11.

[60] Symon L, Pell MF, Habib AH. Radical excision of craniopharyngioma by the temporal route: a review of 50 patients. Br J Neurosurg 1991;5:539–49.

[61] Karavitaki N, Brufani C, Warner JT, et al. Craniopharyngiomas in children and adults: systematic analysis of 121 cases with long-term follow-up. Clin Endocrinol (Oxf) 2005;62: 397–409.

[62] Costine LS, Randall SH, Rubin P, et al. Craniopharyngiomas: fluctuation in cyst size following surgery and radiation therapy. Neurosurgery 1989;24:53–9.

[63] Rajan B, Ashley S, Thomas DG, et al. Craniopharyngioma: improving outcome by early recognition and treatment of acute complications. Int J Radiat Oncol Biol Phys 1997;37: 517–21.

[64] Barloon TJ, Yuh WT, Sato Y, et al. Frontal lobe implantation of craniopharyngioma by repeated needle aspiration. AJNR Am J Neuroradiol 1988;9:406–7.

[65] Malik JM, Cosgrove GR, Van der Berg SR. Remote recurrence of craniopharyngioma in the epidural space. J Neurosurg 1992;77:804–7.

[66] Gupta K, Kuhn MJ, Shevlin DW, et al. Metastatic craniopharyngioma. Am J Neuroradiol 1999;20:1059–60.

[67] Ito M, Jamshidi J, Yamanaka K. Does craniopharyngioma metastasize? Case report and review of the literature. Neurosurgery 2001;48:933–6.

[68] Rajan B, Ashley S, Gorman C, et al. Craniopharyngioma—long-term results following limited surgery and radiotherapy. Radiat Oncol 1993;26:1–10.

[69] Hetelekidis S, Barnes PD, Tao ML, et al. 20-Year experience in childhood craniopharyngioma. Int J Radiat Oncol Biol Phys 1993;27:189–95.

[70] Wen BC, Hussey DH, Staples J, et al. A comparison of the roles of surgery and radiation therapy in the management of craniopharyngiomas. Int J Radiat Oncol Biol Phys 1989;16: 17–24.

[71] Flickinger JC, Lunsford LD, Singer J, et al. Megavoltage external beam irradiation of craniopharyngiomas: analysis of tumour control and morbidity. Int J Radiat Oncol Biol Phys 1990;19:177–2.

[72] Sung DI, Chang CH, Harisiadis L, et al. Treatment results of craniopharyngiomas. Cancer 1981;47:847–52.

[73] Regine WF, Kramer S. Pediatric craniopharyngiomas: long-term results of combined treatment with surgery and radiation. Int J Radiat Oncol Biol Phys 1992;24:611–7.

[74] Varlotto JM, Flickinger JC, Kondziolka D, et al. External beam irradiation of craniopharyngiomas: long-term analysis of tumour control and morbidity. Int J Radiat Oncol Biol Phys 2002;54:492–9.

[75] Hoff JT, Patterson RH. Craniopharyngiomas in children and adults. J Neurosurg 1972;36: 299–302.

[76] Pemberton LS, Dougal M, Magee B, et al. Experience of external beam radiotherapy given adjuvantly or at relapse following surgery for craniopharyngioma. Radiother Oncol 2005; 77:99–104.

[77] Tomita T, Bowman RM. Craniopharyngiomas in children: surgical experience at Children's Memorial Hospital. Childs Nerv Syst 2005;21:729–46.

[78] Szeifert GT, Sipos L, Horvath M, et al. Pathological characteristics of surgically removed craniopharyngiomas: analysis of 131 cases. Acta Neurochir (Wien) 1993;124:139–43.

[79] Nishi T, Kuratsu J, Takeshima H, et al. Prognostic significance of the MIB-1 labeling index for patients with craniopharyngioma. Int J Mol Med 1999;3:157–61.

[80] Duo D, Gasverde S, Benech F, et al. MIB-1 immunoreactivity in craniopharyngiomas: a clinic-pathological analysis. Clin Neuropathol 2003;22:229–34.

[81] Raghavan R, Dickey WT, Margraf LR, et al. Proliferative activity in craniopharyngiomas: clinicopathological correlations in adults and children. Surg Neurol 2000;54:241–8.

[82] Losa M, Vimercati A, Acerno S, et al. Correlation between clinical characteristics and proliferative activity in patients with craniopharyngioma. J Neurol Neurosurg Psychiatry 2004;75:889–92.

[83] Vidal S, Kovacs K, Lloyd RV, et al. Angiogenesis in patients with craniopharyngiomas. Correlation with treatment and outcomes. Cancer 2002;94:738–45.

[84] Xu J, Zhang S, You C, et al. Microvascular density and vascular endothelial growth factor have little correlation with prognosis of craniopharyngiomas. Surg Neurol 2006; 66(Suppl 1):S30–4.

[85] Lefranc F, Chevalier C, Vinchon M, et al. Characterization of the levels of expression of retinoic acid receptors, galectin-3, macrophage migration inhibiting factor, and p53 in 51 adamantinomatous craniopharyngiomas. J Neurosurg 2003;98:145–53.

[86] Lubansu A, Ruchoux M-M, Brotchi J, et al. Cathepsin B, D and K expression in adamantinomatous craniopharyngiomas relates to their levels of differentiation as determined by the patterns of retinoic acid receptor expression. Histopathology 2003;43:563–72.

[87] Kalapurakal JA, Goldman S, Hsieh YC, et al. Clinical outcome in children with recurrent craniopharyngioma after primary surgery. Cancer J 2000;6:388–93.

[88] Gutin DH, Klemme WM, Lagger RI, et al. Management of unresectable cystic craniopharyngioma by aspiration through an Ommaya reservoir drainage system. J Neurosurg 1980; 52:36–40.

[89] Backlund EO. Studies on craniopharyngiomas III. Stereotactic treatment with intracystic yttrium-90. Acta Chir Scand 1973;139:237–47.

[90] Pollock BE, Lunsford LD, Kondziolka D, et al. Phosphorus-32 intracavitary irradiation of cystic craniopharyngiomas: current technique and long-term results. Int J Radiat Oncol Biol Phys 1995;33:437–46.

[91] Voges J, Sturm V, Lehrke R, et al. Cystic craniopharyngioma: long-term results after intracavitary irradiation with stereotactically applied colloidal beta-emitting radioactive sources. Neurosurgery 1997;40:263–70.

[92] Bond WH, Richards D, Turner E. Experiences with radioactive gold in the treatment of craniopharyngioma. J Neurol Neurosurg Psychiatry 1965;28:30–8.

[93] Van den Berge JH, Blaauw G, Breeman WA, et al. Intracavitary brachytherapy of cystic craniopharyngiomas. J Neurosurg 1992;77:545–50.

[94] Hasegawa T, Kondzilka D, Hadjipanayis CG, et al. Management of cystic craniopharyngiomas with phosphous-32 intracavitary irradiation. Neurosurgery 2004;54:813–22.

[95] Blackburn TPD, Doughty D, Plowman PN. Stereotactic intracavitary therapy of recurrent cystic craniopharyngioma by installation of [90]yttrium. Br J Neurosurg 1999;14(4):359–65.

[96] Takahashi H, Yamaguchi F, Teramoto F. Long-term outcome and reconsideration of intracystic chemotherapy with bleomycin for craniopharyngioma in children. Childs Nerv Syst 2005;21:701–4.

[97] Hader WJ, Steinbok P, Hukin J, et al. Intratumoral therapy with bleomycin for cystic craniopharyngiomas in children. Pediatr Neurosurg 2000;33:211–8.

[98] Frank F, Fabrizi AP, Frank G, et al. Stereotactic management of craniopharyngiomas. Stereotact Funct Neurosurg 1995;65:176–83.

[99] Caceres A. Intracavitary therapeutic options in the management of cystic craniopharyngioma. Childs Nerv Syst 2005;21:705–18.

[100] Leber KA, Bergloeff J, Pendl G. Dose response tolerance of the visual pathways and cranial nerves of the cavernous sinus to stereotactic radiosurgery. J Neurosurg 1998;88:43–50.

[101] Mokry M. Craniopharyngiomas: a six years experience with gamma knife radiosurgery. Stereotact Funct Neurosurg 1999;72(S1):140–9.

[102] Chung WY, Pan DH, Shiau CY, et al. Gamma knife radiosurgery for craniopharyngiomas. J Neurosurg 2002;93(Suppl 3):47–56.

[103] Chiou SM, Lunsford LD, Niranjan A, et al. Stereotactic radiosurgery of residual or recurrent craniopharyngioma after surgery with or without radiation therapy. Neuro Oncol 2001;3:159–66.

[104] Kobayashi T, Kida Y, Mori Y, et al. Long-term results of gamma knife surgery for the treatment of craniopharyngiomas in 98 consecutive cases. J Neurosurg 2005; 103(6 Suppl):482–8.

[105] Yu X, Liu Z, Li S. Combined treatment with stereotactic intracavitary irradiation and gamma knife surgery for craniopharyngiomas. Stereotact Funct Neurosurg 2000;75: 117–22.

[106] Schulz-Ertner D, Frank C, Herfarth KK, et al. Fractionated stereotactic radiotherapy for craniopharyngiomas. Int J Radiat Oncol Biol Phys 2002;54:114–20.

[107] Minniti G, Saran F, Traish D, et al. Fractionated stereotactic conformal radiotherapy following conservative surgery in the control of craniopharyngiomas. Radiother Oncol 2007; 82:90–5.

[108] Ahmed S, Elsheikh M, Stratton IM, et al. Outcome of transsphenoidal surgery for acromegaly and its relationship to surgical experience. Clin Endocrinol 1999;50:561–7.

[109] Paja M, Lucas T, Garcia-Uria F, et al. Hypothalamic-pituitary dysfunction in patients with craniopharyngioma. Clin Endocrinol 1995;42:467–73.

[110] Weiss M, Sutton L, Marcial V, et al. The role of radiation therapy in the management of childhood craniopharyngioma. Int J Radiat Oncol Biol Phys 1989;17(6):1313–21.

[111] Thomsett MJ, Conte FA, Kaplan SL. Endocrine and neurologic outcome in childhood craniopharyngioma: review of effect of treatment in 42 patients. J Pediatr 1980;97: 728–35.

[112] Honegger J, Buchfelder M, Fahlbusch R. Surgical treatment of craniopharyngiomas: endocrinological results. J Neurosurg 1999;90:251–7.

[113] Zahmann M, Illig R. Precocious puberty after surgery for craniopharyngioma. J Pediatr 1979;95:86–8.

[114] Cabezudo JM, Perez C, Vaquero J, et al. Pubertas praecox in craniopharyngioma. J Neurosurg 1981;55:127–31.

[115] Geffner ME. The growth without growth hormone syndrome. Endocrinol Metab Clin North Am 1996;25(3):649–63.

[116] Verhelst J, Kendal-Taylor P, Erfurth EM, et al. Baseline characteristics and response to 2 years of growth hormone (GH) replacement of hypopituitary patients with GH deficiency due to adult-onset craniopharyngiomas in comparison with patients with non-functioning pituitary adenoma: data from KIMS (Pfizer International Metabolic Database). J Clin Endocrinol Metab 2005;90:4636–43.

[117] Price DA, Wilton P, Jonsson P, et al. Efficacy and safety of growth hormone treatment in children with prior craniopharyngioma: an analysis of Pharmacia and Upjohn International Growth Database (KIGS) from 1988 to 1996. Horm Res 1998;49:91–7.

[118] Abs R, Bengtsson B-A, Hernberg-Stahl E, et al. GH replacement in 1034 growth hormone deficient hypopituitary adults: demographic and clinical characteristics, dosing and safety. Clin Endocrinol 1999;50:703–13.

[119] Karavitaki N, Warner JT, Marland A, et al. GH replacement does not increase the risk of recurrence in patients with craniopharyngiomas. Clin Endocrinol 2006;64(5):556–60.

[120] Darendeliler F, Karagiannis G, Wilton P, et al. Recurrence of brain tumours in patients treated with growth hormone: analysis of KIGS (Pfizer International Growth Database). Acta Paediatr 2006;95:1284–90.

[121] Abrams LS, Repka MX. Visual outcome of craniopharyngioma in children. J Pediatr Ophthalmol Strabismus 1997;34(4):223–4.

[122] Cabezudo Artero JM, Vaquero Crespo J, Bravo Zabalgoitia G. Status of vision following surgical treatment of craniopharyngiomas. Acta Neurochir (Wien) 1984;73:165–77.

[123] Harris JR, Levene MB. Visual complications following irradiation for pituitary adenomas and craniopharyngiomas. Radiology 1976;120:167–71.

[124] De Vile CJ, Grant DB, Hayward RD, et al. Growth and endocrine sequelae of craniopharyngioma. Arch Dis Child 1996;75:108–14.

[125] Smith D, Finucane F, Phillips J, et al. Abnormal regulation of thirst and vasopressin secretion following surgery for craniopharyngioma. Clin Endocrinol 2004;61:273–9.

[126] Pereira AM, Scmid EM, Schutte PJ, et al. High prevalence of long-term cardiovascular, neurological and psychosocial morbidity after treatment for craniopharyngiomas. Clin Endocrinol 2005;62:197–204.

[127] Bulow B, Attewell R, Hagmar L, et al. Postoperative prognosis in craniopharyngioma with respect to cardiovascular mortality, survival, and tumour recurrence. J Clin Endocrinol Metab 1998;83:3897–904.

[128] Van Effenterre R, Boch AL. Craniopharyngioma in adults and children. J Neurosurg 2002; 97:3–11.

[129] Stripp DC, Maity A, Janss AJ, et al. Surgery with or without radiation therapy in the management of craniopharyngiomas in children and young adults. Int J Radiat Oncol Biol Phys 2004;58:714–20.

[130] Tomlinson JW, Holden N, Hills RK, et al. Association between premature mortality and hypopituitarism. Lancet 2001;357:425–31.
[131] Lyen KR, Grant DB. Endocrine function, morbidity, and mortality after surgery for craniopharyngioma. Arch Dis Child 1982;57:837–41.
[132] Tarbell NJ, Barnes P, Scott RM, et al. Advances in radiation therapy for craniopharyngiomas. Pediatr Neurosurg 1994;21(Suppl 1):101–7.

ELSEVIER
SAUNDERS

Endocrinol Metab Clin N Am
37 (2008) 195–211

ENDOCRINOLOGY
AND METABOLISM
CLINICS
OF NORTH AMERICA

Rare Sellar Lesions

Andrea Glezer, MD,
Diane Belchior Paraiba, MD,
Marcello Delano Bronstein, MD*

*Neuroendocrine Unit, Division of Endocrinology and Metabolism,
Hospital das Clinicas, University of Sao Paulo Medical School, Avenida 9 de Julho,
3858 CEP 01406-100 Sao Paulo – SP, Brazil*

Pituitary adenomas represent 10% of all intracranial neoplasms and make up more than 90% of all sellar masses [1]. The differential diagnosis of nonpituitary sellar masses is broad and includes inflammatory and infectious diseases, cell rest tumors, germ cell tumors, gliomas, meningiomas, metastatic tumors, and vascular lesions [2]. Nonadenomatous pituitary lesions can be classified as shown in Table 1 and as described later [3]. Craniopharyngioma is described in the article by Karavitaki and Wass elsewhere in this issue.

Clinical presentation

Nonadenomatous sellar lesions do not present with any hypersecretory syndrome but rather with neurologic or hypopituitary symptoms as a result of the mass-effect mechanism.

Neurologic symptoms include headache, visual disturbance, cranial neuropathy, hydrocephalus, and mental changes. Hypopituitarism most often is characterized by growth hormone deficiency and gonadal dysfunction, followed by secondary hypothyroidism and adrenal insufficiency. Hyperprolactinemia secondary to stalk compression is a common cause of hypogonadism. Diabetes insipidus is highly suggestive of nonadenomatous sellar lesions, especially in sarcoidosis and in metastatic sellar involvement.

---

* Corresponding author.
E-mail address: mdbronstein@uol.com.br (M.D. Bronstein).

0889-8529/08/$ - see front matter © 2008 Elsevier Inc. All rights reserved.
doi:10.1016/j.ecl.2007.10.003

Table 1
Classification of rare intrasellar nonadenomatous lesions

Tumors	Inflammatory diseases
Cell rest tumors	Sarcoidosis
Rathke's cleft cyst	Wegener's granulomatosis
Epidermoid and dermoid cysts	Mucocele
Chordoma	Langerhans' cell histiocytosis
Colloid cyst	Hypophysitis
Primitive germ cell tumors	Infectious diseases
Germinoma	Pituitary abscess
Teratoma and atypical teratoma	Tuberculosis
(dysgerminoma)	
Other tumors	Vascular lesions
Meningioma	Carotid aneurysm
Gliomas	Apoplexy
Ependymoma	Miscellaneous
Astrocytoma	Arachnoid cyst
Lymphoma	Secondary pituitary hyperplasia
Metastatic tumors	Double pituitary

Specific lesions

Neoplastic/developmental lesions

Cell rest tumors
Rathke's cleft cyst. Cysts derived from Rathke's pouch are found between the pars anterior and the infundibular process in 13% to 22% of the pituitary glands [4]. Typically, Rathke's cleft cysts are small and asymptomatic. Symptomatic cysts can occur at any age but more frequently between ages 40 and 60. This lesion usually is intrasellar and may present with impaired vision, hypopituitarism, and headache.

On CT scanning, cysts usually are hypodense and not enhanced by contrast. The lack of calcification is important to differentiate them from craniopharingioma. In MRI, the cyst signal often is similar to cerebrospinal fluid on T_1- and T_2-weighted images [2].

Surgical approach is recommended when a cyst is large enough to cause symptoms. Transsphenoidal approach can drain a cyst effectively but if it recurs, a transcranial approach may be needed to resect the cyst wall. Cyst content may be clear and colorless, oily, or milky [4].

Epidermoid and dermoid cysts. Epidermoid and dermoid cysts result from the inclusion of epithelial elements during neural tube closure. The contents of dermoid lesions are desquamated epithelium, sebaceous material, and, sometimes, dermal appendages, whereas epidermoid cysts contain a white cheesy material (keratin) within a thin capsule. They appear as hypodense cysts with no enhancement in CT or MRI [4].

Chordomas. Chordomas are rare, slow-growing tumors of midline, representing 1% of all malignant bone tumors and 0.1% to 0.2% of all intracranial neoplasms. They arise from notochordal remnants in the clivus, usually producing sphenoid basis destruction. Chordomas involving the sellar region are rare and fewer than 30 cases are described in the literature [5]. The most common symptoms are headaches, visual deficits, neck pain, diplopia, and nasopharyngeal obstruction.

Bone destruction and calcification are common, occurring in more than 50% of cases and are seen better on CT than on MRI. Chordomas may extend along the entire skull base and the sella usually is destroyed instead of ballooned as often seen in pituitary adenomas. The location, bone destruction, and calcification usually make the differential diagnosis with pituitary adenomas easier. Fig. 1 shows an MRI of a parasellar chordoma.

Surgery is the treatment of choice; however, because of bone invasiveness, total excision generally is not possible. Radiotherapy can be recommended as adjunctive therapy [2,4].

Primitive germ cell tumors

Germinomas. Germinomas are malignant intracranial tumors with peak incidence in children and adolescents. Their usual localizations are the midline central nervous system structures, most frequently the pineal gland. Three patterns are described: germinomas of the ventral hypothalamus associated with germinoma in the pineal region; germinomas in the anterior third ventricle that can involve the pituitary fossa as extension; and intrasellar germinoma mimicking an intrasellar adenoma. The most common symptom is diabetes insipidus, seen in more than 80% of cases, followed by visual disturbances and obesity. CT scanning depicts isodense or hyperdense mass, sometimes multicentric, that can be enhanced markedly. Although only 5% of pure germinomas present with high values of β-chorionic gonadotropin

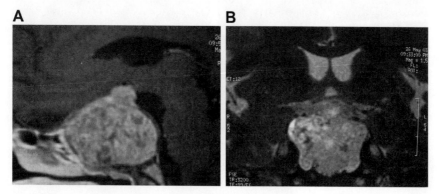

Fig. 1. Sellar chordoma: sagittal T_1-weighted image (*A*) and coronal T_2-weighted image (*B*) depicting a mass invading sphenoid sinus and eroding sellar bone.

and α-fetoprotein in cerebrospinal fluid or serum, these markers are present in approximately 30% of dysgerminomas that contain other malignant components. Histologic examination shows a granulomatous infiltrate around germ cells. Lymphocytic infiltrate can make the diagnosis more difficult. Because of a germinoma's localization and multicentricity, surgery rarely is curative and shunting often indicated.

Germinomas usually respond well to chemotherapy and radiotherapy. Remission is achieved in 75% to 80% of cases. As germinomas are sensitive to radiotherapy, a therapeutic trial with a fractionated dose of 1500 cGy can be performed, a positive response indicative of germinoma (Fig. 2) [2,6].

Teratoma. Teratomas are benign tumors derived from the pluripotential cells from all three embryologic layers: ectoderm, mesoderm, and endoderm. Intracranial teratomas are rare, comprising approximately 0.5% of all intracranial tumors. Mature teratoma is characterized by one or two fully differentiated embryologic layers; immature teratoma is formed by embryonic elements from one or more layers. These tumors are found most commonly in the pineal region, followed by the suprasellar and hypothalamic regions, and rarely in the sellar region. They occur more frequently in children and young adults. Teratomas can involve the pituitary gland primarily or secondarily, by invasion. Pituitary dysfunction is seen commonly and depends on tumor growth.

Teratoma appears in imaging assessments as a well-delineated mixed cyst with calcification. This tumor can undergo ossification, teeth formation, or malignant transformation.

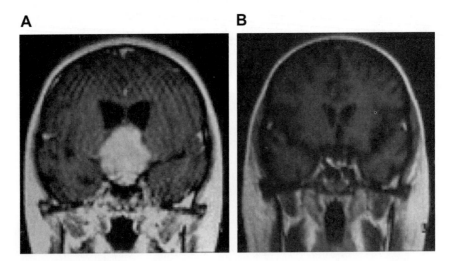

Fig. 2. Coronal MRI sellar T_1-weighted images depicting a germinoma: pretreatment (*A*) and after radiotherapy (*B*).

Mature teratomas are benign and usually radioresistant; therefore, surgery is recommended. Immature teratomas, in contrast, are aggressive and have metastatic potential [7].

Other tumors

Meningioma. Meningiomas are benign tumors originating from arachnoid cells and frequently adhere to the dura mater. They account for 20% of all intracranial tumors. Meningiomas that arise from tuberculum sella, the planum sphenoidale, or the diaphragma sella can appear as suprasellar mass. Intrasellar meningioma is rare and originates from arachnoid tissue in a herniated pouch. They are more common in 40 to 50 year olds and they predominate in women. Visual loss is the most common symptom.

CT shows a hyperdense lesion originating from the tuberculum sella, planum sphenoidale, or sphenoidal ridge with hyperostosis. In MRI, meningiomas typically appear as isointense on precontrast T_1-weighted images and with a bright enhancement after gadolinium contrast. A dural tail sign, which is a thickening of the dura in continuity with convexity on contrast T_1 images, is suggestive of meningioma [8].

For patients who have benign meningiomas that are resectable with minimal morbidity or that have significant mass effect, excision is the treatment of choice, occasionally followed by fractionated radiotherapy [9].

Glioma. Optic nerve gliomas are rare and comprise 3.5% of intracranial tumors in children and 1% of intracranial tumors in adults, in whom they have malignant behavior. Approximately 30% are associated with von Recklinghausen's disease (neurofibromatosis type 1).

In children, the most common symptoms are visual loss, headache, and proptosis, whereas in adults, the initial symptom is impaired vision and retroorbital pain. Diencephalic syndrome, characterized by failure to gain weight, diabetes insipidus, and visual loss, occurs if there is hypothalamic tumoral invasion [2]. Imaging examinations show a tumor with origin in chiasm or optic nerve, classically a hypointense lesion on T_1 images with contrast enhancement.

Most optic gliomas in children are low-grade astrocytomas; high-grade lesions are seen more commonly in adults.

Radiotherapy plays a primary role in management. Surgery can be performed on exophytic chiasmal tumors causing mass effect or hydrocephalus. Chemotherapy can delay other aggressive therapies, such as radiation or surgery, in young children until they progress neuropsychologically [10].

Ependymoma. Ependymomas are glial neoplasms arising from the ependyma of cerebral ventricules, the spinal cord central canal, or cells of the terminal ventricle in the terminal filum. Pituitary fossa is a rarely documented site of these tumors and only four cases are described in the literature.

Ependymomas appear as hyperdense lesions in CT with low-density areas suggestive of cystic or necrotic regions. These areas are seen as low-attenuation regions in MRI. There are no specific features in imaging examinations.

Surgical removal is the treatment of choice. Some investigators suggest radiotherapy [11].

Astrocytoma. Hypophyseal stalk and posterior pituitary can be a host to all tumors that originate from glial cells. Pituicytoma is a rare primary tumor of the neurohypophysis that also can be located at the pituitary stalk. Pituicytoma usually occurs in young to middle-aged women and the most common symptoms are headache and hypopituitarism. Visual loss is described infrequently. On MRI, lesions with low intensity on T_1-weighted images with homogeneous enhancement and low to intermediate intensity on T_2- weighted images usually are found. Special attention to the posterior pituitary is the key in diagnosis. Although histologically benign, the location and vascular nature of these tumors can make surgical resection difficult. Cure can be achieved by total excision [12,13].

Lymphoma. Lymphomas can involve the pituitary gland primarily or secondarily, by metastatic spread. Primary pituitary lymphomas are rare [14].

Giustina and colleagues [15], in 2001, described 14 cases of primary pituitary lymphomas. The investigators observed that primary pituitary lymphomas are twice as common in men and occur most often around the sixth decade of life. Pituitary adenomas, lymphocytic hypophysitis, and AIDS are considered pituitary lymphoma risks. Patients can present with hypopituitarism, diabetes insipidus, and other neurologic signs due to mass effect.

Surgery, radiotherapy, and chemotherapy can be used to treat these tumors.

Metastatic tumors. Metastasis to the pituitary is an infrequent clinical problem with surgical prevalence less than 1% of sellar and parasellar masses.

Usually, metastic tumors affect patients in the sixth or seventh decade of life with no gender predominance. Breast and lung cancer are the most common primary neoplasms, accounting for two thirds of the cases, followed by gastrointestinal and prostate cancer, but virtually any neoplasm can metastasize to pituitary. Confirming these data, in 380 cases of metastases to pituitary, 39.7% had primary tumor origin in the breast, 23.7% in the lungs, 6.3% in the gastrointestinal system, and 5% in the prostate [16]. In general, there are other metastatic sites at the time of diagnosis, and pituitary metastasis is not the first manifestation. Pituitary metastasis was a presenting sign of extrapituitary malignancy in 43.7% of cases, however, in a series of 190 cases compiled by Komminos and colleagues [16].

In patients who have metastasis to the pituitary, the most common symptoms are diabetes insipidus in 45.2%, visual deficiency in 27.9%, anterior pituitary deficiency in 23.6%, other cranial nerve paresis in 21.6%, and headache in 15.8% [16]. Syndrome of inappropriate antidiuretic hormone secretion or diabetes insipidus also is described. Hyperprolactinemia resulting from stalk compression is encountered in 6% of cases. There are no specific radiologic findings in radiologic assessment.

A rapidly growing sellar tumor or a sudden onset of diabetes insipidus, ophthalmoplegia, or headaches in patients over age 50 suggests metastases to the pituitary. Diagnosis is important to avoid unnecessary surgery in patients who are severely compromised and prognosis is determined by the primary tumor.

Extremely rare nonadenomatous pituitary tumors. Hypothalamic hamartomas can occur in sellar regions. They are associated with precocious puberty. Gangliocytomas are benign tumors composed of neuronal tissue that can originate in sellar or parasellar areas. They sometimes are associated with functioning pituitary adenomas [3]. Other tumors, such as schwanommas [17], melanocytic tumor [18], chondrosarcoma [19], and plasmacytoma [20], are rare and appear as case reports in literature.

Inflammatory lesions

Sarcoidosis

Sarcoidosis is a chronic granulomatous disease of unknown origin affecting mainly young and middle-aged adults. The organs involved most commonly are the lungs, skin, and lymph nodes [21]. This disorder can affect individuals of both genders and almost all ages [22]. Endocrine disease is rare in sarcoidosis; hypothalamus and pituitary are the glands affected most commonly [23].

Diabetes insipidus is reported in approximately 25% to 33% of all neurosarcoidosis cases [24]. Hyperprolactinemia also occurs commonly as the result of loss of dopaminergic inhibition [23]. Anterior pituitary deficiency, mainly hypogonadism, can be present. Other hypothalamic disturbances may occur less frequently. These disturbances are attributed to granulomatous invasion of the hypothalamus-pituitary axis. Visual field defects can occur with mass expansion [21]. Psychiatric disturbances and seizures can occur. Rarely, multiple lesions mimicking multiple sclerosis, spinal cord abnormalities, and peripheral neuropathy may be present. Symptoms of neurosarcoidosis often occur after more common manifestations, such as lungs and lymph nodes involvement [22]. In patients suspected of neurosarcoidosis, cerebrospinal fluid examination, including angiotensin-converting enzyme, cytology, and tumor markers, is indicated [25].

MRI findings can show the absence of normal hyperintense signal of the neurohypophysis on T_1-weighted views. The pathologic lesions are isointense on T_1-weighted images and enhance with gadolinium [3,21,23]. In some patients, the diagnosis is made only by biopsy of the granulomatous lesion [25].

Corticosteroids are the therapy of choice, but various adjuvant immuno-suppressants are used [21,23,25].

Wegener's granulomatosis

Wegener's granulomatosis (WG) is a multisystemic disorder character-ized by systemic vasculitis and necrotizing granulomas in the respiratory tract and the kidney. They also can be present in the orbits, heart, skin, and joints [26,27]. Pituitary involvement is rare and affects predominantly the posterior pituitary as central diabetes insipidus; that usually occurs after pulmonary or kidney lesions [28,29]. Rarely, partial or total anterior pitui-tary abnormality can be present. The suggested causes of this complication include vasculitis of pituitary blood vessels, granulomatous lesions in situ, or encroachment on the nervous system by adjacent nasal or paranasal granu-loma [27]. A combination of respiratory tract involvement, positive antineu-trophil cytoplasmic antibodies (ANCA), and increased proteinase 3-ANCA suggests a diagnosis of WG [27].

MRI usually shows an enlarged pituitary gland with homogeneous enhancement and thickening of infundibulum, especially in the superior portion [26].

The majority of patients respond to medical management, such as corti-costeroids and immunosuppressors associated with hormonal replacement. Several cases show complete resolution of diabetes insipidus and control of WG. Others patients have demonstrated persistent diabetes insipidus in spite of improvement of peripheral manifestations of the disease and even diminution in hypothalamic granulomatous lesions [27–29].

Sphenoidal sinus mucocele

Mucocele of the sphenoid sinus is a lesion resulting from a chronic obstruction of the sinus that leads to accumulation and dehydration of secretions [30]. Congenital anomaly, trauma, inflammatory conditions, and previous surgery of sphenoid sinus may predispose to mucocele devel-opment [31].

Rarely, mucocele can extend to the pituitary fossa, parasellar and supra-sellar regions, nasopharynx, orbits, clivus, or ethmoid air cells [31] . Head-ache frequently is present and can be severe. Visual impairment resulting from direct nerve compression and ocular palsies can occur. Exophthalmos is common, present in approximately half of patients [3]. Hypopituitarism is less common, but hyperprolactinemia is described [32].

Because of its high protein content, the most characteristic mucocele appearance on MRI is a mass with a homogeneously hyperintense T_1 signal [30]. Contrast enhancement usually is absent or there may be a thin peripheral rim (Fig. 3). Erosion of the walls of the sphenoid bone occasionally may be present [3,30]. Transsphenoidal surgery offers excellent prognosis.

Langerhans' cell histiocytosis

Langerhans' cell histiocytosis or class I histiocytosis is a rare disease that affects the reticuloendothelial tissue [33] and is characterized by aberrant proliferation of specific dendritic cells, called Langerhans' cells, belonging to the monocyte-macrophage system; these cells can infiltrate and destroy many sites, such as bone, lung, skin, hypothalamic-pituitary axis, and, less frequently, liver, spleen, and lymph nodes [34]. The pathogenesis still is unclear, but some investigators have demonstrated clonal proliferation, suggesting a neoplasic disorder. Immunohistochemical features, such as S-100 protein, a CD1a antigen, are characteristic of Langerhans' cells [35]. The incidence is 3 to 4 cases per million per year in children younger than 15 years old and with prevalence 2 times more frequent in men than in women [33]. Only 30% of the cases reported are in adults [34]. Diabetes insipidus is a common symptom and the most prevalent endocrinopathy in these patients, occurring in 10% to 50% of cases; it nearly always occurs concomitant to or after other manifestations of this disease, but it can be the first or an isolated symptom [33,34,36]. In childhood, Langerhans' cells histiocytosis is the second most common cause of diabetes; this diagnosis needs to be sought actively in childhood-onset diabetes insipidus [37]. Anterior pituitary dysfunction is less frequent [38]. On MRI, pituitary stalk thickening (>3.5 mm) and the absence of the hyperintense signal of the normal posterior pituitary gland (bright spot) are the most common findings. An isolated hypothalamic lesion can be present [37,38]. Pituitary stalk biopsy is not recommended routinely in lesions smaller than 7 mm because of the risks [37]. The diagnosis may be based on the symptoms, imaging techniques, and surgical biopsy of other involved sites. There are reports

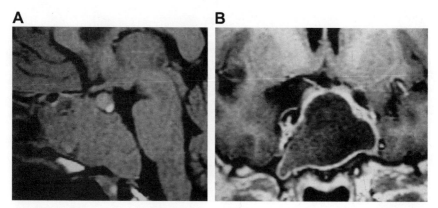

Fig. 3. Mucocele: sagittal T_1-weighted MRI (*A*) and contrast-enhanced coronal T_1-weighted MRI (*B*) depicting a thin peripheral and regular rim.

of spontaneous resolution of Langerhans' cell histiocytosis; therefore, simple observation can be reasonable. Radiotherapy may be useful in some cases of diabetes insipidus and to control mass growth. High doses of corticosteroids and chemotherapic agents, such as vincristina, vinblastina, etoposide, and cyclosporine, can yield partial response or decrease the progression of disease. Surgery is limited to lesions with rapid progression and compression of neural structures.

Hypophysitis

Primary hypophysitis is an unusual disorder characterized by focal or diffuse inflammatory infiltration and varying degrees of pituitary gland destruction [39]. The natural history still is not understood completely, and the incidence of this disease is unknown. The number of published case reports recently has increased, probably because of the widespread use of MRI and transsphenoidal surgical biopsies [40].

Clinically, primary inflammatory hypophysitis is classified into three types: lymphocytic hypophysitis, granulomatous hypophysitis, and xanthomatous hypophysitis [40].

Lymphocytic hypophysitis, often referred to as autoimmune hypophysitis, is an inflammatory disorder and the most common among the primary cases of hypophysitis (Fig. 4) [40,41]. This type may be subclassified into three types: lymphocytic adenohypophysitis, lymphocytic infundibuloneurohypophysitis, and lymphocytic panhypophysitis. Histologic assessment shows adenohypophyseal and neutohypophyseal infiltration by lymphocytes and fibrosis [40]. In granulomatous hypophysitis, the pituitary presents diffuse collections of multinucleated giant cells, histiocytes, lymphocytes, and plasma cells [42]. As granulomatous hypophysitis and autoimmune hypophysitis can occur together, some investigators suggest that the two disorders represent a spectrum of autoimmune manifestation [40].

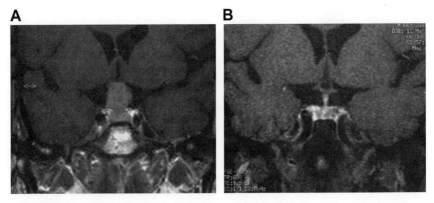

Fig. 4. Contrast-enhanced coronal T_1-weighted MRI from a male patient who had lymphocytic hypophysitis (*A*) shows almost complete shrinkage of mass after high glucocorticoid dose (*B*).

Xanthomatous hypophysitis is rare. Cystic-like areas of liquefaction, infiltrated by lipid-rich foamy histiocytes and lymphocytes, are present in the pituitary gland. Xanthomatous hypophysitis can be considered an inflammatory response to ruptured cysts components [43]. Necrotizing hypophysitis is a rare entity, having been demonstrated histologically only in two patients. The pituitary is destroyed by diffuse necrosis with lymphocytes, plasma cells, and eosinophile infiltration [40].

Clinical presentation is variable and can be similar to symptoms observed in clinically nonfunctioning pituitary adenoma. Therefore, visual impairment and severe headache due to expanding lesion are the most common and usually the initial complaints [39,40].

Ophthalmologic disturbances include visual field impairment and decreased acuity secondary to compression of the optic chiasm by suprasellar mass expansion. Parasellar expansion is less frequent, leading to paresis or palsy of the III, IV, and VI cranial nerves [42]. Partial or complete hypopituitarism may present initially as corticotropin deficiency, followed by thyrotropin, gonadotropins, growth hormone, and prolactin [40,41]. The primary inflammatory hypophysitis with involvement of posterior pituitary and infundibular stem is present with diabetes insipidus [44]. In contrast to other cases of hypophysitis, lymphocytic adenohypophysitis is strikingly associated with pregnancy, for unknown reasons [41]. Pituitary apoplexy in patients who have lymphocytic hypophysitis is described in the literature [45].

MRI often shows symmetric enlargement of the pituitary gland with homogeneous contrast enhancement. Thickened infundibular stalk and loss of the hyperintense bright spot signal of the posterior pituitary often are seen [39,40,46]. The definitive diagnosis is obtained only by microscopic examination of the pituitary tissue.

High doses of corticosteroids are described to elicit response (see Fig. 4), but when the dose is tapered, the risk for recurrence is high. Transsphenoidal surgery may be indicated in cases of mass effect or corticosteroids therapy failure [39,41]. Successful stereotactic radiotherapy in two resistant cases was published [47].

Infectious lesions

Pituitary abscess

Pituitary abscesses are a rare but potentially life-threatening disease comprising less than 1% of all pituitary diseases and 0.27% of pituitary surgeries. Primary abscesses comprise two thirds of the cases and occur in a previously normal pituitary, whereas secondary abscesses arise in an already compromised pituitary gland (adenoma or Rathke's cleft cyst). Clinical manifestations are nonspecific and diabetes insipidus appears in half of the patients [48,49].

Fever and leukocytosis are seen in only one third of cases, and predisposing factors, such as sinusitis, cavernous sinus thrombophlebitis, or pituitary surgery, usually are absent [50,51]. The most common clinical feature is headache, followed by visual complaints and hypopituitarism.

On MRI, a round sellar cystic lesion, hypo- or isointense on T_1 precontrast imaging and hyper- or isointense on T_2 imaging with peripheral gadolinium enhancement, is compatible with pituitary abscess.

Diagnosis usually is made during surgical exploration when pus is found in a cystic lesion. Culture of the abscess material identifies pathogens in only one half of the cases. The most common pathogens are gram-positive bacteria, but gram-negative bacteria, anaerobic bacteria, and fungus also can be found. The source of infection can be hematogenous spread or contiguous infection, although the infection source cannot be identified in all cases. Mortality can reach 30% to 50% of cases when it is complicated by meningitis.

Treatment consists of surgical drainage and antibiotic administration for 2 to 6 weeks. Transsphenoidal approach avoids cerebral contamination and for this reason is the preferred approach. Surgical drainage and antibiotics diminish mortality to less than 10% [52].

Tuberculosis

Intracranial tuberculosis accounted for 30% to 50% of intracranial lesions before the arrival of antibiotic therapy; however, nowadays, it accounts for 0.15% to 4% of the cases. Pituitary tuberculomas are rare. Most patients have other signs of active tuberculosis, but this not always is true. Patients are affected at any age and there is female predominance. Visual loss and headache are the most common symptoms.

MRI shows thickening of pituitary stalk in some cases. Biopsy shows caseating necrosis, and specific antibiotic therapy is mandatory [53].

Other infections

Fungal infections (aspergillosis and coccidiomycosis) [54], cysticercosis [55], and neurosyphilis [56] are rare.

Vascular lesions

Intrasellar aneurysms

Intrasellar aneurysm can mimic pituitary adenoma and imaging techniques are essential for distinguishing between the two disorders before surgery. Intense homogeneous blush on CT images with contrast suggests an aneurysm [3]. On conventional spin-echo MRI, the aneurysm appears black because of flow void, has well-defined margins, and is contiguous to vessel [57].

There are different surgical approaches to the intrasellar aneurysm, such as endovascular coiling.

Pituitary apoplexy

Pituitary apoplexy is a life-threatening condition caused by infarction or hemorrhage into a growing pituitary adenoma [58,59].

Pituitary apoplexy usually occurs in macroadenomas of any histologic subtype [60] and rarely is described in the normal pituitary gland, craniopharyngiomas, or lymphocytic hypophysitis [45,59].

Precipitating factors [60] may include reduced pituitary blood flow (hypotension or hemodialysis, angiography, or spinal anesthesia resulting from decreased intracranial pressure) or radiotherapy resulting from vascular damage. Myocardial infarction, anticoagulants, infection, stimulation of pituitary gland as happens in increased estrogen milieu, dynamic testing using gonadotropin-releasing hormone or thyrotropin-releasing hormone, and the use of bromocriptine all are implicated [58,60]. There is no evidence that hypertension and diabetes are more prevalent in patients who have pituitary apoplexy.

Clinical presentation is variable and sometimes apoplexy is asymptomatic [58]. Headache is the most prevalent complaint (76% to 87%); visual deficits are present in 56% to 62% of cases, ocular palsies in 40% to 45% [45,59], and diabetes insipidus in 8% [60]. Pituitary hypersecretion can be "cured" [61,62].

CT is the most important tool in the acute setting (24–48 hours), after contrast administration showing a high-intensity or heterogeneous gland with or without evidence of subarachnoid hemorrhage [63]. On a recent MRI, pituitary hemorrhage appears hypointense in T_1- and T_2-weighted images, but after a week, high signal intensity is evident on T_1-weighted images [64].

Medical treatment with stress doses of glucocorticoids is mandatory [58]. Patients presenting with visual loss or consciousness impairment must be operated on immediately, with better results achieved when the surgery is done fewer than 7 days after the complaints started. In some cases, patients can be managed conservatively with corticosteroids and close clinical and imaging observation [65].

Miscellaneous

Arachnoid cyst

A true intrasellar arachnoid cyst is rare. It is believed to arise from an arachnoid herniation into the pituitary fossa as a result of incompetence of the diaphragma sellae after trauma or as a result of an adhesive arachnoiditis secondary to infection. On MRI, signal intensity is similar to cerebrospinal fluid and contrast enhancement of the cyst wall usually is not found [2–4].

Pathologic pituitary hyperplasia

Physiologic enlargement of the pituitary may be observed during puberty and pregnancy. Primary hypothyroidism can cause pituitary hyperplasia, reverted with levothyroxine replacement. In patients who have symmetric pituitary enlargement and hypothyroidism, finding of high thyrotropin establishes the diagnosis. Growth hormone–releasing hormone and

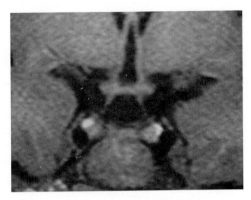

Fig. 5. Coronal T$_1$-weighted MRI shows double anterior and posterior pituitary gland with duplication of pituitary stalk.

corticotropin-releasing hormone neoplasias also are causes of pituitary hyperplasia [3].

Double pituitary

Duplication of the pituitary is rare and few cases are reported in the literature. Its pathogenesis is considered to result from notochordal anomaly and can be associated with other malformations, such as absence of corpus callosum and of midline commissures in both cerebral hemispheres, frequently being incompatible with life [66]. Double pituitary may occur, however, as an isolated anomaly and without symptoms, as just an incidental finding (Fig. 5) [67].

Acknowledgments

The authors would like to thank Drs. Luiz Roberto Salgado, Sergio Koidara, Aldo Stamm, Jozélio Freire Carvalho, and Diego Rodrigo Hermann for kindly providing some magnetic resonance images.

References

[1] Huang BY, Castilo M. Nonadenomatous tumors of the pituitary and sella turcica. Top Magn Reson Imaging 2005;16(4):289–99.

[2] Post KD, McCormick PC, Bello JA. Differential diagnosis of pituitary tumors. Endocrinol Metab Clin North Am 1987;16(3):609–45.

[3] Freda PU, Post KD. Differential diagnosis of sellar masses. Endocrinol Metab Clin North Am 1999;28(1):81–117.

[4] Iqbal J, Kanaan I, Al Homsi M. Non-neoplastic cystic lesions of the sellar region: presentation, diagnosis and management of eight cases and review of the literature. Acta Neurochir (Wien) 1999;141:389–98.

[5] Thodou E, Kontogeorgos G, Scheithauer BW, et al. Intrasellar chordomas mimicking pituitary adenoma. J Neurosurg 2000;92:976–82.

[6] Thorner MO, Vance ML, Laws ER Jr, et al. The anterior pituitary. In: Wilson JD, Foster DA, Kronenberg HM, editors. Williams textbook of endocrinology. 9th edition. Philadelphia: WB Saunders; 1998. p. 249–340.

[7] Muzumdar D, Goel A, Desai K, et al. Mature teratoma arising from the sella-case report. Neurol Med Chir (Tokyo) 2001;41:356–9.

[8] Guermazi A, Lafitte F, Miaux Y, et al. The dural tail sign-beyond meningioma. Clin Radiol 2005;60:171–88.

[9] Goldsmith B, Mc Dermott MW. Meningioma. Neurosurg Clin N Am 2006;17(2):111–20.

[10] Jauraus CD, Tarbell NJ. Optic pathways gliomas. Pediatr Blood Cancer 2006;46(5):586–96.

[11] Mukhida K, Asa A, Gentili F, et al. Ependymoma of the pituitary fossa. Case report and review of the literature. J Neurosurg 2006;105:616–20.

[12] Kowalski RJ, Pravson RA, Mayberg MR. Pituicytoma. Ann Diagn Pathol 2004;8(5):290–4.

[13] Shah B, Lipper MH, Laws ER, et al. Posterior pituitary astrocytoma: a rare tumor of the neurohypophysis: a case report. AJNR Am J Neuroradiol 2005;26:1858–61.

[14] Ogilvie CM, Payne S, Evansosn J, et al. Lymphoma metastasizing to the pituitary: an unusual presentation of a treatable disease. Pituitary 2005;8:139–46.

[15] Giustina A, Gola M, Doga M, et al. Primary lymphoma of the pituitary: an emerging clinical entity. J Clin Endocrinol Metab 2001;86:4567–75.

[16] Komminos J, Vlassopoulo V, Protopapa D, et al. Tumors metastatic to the pituitary gland: case report and literature review. J Clin Endocrinol Metab 2004;89(2):574–80.

[17] Honegger J, Koerbel A, Psaras T, et al. Primary intrasellar schwanomma: clinical, aetiopathological and surgical considerations. Br J Neurosurg 2005;19(5):432–8.

[18] Rousseau A, Bernier M, Kujas M, et al. Primary intracranial melanocytic tumor simulating pituitary macroadenoma: case report and review of the literature. Neurosurgery 2005;57: E369.

[19] Allan CA, Kaltas G, Evanson J, et al. Pituitary chondrosarcoma: an unusual cause of a sellar mass presenting as pituitary adenoma. J Clin Endocrinol Metab 2001;86(1):386–91.

[20] Sinnott BP, Hatipoglu B, Sarne DH. Intrasellar plasmacytoma presenting as non-functional invasive pituitary macroadenoma: case report & literature review. Pituitary 2006;9:65–72.

[21] Tabuena RP, Nagai S, Handa T, et al. Diabetes insipidus from neurosarcoidosis: long-term follow-up for more than eight years. Intern Med 2004;43(10):960–6.

[22] Crystal RG. Sarcoidosis. In: Braunwald E, Fauci AS, Kasper DL, et al, editors. Harrinson's principles of internal medicine. International textbook of medicine. vol. 2. 15th edition. New York: The McGraw Hill Companies; 2001. p. 1969–79.

[23] Loh KC, Green A, Dillon WP Jr, et al. Diabetes insipidus from sarcoidosis confined to the posterior pituitary. Eur J Endocrinol 1997;137:514–9.

[24] Oksanen V. Neurosarcoidosis: clinical presentation and course in 50 patients. Acta Neurol Scand 1986;73:283–90.

[25] Takano K. Sarcoidosis of hypothalamus and pituitary. Intern Med 2004;43(10):894–5.

[26] Murphy JM, Gomez-Anson B, Gillard JH, et al. Wegener granulomatosis: MR imaging findings in brain and meninges. Radiology 1999;213:794–9.

[27] Jianling T, Yi D. Pituitary involvement in Wegener's granulomatosis: a case report and review of the literature. Chin Med J 2003;116(11):1785–8.

[28] Tappouni R, Burns A. Pituitary involvement in Wegener's granulomatosis. Nephrol Dial Transplant 2000;15:2057–8.

[29] Goyal M, Kucharczyk W, Keystone E. Granulomatosis hypophysitis due to Wegener's granulomatosis. AJNR Am J Neuroradiol 2000;21:1466–9.

[30] Bonneville F, Cattin F, Marsot-Dupuch K, et al. T_1 signal hyperintensity in the sellar region: spectrum of findings. Radiographics 2006;26:93–113.

[31] Iqbal J, Kanaan I, Ahmed M, et al. Neurosurgical aspects of sphenoidal sinus mucocele. Br J Neurosurg 1998;12(6):527–30.

[32] Fody EP, Binet EF. Sphenoid mucocele causing hyperprolactinemia: radiologic/pathologic correlation. South Med J 1986;79(8):1017–21.

[33] Horn E, Coons SW, Spetzler RF, et al. Isolated Langerhans cell histiocytosis of the infundibulum presenting with fulminant diabetes insipidus. Childs Nerv Syst 2006;22: 542–4.

[34] Kaltsas GA, Powles TB, Evanson J, et al. Hypothalamo-pituitary abnormalities in adult patients with Langerhans cells Histiocytosis: clinical, endocrinological, and radiological features and response to treatment. J Clin Endocrinol Metab 2000;85:1370–6.

[35] Scolazzi P, Lombardi T, Monnier P, et al. Multisystemim Langerhans' cell histiocytosis (Hand-Schüller-Christian disease) in an adult: a case report and review of the literature. Eur Arch Otorhinolaryngol 2004;261:326–30.

[36] Grois N, Prayer D, Prosch H, et al. Course and clinical impact of magnetic resonance imaging findings in diabetes insipidus associated with Langerhans cell histiocytosis. Pediatr Blood Cancer 2004;43:59–65.

[37] Prosch H, Grois N, Bökkerink J, et al. Central diabetes insipidus: is it Langerhans cell histiocytosis of the pituitary stalk? A diagnostic pitfall. Pediatr Blood Cancer 2006;46(3): 363–6.

[38] Halefoglu AM. Magnetic resonance imaging of thickened pituitary stalk proceeding to Langerhans cell histiocytosis in a child. Australas Radiol 2006;50:175–8.

[39] Leung GKK, Lopes MBS, Thorner MO, et al. Infundibulohypophisitis in a man presenting with diabetes insipidus and a cavernous sinus involvement. J Neurol Neurosurg Psychiatry 2001;71:798–801.

[40] Caturegli P, Newschaffer C, Olivi A, et al. Autoimmune hypophysitis. Endocr Rev 2005; 26(5):599–614.

[41] Breen TL, Post KD, Wardlaw SL. Lymphocytic hypophysitis. Endocrinologist 2004;14(1): 13–8.

[42] Arsava EM, Uluç K, Kansu T, et al. Granulomatous hypophysitis and bilateral optic neuropathy. J Neuroophthalmol 2001;21(1):34–6.

[43] Paulus W, Honegger J, Keyvani K, et al. Xanthogranuloma of the sellar region: a clinicopathological entity different from adamantinomatous craniopharyngioma. Acta Neuropathol (Berl) 1999;97:371–82.

[44] Tubridy N, Saunders D, Thom M, et al. Infundibulohypophisitis in a man presenting with diabetes insipidus and cavernous sinus involvement. J Neurol Neurosurg Psychiatry 2001;71: 798–801.

[45] Lee MS, Pless M. Apopletic lymphocytic hypophysitis. J Neurosurg 2003;98:183–5.

[46] Cheung CC, Ezzat S, Smyth HS, et al. The spectrum and significance of primary hypophysitis. J Clin Endocrinol Metab 2001;86:1048–59.

[47] Selch MT, DeSalles AAF, Kelly DF, et al. Sterotactic radiotherapy for treatment of lymphocytic hypophysitis. J Neurosurg 2003;99:591–6.

[48] Wolandsky LJ, Gallagher JD, Heary RF, et al. MRI of pituitary abscess: two cases and review of literature. J Neuroradiol 1997;39:499–503.

[49] Blackett PR, Bailey JD, Hoffman HJ. A pituitary abscess simulating an intrasellar tumor. Surg Neurol 1980;14:129–31.

[50] Grosskopf D, Chamouard JM, Bosquet F, et al. Pituitary abscess: a study of a case and review of the literature. Neurochirurgie 1987;33:228–31.

[51] Guigui J, Boukobza M, Tamer I, et al. Case report: MRI and CT in a case of pituitary abscess. Clin Radiol 1998;53:777–9.

[52] Yen-Hao S, Chen Y, Sheng-Hong T. Pituitary abscess. J Clin Neurosci 2006;13:1038–41.

[53] Sharma MC, Arora R, Mahapatra AK, et al. Intrasellar tuberculoma—an enigmatic pituitary infection: a series of 18 cases. Clin Neurol Neurosurg 2000;102:72–7.

[54] Scanarini M, Rotilio A, Rigobello L, et al. Primary intrasellar coccidioidomycosis simulating a pituitary adenoma. Neurosurgery 1991;28(5):748–51.

[55] Brutto OH, Guevara J Sotelo J. Intrasellar cysticercosis. J Neurosurg 1988;69:58–60.

[56] Benzick AE, Wirthwein DP, Weinberg A, et al. Pituitary gland gumma in congenital syphilis after failed maternal treatment: a case report. Pediatrics 1999;104:e4.

[57] Johnsen DE, Woodruff WW, Allen IS, et al. MR imaging of the sellar and juxtasellar regions. Radiographics 1991;11:727–58.

[58] Rolih CA, Ober KP. Pituitary apoplexy. Endocrinol Metab Clin North Am 1993;22: 291–302.

[59] Semple PL, Webb MK, Villiers JC, et al. Pituitary apoplexy. Neurosurgery 2005;56:65–73.

[60] Biousse V, Newman NJ, Oyesiku NM. Precipitating factors in pituitary apoplexy. J Neurol Neurosurg Psychiatry 2001;71:542–5.

[61] Findling JW, Tyrrell JB, Aron DC, et al. Silent pituitary apoplexy: subclinical infarction of an adrenocorticotropin-producing pituitary adenoma. J Clin Endocrinol Metab 1981;52: 95–7.

[62] Kulah A, Erel C, Memis M, et al. Arrested puberty associated with apoplectic prolactinoma in a male adolescent. Childs Nerv Syst 1995;11:124–7.

[63] Fujimoto M, Yoshino E, Uegushi T, et al. Fluid blood density level demonstrated by CT in pituitary apoplexy: report of two cases. J Neurosurg 1981;55(1):143–4.

[64] L'Huillier F, Combes C, Martin N, et al. MRI in the diagnosis of so-called pituitary apoplexy: seven cases. J Neuroradiol 1989;16(3):221–37.

[65] Maccagnan P, Macedo CLD, Kayath MJ, et al. Conservative management of pituitary apoplexy: a prospective study. J Clin Endocrinol Metab 1995;80:2190–7.

[66] Hori A, Schimidt D, Kuebber S. Immunohistochemical survey of migration of human anterior pituitary cells in development, pathological, and clinical aspects: a review. Microsc Res Tech 1999;46(1):59–68.

[67] Bagherian V, Graham M, Gerson LP, et al. Double pituitary glands with partial duplication of facial and fore brain structures with hydrocephalus. Comput Radiol 1984;8(4):203–10.

ELSEVIER
SAUNDERS

Endocrinol Metab Clin N Am
37 (2008) 213–234

ENDOCRINOLOGY
AND METABOLISM
CLINICS
OF NORTH AMERICA

Disorders of Water and Salt Metabolism Associated with Pituitary Disease

Jennifer A. Loh, MD, Joseph G. Verbalis, MD*

*Georgetown University Hospital, Endocrinology Division, 232 Building D,
4000 Reservoir Road, Washington, DC 20037, USA*

Disorders of water and sodium homeostasis are very common problems encountered in clinical medicine. Disorders of water metabolism are divided into hyperosmolar and hypoosmolar states, with hyperosmolar disorders characterized by a deficit of body water in relation to body solute, and hypoosmolar disorders characterized by an excess of body water in relation to total body solute. Because sodium is the main constituent of plasma osmolality, these disorders are typically characterized by hypernatremia and hyponatremia, respectively. Hyponatremia is far more common, occurring at prevalences as high as 6% to 22% of hospitalized patients [1], and has been associated with mortality rates from 0% to 50%, depending on the acuteness and severity of the hyponatremia. Hypernatremia has a prevalence of only 1% of hospitalized patients, but is associated with high mortality rates, from 42% to 60% [2].

In the setting of intrasellar and suprasellar lesions, excessive water loss from diabetes insipidus is more likely than inappropriate water retention from the syndrome of inappropriate antidiuretic hormone secretion (SIADH), although both can occur following surgical resection of these lesions. This article briefly reviews the physiology of hyperosmolar and hypoosmolar syndromes, then focuses on a discussion of the pathophysiology, evaluation, and treatment of specific pre- and postoperative disorders of water metabolism in patients with pituitary lesions.

Overview of normal water metabolism

Water metabolism is controlled primarily by arginine vasopressin (AVP), a nonapeptide that is synthesized in the neurohypophyseal magnocellular

---

* Corresponding author.
E-mail address: verbalis@georgetown.edu (J.G. Verbalis).

0889-8529/08/$ - see front matter © 2008 Elsevier Inc. All rights reserved.
doi:10.1016/j.ecl.2007.10.008   *endo.theclinics.com*

neurons of the supraoptic and paraventricular nuclei of the hypothalamus. The newly synthesized AVP prohormone is packaged into neurosecretory granules and then transported down the supraopticohypophyseal tract to the posterior pituitary, during which it is enzymatically cleaved into AVP, neurophysin, and a C-terminal glycopeptide. When release is stimulated, circulating AVP binds to AVP V2 receptors in the collecting duct of the kidney, activating a cyclic AMP-mediated signal transduction pathway that stimulates insertion of aquaporin-2 (AQP2) water channels into the apical membrane of the collecting duct epithelial cells. The AQP2 channels render the collecting duct permeable to water, which facilitates passive reabsorption of water along osmotic gradients. This reabsorption of water, or antidiuresis, is dependent on the presence of interstitial hyperosmolality in the inner medulla of the kidney established by the countercurrent multiplier mechanism [3].

Secretion of AVP is stimulated by osmotic and nonosmotic factors, with changes in plasma osmolality serving as the primary stimulus for AVP release. Osmoreceptors located in the anterior hypothalamus are exquisitely sensitive to even small increases in plasma osmolality. There is a discrete osmotic threshold for AVP secretion, which usually occurs when plasma osmolality reaches 282 milliosmole (mOsm)/kg H_2O to 285 mOsm/kg H_2O, above which a linear relationship between plasma osmolality and AVP levels occurs. In general, each 1 mOsm/kg H_2O increase in plasma osmolality causes an increase in plasma AVP levels from 0.4 picogram (pg)/mL to 0.8 pg/mL, with a corresponding renal concentrating response [4]. Thus, changes of 1% or less in plasma osmolality will trigger an increase in plasma AVP levels and urine osmolality.

Baroreceptors located in the carotid arteries and aortic arch also stimulate AVP release in response to decreases in blood volume and arterial pressure. The resulting urinary concentration and renal water conservation is an appropriate physiologic response to the volume depletion. However, AVP secretion is much less sensitive to small changes in blood pressure and volume than to changes in osmolality [5]. As a result, modest changes in blood volume and pressure are relatively weak stimuli for AVP release.

AVP secretion is also influenced by multiple other factors. Many of these can stimulate AVP release, including nausea, pain, medications, angiotensin II, histamine, dopamine, bradykinin, and acetylcholine. Many others can inhibit AVP release, including nitric oxide, atrial natriuretic peptide, and opioids [6,7]. Because AVP secretion is influenced by many different factors, any defects in the normal regulation of AVP secretion can lead to problems with either water conservation or water excretion.

Hyperosmolality and hypernatremia

Hyperosmolality indicates a deficiency of water relative to solute in the extracellular fluid. Because water moves freely between the extracellular

(ECF) and intracellular (ICF) fluid, this also indicates a deficiency of total body water relative to total body solute. In evaluating hypernatremia, it is helpful to classify it broadly by etiology: hypervolemic, inadequate water intake, and increased free water losses.

Hypervolemic hypernatremia

Hypervolemic hypernatremia is caused by an excess of body sodium with normal or expanded body water. Although uncommon, it can occur in the postoperative or hospital setting from the infusion of hypertonic fluids or from enteral feedings without adequate free water administration [8]. More rarely, cases of true sodium chloride (NaCl) intoxication have been reported [9].

Inadequate fluid intake

Hypernatremia from inadequate fluid intake is usually seen in the hospital or postoperative setting in patients who have an intact thirst mechanism, but are unable to obtain or ingest fluids. This usually occurs when the patient has a depressed sensorium because of illness or medications, or during recovery from anesthesia in the postoperative setting. Less commonly, inadequate fluid intake can be caused by defects in the thirst mechanism resulting from surgical damage to the anterior hypothalamus, causing hypodipsia [10].

Increased water losses

Hypernatremia from increased water losses occurs commonly, with hyperglycemia and resultant glucosuria being the most common etiology. Other forms of solute diuresis, gastrointestinal water losses, intrinsic renal disease, hypercalcemia, and hypokalemia can all cause increased free water losses. When not a result of any of these causes, excessive free water loss is usually caused by a deficiency of AVP secretion or impaired AVP effects in the kidney [11].

Diabetes insipidus

Diabetes insipidus (DI) is the most well-known manifestation of a deficiency in AVP secretion or abnormal renal response to AVP. Central DI is caused by a variety of acquired or congenital anatomic lesions that disrupt the hypothalamic-posterior pituitary axis, and include some types of tumors, trauma, hemorrhage, thrombosis, infarction, granulomatous disease, and pituitary surgery. It is unusual for pituitary adenomas to present with DI. This is because synthesis of AVP occurs in the supraoptic and paraventricular nuclei of the hypothalamus, rather than in the posterior pituitary. Even large intrasellar masses usually grow slowly over long periods of time, and this allows an adaptation of neurohypophyseal function to occur. In such cases, the site of AVP release shifts from the posterior pituitary to the median eminence, which sometimes can be detected by an upward migration of the posterior bright spot by MRI [12].

Incidence

DI complicates the postoperative course in as many as 30% of patients undergoing pituitary surgery, although the disease is transient and relatively benign in the majority of cases [13]. Chronic postoperative DI has been reported in from 0.5% to 15% in neurosurgic reviews. It is relatively uncommon because experimental studies have shown that more than 90% of the magnocellular AVP neurons in the supraoptic and paraventricular nuclei must degenerate bilaterally before permanent DI occurs [14].

Diagnosis

The diagnosis of DI should be considered when a neurosurgical patient excretes large volumes of dilute urine in the postoperative period, typically more than 2.5 mL/kg body weight to 3.0 mL/kg body weight per hour. When such postoperative polyuria is noted, it is important to consider several other potential clinical scenarios before a diagnosis of DI is concluded. First, patients who undergo surgery in the suprasellar region very frequently receive stress doses of glucocorticoids to prevent secondary adrenal insufficiency. In cases where steroid-induced insulin resistance produces hyperglycemia, the resulting osmotic diuresis from glucosuria can be confused with DI. Therefore, urine and blood glucose should be measured and any elevated glucose levels brought under control to eliminate an osmotic diuresis as a cause of the polyuria. Second, excess fluids are sometimes administered intravenously during the perioperative period, which are then excreted appropriately postoperatively. If this large postoperative diuresis is matched with continued intravenous fluid infusions, an incorrect diagnosis of DI may be made based on the resulting hypotonic polyuria. Therefore, if the serum [Na^+] is not elevated concomitantly with the polyuria, the rate of parenterally administered fluid should be slowed with careful monitoring of the serum [Na^+] and urine output until a diagnosis of DI can be confirmed by continued hypotonic polyuria in the presence of hypernatremia or hyperosmolality [15].

The diagnosis of DI in the postoperative setting is made based on both clinical and biochemical data. Patients characteristically complain of an abrupt onset of polyuria and polydipsia, which typically is manifest in the first 24 to 48 hours following neurosurgery. This precipitous onset reflects the fact that patients are able to maintain urinary concentration fairly well until the number of AVP-producing neurons in the hypothalamus decreases to 10% to 15% of normal, after which plasma AVP levels decrease to the range where urine output increases dramatically [14]. Patients with DI often describe a craving for ice-cold water, which better quenches osmotically-stimulated thirst [16]. Urine studies should reveal a hypotonic (ie, dilute) urine, with specific gravity less than 1.005 or urine osmolality greater than 200 mOsm/kg H_2O. Urine output is often voluminous, ranging from 4 to18 liters per day [17]. Serum hyperosmolality and hypernatremia also strongly support the diagnosis of DI. However, most patients with DI generally have intact thirst mechanisms; therefore, as long as they are allowed free access to oral fluids, they usually do not present with either hyperosmolality or hypernatremia. Consequently, it is often necessary to limit fluid intake until either hyperosmolality or hypernatremia develop in order to confirm a diagnosis of DI. Diagnostic criteria for a diagnosis of DI are summarized in Box 1.

MRI has been explored as a diagnostic tool for DI, as a bright spot in the sella can be visualized on T1-weighted images when stored vasopressin and oxytocin are present in neurosecretory granules of the posterior pituitary. Absence of this bright spot is characteristic of DI, [18] although a persistence of the bright spot has been reported in patients with clinical evidence of DI [19]. This does not exclude a diagnosis of DI, and can be explained by the presence of the bright spot early in the disease process, when partial DI is more likely to be present, with subsequent disappearance as the severity of DI progresses. Alternatively, the presence of oxytocin in the pituitary may be responsible for some cases of DI despite a normal bright spot. Additionally, while many small studies have reported the presence of a bright spot in all normal subjects, larger studies have noted the absence of the bright spot in some clinically normal patients, particularly with increasing age [20]. Thus, neither the absence nor the presence of a posterior pituitary bright spot is diagnostic of DI or its absence.

Box 1. Diagnosis of postoperative diabetes insipidus

Rule out osmotic diuresis or fluid overload
Clinical signs and symptoms
- Polyuria, high volumes (4 L/day–18 L/day), with abrupt onset, typically within 24–48 hours postoperatively
- Polydipsia, with craving for cold fluids
- With/without hypovolemia, depending on whether the patient has an intact thirst mechanism

Laboratory data
- Dilute urine (specific gravity less than1.005, urine osmolality less than 200 mOsm/kg H_2O)
- Normal to increased serum osmolality
- Serum $[Na^+]$ greater or equal to 145 milliequivalent/L with continued diuresis of hypotonic urine

Postoperative clinical course

The postoperative course of DI can be transient, permanent, or triphasic, as described in classic studies of pituitary stalk transection [21]. Transient DI almost always begins within 24 to 48 hours of surgery and usually abates within several days. Both transient DI and the first phase of the triphasic pattern are thought to be caused by temporary dysfunction of AVP-producing neurons, secondary to severing of the neuronal connections between the magnocellular cell bodies and the nerve terminals in the posterior pituitary, or axonal shock from perturbations in the vascular supply to the pituitary stalk and posterior pituitary. Transient DI usually resolves as the vasopressinergic neurons regain full function. Less commonly, persistent DI may follow as preformed stores of AVP are depleted and no additional AVP is synthesized. Previous studies showed that the major determinant of permanent DI, following pituitary stalk sectioning, was related to the level of the lesion: the closer the lesion to the magnocellular cell bodies in the hypothalamus, the more likely that the hypothalamic cell bodies will degenerate, resulting in permanent DI. In a series of 24 patients receiving a low pituitary stalk section at the level of the diaphragm sella, only 62% developed permanent DI [22], compared to an incidence of 80% to 100% with higher stalk injury [23].

In the triphasic pattern, the first phase of DI typically lasts 5 to 7 days, and then transitions into a second antidiuretic phase of SIADH (Fig. 1A). The second phase of the triphasic response is caused by the uncontrolled release of AVP from degenerating posterior pituitary tissue, or from the remaining magnocellular neurons whose axons have been severed [14,21]. In this phase, the urine quickly becomes concentrated in response to the elevated plasma AVP levels and urine output markedly decreases. Continued administration of excess water during this period can quickly lead to hyponatremia and hypoosmolality. The duration of the second phase is highly variable, and can last from 2 to 14 days [14]. After the AVP stores are depleted from the degenerating posterior pituitary, the third phase of chronic DI then typically ensues, although not always [24]. In this phase, there are insufficient remaining AVP neurons capable of synthesizing additional AVP, thereby resulting in permanent DI.

Treatment

Treatment of postoperative DI is summarized in Box 2, and should be individualized to each patient. Optimally, patients should be monitored in an expectant fashion for the development of polyuria or hypoosmolality. Fluid intake and output should be carefully recorded, and patients questioned regarding symptoms of thirst. Once a diagnosis of DI has been verified as described above, antidiuretic hormone therapy should be initiated. Because of the alternative reasons for a postoperative diuresis discussed in the previous section, it is important not to begin antidiuretic therapy until the presence of

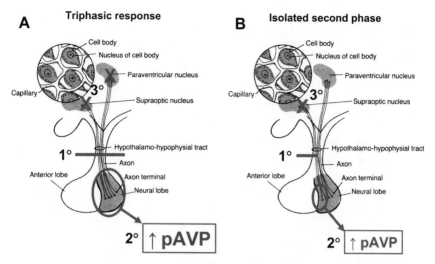

Fig. 1. Mechanisms underlying the pathophysiology of the triphasic pattern of diabetes insipidus and the isolated second phase. (*A*) In the triphasic response, the first phase of DI is initiated following a partial or complete pituitary stalk section, which severs the connections between the AVP neuronal cell bodies in the hypothalamus and the nerve terminals in the posterior pituitary gland, thus preventing stimulated AVP secretion (1°). This is followed in several days by the second phase of SIADH, which is caused by uncontrolled release of AVP into the bloodstream from the degenerating nerve terminals in the posterior pituitary (2°). After all of the AVP stored in the posterior pituitary gland has been released, the third phase of DI returns if greater than 80% to 90% of the AVP neuronal cell bodies in the hypothalamus have undergone retrograde degeneration (3°). (*B*) In the isolated second phase, the pituitary stalk is injured, but not completely cut. Although maximum AVP secretory response will be diminished as a result of the stalk injury, DI will not result if the injury leaves intact at least 10% to 20% of the nerve fibers connecting the AVP neuronal cell bodies in the hypothalamus to the nerve terminals in the posterior pituitary gland (1°). However, this is still followed in several days by the second phase of SIADH, which is caused by uncontrolled release of AVP from the degenerating nerve terminals of the posterior pituitary gland that have been injured or severed (2°). Because a smaller portion of the posterior pituitary is denervated, the magnitude of AVP released as the pituitary degenerates will be smaller and of shorter duration than with a complete triphasic response. After all of the AVP stored in the damaged part of the posterior pituitary gland has been released, the second phase ceases, but clinical DI will not occur if less than 80% to 90% of the AVP neuronal cell bodies in the hypothalamus undergo retrograde degeneration (3°).

DI is confirmed by continued hypotonic polyuria despite hyperosmolality. However, the criteria for subsequent redosing need not be as stringent, and can be based simply on the redevelopment of polyuria [14].

Desmopressin (1-deamino-8-D-arginine-vasopressin) is the drug of choice for acute and chronic treatment of central DI [25]. Postoperatively, desmopressin may be given in a dose of 1 to 2 micrograms subcutaneously, intramuscularly, or intravenously. Parenteral routes are preferable, because this obviates any concern about absorption, causes no significant pressor effects, and has the same total duration of action as the other routes. Treatment generally results in a prompt reduction in urine output and the

---

Box 2. Treatment of postoperative diabetes insipidus

Expectant monitoring
Accurate recording of fluid intake and output
Urine osmolality or specific gravity every 4 to 6 hours,
    until resolution or stabilization
Serum [Na⁺] every 4 to 6 hours, until resolution or stabilization

Antidiuretic hormone therapy
Desmopressin, initial dose of 1 μg to 2 μg intravenously
    or subcutaneously
Redose when urine output 200 mL to 250 mL per hour for greater
    than or equal to 2 hours, with urine specific gravity less than
    1.005 or urine osmolality less than 200 mOsm/kg H_2O

Maintenance of fluid balance
Allow patient to drink according to thirst
Supplement hypotonic intravenous fluids (D_5W to $D_5$1/2NSS)
    if patient is unable to maintain a normal plasma osmolality
    and serum [Na⁺] through drinking

Monitor for resolution of transient DI or triphasic response
Positive daily fluid balance greater than 2 L suggests possibility
    of inappropriate antidiuresis
Antidiuretic hormone therapy should be held and fluids restricted
    to maintain serum [Na⁺] within normal ranges

Manage anterior pituitary insufficiency
Cover with stress dose corticosteroids (hydrocortisone 100 mg
    intravenously every 8 hours, tapered to 15 mg to 30 mg by mouth
    daily) until anterior pituitary function can be fully evaluated

---

duration of antidiuresis is approximately 6 to 12 hours. It is important to follow urine osmolality and volume, and serum [Na⁺] at frequent intervals to ensure improvement in hypernatremia and to determine when redosing should occur. In order to avoid fluid retention and hyponatremia, each dose of desmopressin should be given after the recurrence of polyuria, but before the patient actually becomes hyperosmolar. In general, excretion of 200 mL to 250 mL per hour of urine with an osmolality less than 200 mOsm/kg H_2O or specific gravity less than 1.005 affirms the need for retreatment with desmopressin [16]. Dosing desmopressin on an as needed basis, rather than on a fixed schedule, also has the benefit of allowing the detection of return of endogenous AVP secretion, or the start of the second phase of a triphasic response, by a lack of return of polyuria after the effects of the previous desmopressin dose have dissipated. However, even this strategy will not always prevent the occurrence of hyponatremia during the second phase of SIADH. Consequently, it is important to follow the serum [Na$^+$] at frequent intervals in all postoperative patients.

The side effects of desmopressin are uncommon, mild, and generally dose-related. Patients occasionally experience headache, nausea, nasal congestion, flushing and abdominal cramping. Desmopressin has virtually no pressor effects because it selectively binds to the AVP V2 receptors, but not the AVP V1a receptors on vascular smooth muscle cells, thus rendering it safe in patients with coronary or hypertensive cardiovascular disease [25].

Fluid replacement is also important to manage in the setting of postoperative DI. If the patient is awake and has an intact thirst mechanism, the patient's own symptom of thirst is the best guide to water replacement. Increases in plasma osmolality of 2% to 3% triggers the sensation of thirst, which prevents significant hyperosmolality from occurring [26]. If the patient is unable to respond to thirst because of hypothalamic damage to thirst centers or because of decreased consciousness, fluid balance can be maintained by intravenous fluids. The established water deficit may be estimated using the following formula [27]:

$$\text{Water deficit} \ = \ 0.6 \times \text{premorbid weight}$$
$$\times \left[1 - 140/\left(\text{serum}\left[\text{Na}^+\right], \text{mmol/L}\right)\right]$$

where [Na$^+$] is the serum sodium concentration in mmol/L and body weight is in kilograms. However, because this formula does not take into account ongoing water losses, it is at best an estimate of fluid requirements; therefore, serum electrolytes should be measured frequently (eg, every 6 to 8 hours) to ensure that appropriate fluid replacement is occurring.

Patients with chronic DI can be treated with intranasal or oral desmopressin. The nasal spray delivers metered single doses of 0.1 mL (10 micrograms). The reliability of intranasal desmopressin can be diminished in patients with mucosal atrophy, nasal congestion, scarring, or nasal discharge; thus, in general it is advisable to wait until several days postoperatively before using intranasal desmopressin, especially in patients who have nasal packing in place. The duration of action of intranasal desmopressin generally ranges from 6 to12 hours, though occasional patients may exhibit longer responses. Consequently, most patients require twice daily dosing. Treatment should be designed to minimize polyuria and polydipsia, while avoiding hyponatremia from over-treatment. It is often useful to permit intermittent polyuric episodes every 1 to 2 weeks by delaying a dose of desmopressin, thereby verifying continued presence of DI and allowing any retained excess water to be excreted so that normal water balance is maintained.

Oral desmopressin has also been shown to be effective for treatment of central DI. Patients with chronic rhinitis or mucosal scarring may find it to be a more viable option than the intranasal spay. Oral tablets are available in 0.1 mg to 0.2 mg dosing options, with most patients requiring a 20 times higher dose than with the intranasal spray because more than 99% of the orally administered dose of desmopressin is destroyed by gastrointestinal peptidases. Most patients with central DI require on average 200 µg to 600 µg of oral desmopressin times per day to control polyuria [12]. Oral tablets should be taken on an empty stomach to maximize absorption.

Anterior pituitary function

Finally, as a practical consideration, any patient with postoperative DI, and particularly those manifesting a triphasic response, should be assumed to have anterior pituitary insufficiency and covered with corticosteroid replacement. In the postoperative setting, hydrocortisone 50 mg to 100 mg intravenously every 8 hours is generally utilized and then rapidly tapered to daily maintenance doses (15 mg–30 mg per day) until anterior pituitary function can be definitively evaluated.

Hypoosmolality and hyponatremia

Hyponatremia is the most common electrolyte disorder in hospitalized adult patients. The reported incidence of hyponatremia varies depending on the age of hospitalized patients studied, and the definition of hyponatremia used. When hyponatremia is defined as a serum $[Na^+]$ less than 135 mmol/L, incidences of 6% to 22% have been reported [1]. However, when hyponatremia is defined by more stringent criteria of serum $[Na^+]$ less than 130 mmol/L, incidences fall to 1% to 4%. This cutoff likely represents the clinically significant incidence of hyponatremia in the hospital setting, as adverse clinical events are rarely seen unless the serum sodium is less than 130 mmol/L [28,29]. Clinically, hyponatremia is generally categorized based on serum tonicity as isotonic, hypotonic, or hypertonic.

Isotonic hyponatremia

Hyponatremia with a normal plasma osmolality is usually synonymous with pseudohyponatremia, and can be produced by marked elevation of plasma lipids and proteins. In this situation, the concentration of sodium per liter of plasma is decreased because the nonaqueous portion of the plasma that is occupied by lipid or protein is increased, but the concentration of sodium per liter of plasma water is normal.

Hypertonic hyponatremia

Hyponatremia with an elevated plasma osmolality occurs when there are osmotically active solutes in the plasma, such as glucose, mannitol, sorbitol, or radiocontrast agents. These osmotically active particles induce the movement of water from the ICF to the ECF, decreasing the serum [Na^+], even though serum osmolality remains elevated.

Hypotonic hyponatremia

Hyponatremia with corresponding hypotonicity is the most frequent type of hyponatremia encountered in clinical practice, and the most clinically relevant category. It is generally subdivided according to the clinical assessment of the ECF volume status [30].

Hypovolemic hyponatremia

Hypovolemic hyponatremia occurs when there are simultaneous losses of body water and sodium, resulting in ECF volume depletion. The decrease in blood volume and pressure results in secondary stimulated AVP secretion, and ultimately decreased free water excretion by the kidney. Retention of water from ingested or infused fluids can then lead to the development of hyponatremia. Primary solute depletion, from either renal losses (eg, diuretics, mineralocorticoid deficiency, and various nephropathies) or extrarenal losses (eg, vomiting, diarrhea, hemorrhage, and excessive sweating), all can lead to hypovolemic hyponatremia if predominantly water or hypotonic fluids are ingested or infused in response to the body fluid losses [11]. A low urine sodium concentration (U_{Na}) suggests a nonrenal cause of solute depletion, whereas a high U_{Na} suggests renal causes of solute depletion. Diuretic use is the most common cause of hypovolemic hypoosmolality, with thiazides more commonly associated with severe hyponatremia than loop diuretics [31].

Hypervolemic hyponatremia

In hypervolemic hyponatremia, there is an excess of total body water and total body sodium, resulting in clinically evident hypervolemia manifested by edema or ascites. Hyponatremia occurs because the increase in total body water is usually in excess of the increase in total body sodium as a result of potent AVP secretion in response to a decreased effective arterial blood volume (EABV) [32]. Hypoosmolality in these patients suggests a relatively decreased intravascular volume, leading to water retention as a result of elevated plasma AVP levels and decreased distal delivery of glomerular filtrate [32]. Cirrhosis, congestive heart failure, and nephrotic syndrome all share this common pathophysiology. These patients usually have a low U_{Na} because of secondary hyperaldosteronism; however, the U_{Na} can be difficult to interpret if the patient is on concomitant diuretic therapy.

Euvolemic hyponatremia

Euvolemic hyponatremia can be caused by virtually any disorder causing hypoosmolality. The pathogenesis of euvolemic hyponatremia is typically excessive water retention, caused by either impaired water excretion from advanced renal failure, or more likely from increased secretion of AVP. Occasionally, hyponatremia can occur from over-ingestion of water, where the gastrointestinal tract absorbs water faster than the kidney's ability to excrete it. Because clinical assessments of volume status are often not very sensitive, the presence of normal or low serum urea nitrogen and uric acid concentrations can be helpful correlates of normal ECF volume. SIADH, glucocorticoid deficiency, and hypothyroidism are the most common etiologies of euvolemic hyponatremia.

Postneurosurgical hyponatremia

Hyponatremia has been reported as either an early or late complication of pituitary surgery, and can occur as an isolated entity or as the second phase of the triphasic response to postoperative DI. Hyponatremia after any neurosurgical procedure can be life threatening [33]; however, the majority of cases are mild and relatively asymptomatic because the serum [Na$^+$] levels are generally not very low (eg, 130 mmol/L–134 mmol/L). The incidence of hyponatremia appears to be higher after resection of ACTH-secreting adenomas, occurring in as high as 61% of patients with Cushing's disease [33]. This may be because the rapid decrease in serum cortisol, after removal of an ACTH-producing adenoma, can produce relative glucocorticoid deficiency, predisposing patients to hyponatremia. Given that many cases of hyponatremia occur as a late complication of transsphenoidal surgery, it is recommended that serum [Na$^+$] be monitored daily during hospitalization in patients undergoing transsphenoidal surgery [34]. As most patients are discharged within a few days postoperatively, serum [Na$^+$] levels are assessed within a week after discharge, and patients should be cautioned to monitor for the abrupt onset of dilute polyuria.

Transient hyponatremia without preceding or subsequent DI has been reported following transphenoidal surgery for pituitary microadenomas. This generally occurred 5 to 10 days postoperatively in as many as 30% of patients when they were carefully followed in some series [34]. This scenario can be best understood within the framework of the pathophysiology of the triphasic response, except that in these cases only the second phase of inappropriate AVP secretion occurs because the degree of neural lobe or pituitary stalk damage is not sufficient to cause dysfunction or loss of greater than 85% to 90% of AVP neurons, either acutely or chronically (see Fig. 1B). Consequently, this syndrome has been named the "isolated second phase" of the triphasic response, because the first and third phases of DI are absent [35].

When euvolemic hyponatremia occurs after transsphenoidal pituitary surgery, hypothyroidism, and adrenal insufficiency must always be excluded. However, most patients receive stress doses of glucocorticoids intraoperatively and immediately postoperatively, and many days are required for thyroid hormone levels to fall sufficiently to cause hyponatremia after cessation of thyrotropin secretion. Consequently, both of these potential causes of hyponatremia are uncommon in the immediate postoperative setting. In these cases, a diagnosis of SIADH or cerebral salt wasting must be carefully considered. The distinction between these two disorders is important because of the differing nature of their treatments.

Syndrome of inappropriate antidiuretic hormone secretion

SIADH is characterized by hyponatremia in the setting of an inappropriately concentrated urine, increased urine sodium concentration, and evidence of normal or slightly increased intravascular volume. SIADH is primarily caused by inappropriate plasma AVP levels at plasma osmolalities where pituitary AVP secretion is normally inhibited, leading to renal water reabsorption and expansion of the ECF volume. Because the volume expansion is primarily because of water rather than sodium, it is usually not apparent clinically, and patients typically do not have edema or distended neck veins on physical exam. However, modest expansion of the intravascular volume can be measured by increases in the glomerular filtration rate and renal blood flow. These changes can lead to decreased sodium reabsorption from the proximal tubule, leading to an increased urinary sodium excretion that is characteristic of SIADH. Concentrations of uric acid and urea, which are reabsorbed along with sodium in the proximal tubule, are also decreased in the blood [36]. SIADH is a diagnosis of exclusion, and nonhypotonic hyponatremia from pseudohyponatremia or hyperglycemia, as well as other etiologies of euvolemic hyponatremia, such as hypocortisolism and hypothyroidism, must be ruled out before a diagnosis of SIADH can be made (Box 3) [37].

Cerebral salt wasting

In contrast to SIADH, cerebral salt wasting (CSW) is defined as the renal loss of sodium during intracranial disease, ultimately leading to hyponatremia and a decrease in ECF volume [36]. CSW was initially described in the 1950s by Peters and colleagues [38] in a report of three patients with neurologic disorders who presented with hyponatremia, renal salt wasting, and clinical evidence of volume depletion without any obvious disturbances in the hypothalamic-pituitary-adrenal axis. CSW is now being diagnosed with increasing frequency in neurologic and neurosurgical patients [39], although the true incidence of this disorder remains controversial.

Box 3. Criteria for diagnosis of syndrome of inappropriate antidiuretic hormone secretion

Decreased effective osmolality of the extracellular fluid
   (plasma Osm less than 275 mOsm/kg H_2O)
Inappropriate urinary concentration (urine Osm greater than
   100 mOsm/kg H_2O with normal renal function)
Clinical euvolemia
Elevated urinary sodium excretion on a normal salt
   and water diet
Absence of other potential causes of euvolemic hypoosmolality
- Hypothyroidism
- Hypocortisolism
- Diuretic use

The mechanism by which cerebral disease or neurosurgical procedures leads to renal salt wasting is poorly understood. One theory is that it involves disruption of neural inputs to the kidney, causing decreased renal sodium absorption in the proximal nephron. This ultimately leads to a large delivery of sodium to the distal nephron, increased sodium excretion, and a decrease in EABV; the decrease in EABV in turn activates baroreceptor-stimulated AVP release [36]. Another proposed mechanism is that there is a central release of one or more natriuretic factors, such as atrial natriuretic peptide (ANP) or brain natriuretic peptide (BNP). Both of these factors increase urinary excretion of sodium because of a direct inhibitory effect on sodium transport in the inner medullary collecting duct [40]. Ten subjects with subarachnoid hemorrhage, who underwent clipping of an aneurysm, had significantly higher levels of BNP both before surgery and up to 8 days postoperatively, compared to controls, and the BNP concentrations were significantly correlated with both urinary sodium excretion and intracranial pressure [41].

Diagnosis

Distinguishing CSW from SIADH in clinical practice can be difficult, given that both are caused by similar neurologic processes, and their laboratory values in terms of plasma osmolality, urine osmolality and urine sodium can look identical (Table 1). Determination of ECF volume remains the single best method of distinguishing the between the two: ECF volume is normal or increased in SIADH and low in CSW. The presence of orthostatic changes in blood pressure and pulse, dry mucus membranes and flat neck veins, negative fluid balance, and weight loss all support a diagnosis of CSW. Laboratories that suggest hemoconcentration, as evidenced by an increased hematocrit, increased serum albumin, and increased serum

Table 1
Diagnosis of cerebral salt wasting versus syndrome of inappropriate antidiuretic hormone secretion

Symptom	CSW	SIADH
Extracellular fluid volume	Decreased	Normal to increased
Plasma albumin/protein concentration	Increased	Normal
Signs or symptoms of dehydration	Present	Absent
Weight	Decreased	Normal to increased
Central venous pressure	Decreased	Increased or normal
Hematocrit	Increased	Decreased or no change
Osmolality	Increased or normal	Decreased
Serum urea nitrogen to creatinine ratio	Increased	Normal
Serum potassium concentration	Increased or no change	Decreased or no change
Plasma uric acid	Normal	Decreased

bicarbonate concentration, also support a diagnosis of CSW. Uric acid levels are depressed in patients with SIADH, reflecting the slight increase in ECF volume seen in this disorder. One would expect that in CSW the uric acid levels would be high, reflecting the volume contracted state of this disorder. However, reported uric acid levels in CSW are unexpectedly low [42]. Consequently, uric acid levels are not helpful in distinguishing between these two entities. Although individual cases of CSW have been well documented, most studies lack sufficiently rigorous documentation of hypovolemia to justify this diagnosis. It is important to remember that elevations of urine sodium concentration are common in SIADH, and therefore this cannot be viewed as evidence of "salt wasting" by the kidneys in the absence of clinical evidence of volume contraction, which is often lacking. Urine sodium concentrations are particularly difficult to interpret once therapy with isotonic saline has begun, as this markedly elevates U_{Na}, even in normal subjects. Because most postoperative patients are euvolemic unless they have DI, it is likely that the majority of postneurosurgical hyponatremia is caused by SIADH, with relatively fewer cases attributable to CSW.

The possibility that both disorders might coexist should be considered. Ample precedent certainly exists for hyponatremia caused by Na^+ wasting with a secondary antidiuresis in Addison's disease, as well as diuretic-induced hyponatremia. Characteristic of these disorders, normalization of ECF volume with isotonic NaCl infusions restores plasma osmolality to normal ranges by virtue of shutting off the secondary AVP secretion. If hyponatremia in patients with CSW occurred via a similar mechanism, it should also respond to this therapy. However, several studies indicate that it does not. Nineteen patients with subarachnoid hemorrhage (SAH) were treated with large volumes of isotonic NaCl sufficient to maintain plasma volume at normal or slightly elevated levels; but despite removal of any volemic stimulus to AVP secretion, 32% still developed hyponatremia in association with nonsuppressed plasma AVP levels, an incidence equivalent to that found in previous studies of SAH [43]. These types of results support the existence of disordered AVP secretion, as well as a coexisting stimulus to natriuresis in many such patients. It therefore seems most likely that SAH and other intracranial diseases associated with CSW represent a mixed disorder in which some patients have both exaggerated natriuresis and inappropriate AVP secretion. Which effect predominates in terms of the clinical presentation will depend on their relative intensities, as well as the effects of concomitant therapy. Consequently, many cases of postneurosurgical hyponatremia probably entail inappropriate secretion of both AVP and ANP/BNP; in such cases the natriuretic peptides would act to further exacerbate the secondary natriuresis already produced by AVP-induced water retention.

Treatment

In SIADH, fluid restriction is the mainstay of treating hyponatremia, with the goal of maintaining fluid intake at least 500 mL per day below the urine output. However, this degree of fluid restriction is often difficult to maintain, especially in a hospital setting where the obligate fluid requirements for various therapies and parenteral nutrition often exceed this level. In contrast, treatment of hyponatremia in CSW entails volume replacement and maintenance of a positive sodium balance. Intravascular volume can be maintained with intravenous isotonic saline, and once patients are capable of taking oral medications NaCl tablets can be used.

It is important to distinguish between these two disorders, because treatment that is appropriate for one disorder can potentially result in poor outcomes when inappropriately applied to the other [44]. As an example, the potential for fluid restriction to worsen an underlying neurologic condition in the setting of CSW was suggested in a retrospective study of patients with SAH, where 44 of 134 patients were found to have developed hyponatremia between 2 to 9 days following their hemorrhage; 21 of 44 patients treated with fluid restriction developed a cerebral infarction, including 15 of 17 patients who clinically met the criteria for SIADH. This suggests that the fluid restriction aggravated an already decreased plasma volume, thereby leading to cerebral ischemia as a result of vasospasm, as well as potentially decreasing cerebral blood flow by increasing blood viscosity and decreasing cardiac output [44].

Conversely, when intravenous isotonic NaCl is infused in patients with SIADH, this can potentially cause a further lowering of serum sodium concentrations, resulting in the development of symptomatic hyponatremia [45,46].

Reeder and Harbaugh [47] have advocated the use of urea and saline in patients with hyponatremia caused by intracranial disease, where it is unclear whether SIADH or CSW is the diagnosis, or where there is the possibility that both coexist. Urea induces a mild osmotic diuresis and depresses urinary sodium excretion, and supplemental NaCl restores sodium deficits. In their retrospective review of 48 neurosurgical patients treated with urea and saline, mean serum [Na$^+$] increased by 8 mmol/L without treatment complications. Randomized controlled trials of this and other therapies will be necessary before definitive recommendations can be made.

Evidence-based guidelines for treatment of hyponatremia are lacking, but a recent consensus statement summarizes areas of general agreement concerning the treatment of various types of hyponatremia [48]. The neurologic sequelae associated with acute hyponatremia are caused when there is a rapid, osmotic influx of water along osmotic gradients into the central nervous system, leading to brain edema. The brain has an early adaptive mechanism to decrease edema by extruding inorganic solutes, and thus water. A later more effective adaptive mechanism occurs whereby the brain regulates its volume by extruding small organic molecules called osmolytes [49]. Once brain edema decreases via this adaptive process, neurologic symptoms generally abate, explaining why patients with chronic hyponatremia may be relatively asymptomatic, despite very low serum [Na$^+$] [50].

Several studies have shown that the rate of decrease of serum [Na$^+$] is more strongly correlated with morbidity and mortality than is the actual magnitude of the hyponatremia [51]. This is because of the fact that the volume adaptation process takes a finite period of time to complete: the more rapid the fall in serum [Na$^+$], the more brain edema will be accumulated before the brain is able to lose solute, and along with it part of the increased water content [4]. Acute hyponatremia, defined as lasting less than 48 hours in duration, can result in sufficient brain edema to cause seizures, tentorial herniation, respiratory arrest, irreversible brain damage and, in severe cases, death. Chronic hyponatremia, defined as lasting more than 48 hours, produces more subtle symptoms, including headache, lethargy, disorientation, and nausea, or may even be asymptomatic if complete brain volume regulation has occurred [52].

It is important for clinicians to understand how the brain volume adapts in response to hyponatremia in order to correct serum [Na$^+$] safely. In both animal and human studies, brain demyelination has clearly been shown to be associated with correction of existing hyponatremia, rather than simply with the presence of severe hyponatremia itself [53]. It is generally agreed that treatment of symptomatic hyponatremia is necessary, regardless of the etiology, but some debate remains as to how quickly the serum [Na$^+$] can be corrected without risk of precipitating pontine and extrapontine myelinolysis, also called the osmotic demyelination syndrome (ODS). Rapid correction of hyperacute hyponatremia (occurring in less than 24 hours), rarely if ever leads to ODS, and rates of serum [Na$^+$] increase can safely exceed 2 mmol/L per hour in such cases [54]. However, in patients with chronic hyponatremia, correction rates must be lower in order to prevent potential demyelination. It is generally accepted that a correction of 12 mmo/L in the first 24 hours, and 18 mmol/L in the first 48 hours, is generally safe [53], but there have been a few case reports of osmotic demyelination that appear to have occurred with corrections slower than 12 mmol/L per 24 hours [55,56]. Thus, in cases of known chronic hyponatremia or hyponatremia of unknown duration, and particularly in patients with other known risk factors for pontine and extrapontine demyelination (eg, alcoholism, malnutrition, liver failure), a more prudent approach would be to aim for a rate of correction of no faster than 8 mmol/L per 24 hours [54].

New developments in water homeostasis

Vasopressin receptor antagonists

A new class of agents, AVP receptor antagonists, have been recently introduced as a method of correcting hyponatremia by blocking the binding of AVP to V2 receptors in the kidney. AVP receptor antagonists are highly effective in producing a safe and predictable increased excretion of free water that increases the serum [Na^+] in hyponatremic patients. Because these agents induce excretion of free water without accompanying natriuresis or kaliuresis, this effect has been termed "aquaresis," to differentiate it from the increased water and solute excretion produced by traditional diuretic agents [57].

Several AVP receptor agonists are under clinical investigation for use in euvolemic hyponatremia: conivaptan (YM-087), lixivaptan (VPA-985), satavaptan (SR-121463), and tolvaptan (OPC-41061). All drugs in this class carry the suffix "vaptan," so as a group they are often referred to as "the vaptans." All four of the current vaptans increase urine volume and decrease urine osmolality, but have no effect on 24-hour sodium excretion [58]. Conivaptan has antagonist activity at both the V1a and V2 AVP receptors, whereas the other three vaptans are selective V2 receptor antagonists [59]. Conivaptan is currently Food and Drug Administration-approved for the treatment of euvolemic and hypervolemic hyponatremia in hospitalized patients. There are several recent reviews for more detailed summaries of clinical trials of various vaptans [58].

Conivaptan is currently the only available agent for treatment of hyponatremia. Phase 3 studies show that it reliably raises serum [Na^+], beginning as early as 1 to 2 hours after administration. In most patients, the serum [Na^+] normalizes over a 4-day continuous infusion, with the greatest increase in serum [Na^+] during the first 24 to 48 hours of treatment. It is interesting to note that no cases of osmotic demyelination have occurred during clinical trials of any of the vaptans [60]. In part, this is because the dosing employed in the clinical protocols infrequently caused increases in serum [Na^+] greater than 12 mmol/L in any 24-hour period. However, it is also because the protocols were constructed to include monitoring of the serum [Na^+] frequently (at least every 6 hours) during active corrections of hyponatremia, and the drug was discontinued if set limits of correction rate were exceeded. Consequently, analogous guidelines should be employed with clinical use of these agents to avoid correcting the serum [Na^+] at a rate faster than 8 mmol/L to 12 mmol/L per 24 hours. Although all of the vaptans have a half-life of less than 12 hours, which should allow dose titration to avoid over-correction, an occasional patient may continue to increase the serum [Na^+] for several hours after discontinuation of the drug, in which case free water should be given to the patient to prevent further correction and clamp the serum [Na^+] at a safe level.

The clearest indication for conivaptan use is in patients with symptomatic euvolemic hyponatremia and mild to moderate neurologic symptoms, such as impaired cognition, confusion, and disorientation. Conivaptan is known to reliably increase serum [Na^+] by several mmol/L within 5 hours at the 20-mg and 40-mg doses, and 6 mmol/L to 9 mmol/L within 24 hours after initiation of therapy [61]. The induced free water aquaresis should resolve such neurologic symptoms promptly by decreasing cerebral edema, with no risk of worsening the hyponatremia. Importantly, in severely symptomatic hyponatremic patients with seizures, obtundation, coma, and respiratory distress, hypertonic saline should still be used as first-line therapy. The vaptan clinical trials excluded patients with symptomatic hyponatremia for ethical reasons of not potentially randomizing critically ill patients to a placebo arm of a double-blinded protocol. Thus, it is not currently known whether sufficiently rapid correction can be achieved with conivaptan alone to prevent herniation and respiratory arrest in patients with severe hyponatremic encephalopathy. Therefore, these patients should receive the current standard of care, which is infusion of hypertonic (3%) NaCl or mannitol [53]. Theoretically, combined treatment with both hypertonic NaCl and conivaptan should be complementary [62], but clinical trials with such protocols will be necessary before their efficacy and safety can be determined.

In the postoperative setting following neurosurgery for sellar lesions, many patients have a transient form of SIADH, either as part of a triphasic response or an isolated second phase, and in such case a short, several-day course of a V2 receptor antagonist can help to resolve the hyponatremia quickly, without need for more chronic therapy. Vaptans theoretically should not be used in patients with CSW, because these patients are by definition hypovolemic and the resultant aquaresis would cause further intravascular volume depletion. However, as previously discussed, many patients who are labeled as having CSW are actually clinically euvolemic, and more likely have SIADH. Furthermore, patients with subarachnoid hemorrhage are generally aggressively volume expanded with hypervolemic-hypertensive therapy to prevent cerebral vasospasm; in this situation, the use of a vaptan can be helpful to prevent further hyponatremia, resulting from continuous administration of large volumes of isotonic saline, as also discussed earlier. The free water aquaresis should normalize the serum [Na^+], thus decreasing cerebral edema caused by hyponatremia and simultaneously allowing continued concurrent infusion of large volumes of isotonic saline to prevent vasospasm.

Some significant side effects with the use of conivaptan have become apparent, including drug interactions via interference with CYP3A4-mediated hepatic metabolism and a high occurrence of infusion site reactions caused by the need to use polypropylene glycol to achieve solubility [61]. Despite the need for cautious use, as with any new class of therapeutic agents, it is abundantly clear that the availability of potent AVP receptor antagonists heralds the beginning of a new era in the treatment of hyponatremia.

References

[1] Rai A, Whaley-Connell A, McFarlane S, et al. Hyponatremia, arginine vasopressin dysregulation, and vasopressin receptor antagonism. Am J Nephrol 2006;26(6):579–89.

[2] Palevsky PM, Bhagrath R, Greenberg A. Hypernatremia in hospitalized patients. Ann Intern Med 1996;124(2):197–203.

[3] Knepper MA. Molecular physiology of urinary concentrating mechanism: regulation of aquaporin water channels by vasopressin. Am J Physiol 1997;272(1 Pt 2):F3–12.

[4] Verbalis JG. Ten essential points about body water homeostasis. Horm Res 2007; 67(Suppl 1):165–72.

[5] Robertson GL. Antidiuretic hormone. Normal and disordered function. Endocrinol Metab Clin North Am 2001;30(3):671–94.

[6] Sklar AH, Schrier RW. Central nervous system mediators of vasopressin release. Physiol Rev 1983;63(4):1243–80.

[7] Sladek CD. Regulation of vasopressin release by neurotransmitters, neuropeptides and osmotic stimuli. Prog Brain Res 1983;60:71–90.

[8] Verbalis JG. Management of disorders of water metabolism in patients with pituitary tumors. Pituitary 2002;5(2):119–32.

[9] Moder KG, Hurley DL. Fatal hypernatremia from exogenous salt intake: report of a case and review of the literature. Mayo Clin Proc 1990;65(12):1587–94.

[10] Smith D, Finucane F, Phillips J, et al. Abnormal regulation of thirst and vasopressin secretion following surgery for craniopharyngioma. Clin Endocrinol (Oxf) 2004;61(2): 273–9.

[11] Adler SM, Verbalis JG. Disorders of body water homeostasis in critical illness. Endocrinol Metab Clin North Am 2006;35(4):873–94.

[12] Robinson AG, Verbalis JG. The posterior pituitary. In: Larsen PR, Kronenberg HM, Melmed S, et al, editors. Williams textbook of endocrinology. 10th edition. Philadelphia: W.B. Saunders; 2003. p. 281–329.

[13] Nemergut EC, Zuo Z, Jane JA Jr, et al. Predictors of diabetes insipidus after transsphenoidal surgery: a review of 881 patients. J Neurosurg 2005;103(3):448–54.

[14] Verbalis JG, Robinson AG, Moses AM. Postoperative and post-traumatic diabetes insipidus. In: Czernichow P, Robinson AG, editors. Diabetes insipidus in man. Basel (Germany): Karger; 1984. p. 247–65.

[15] Verbalis JG. Diabetes insipidus. Rev Endocr Metab Disord 2003;4(2):177–85.

[16] Robinson AG. Disorders of antidiuretic hormone secretion. Clin Endocrinol Metab 1985; 14:55–88.

[17] Singer I, Oster JR, Fishman LM. The management of diabetes insipidus in adults. Arch Intern Med 1997;157(12):1293–301.

[18] Tien R, Kucharczyk J, Kucharczyk W. MR imaging of the brain in patients with diabetes insipidus. AJNR Am J Neuroradiol 1991;12:533–42.

[19] Maghnie M, Genovese E, Bernasconi S, et al. Persistent high MR signal of the posterior pituitary gland in central diabetes insipidus. AJNR Am J Neuroradiol 1997;18(9):1749–52.

[20] Brooks BS, el Gammal T, Allison JD, et al. Frequency and variation of the posterior pituitary bright signal on MR images. AJNR Am J Neuroradiol 1989;10(5):943–8.

[21] Hollinshead WH. The interphase of diabetes insipidus. Mayo Clin Proc 1964;39:92–100.

[22] Sharkey PC, Perry JH, Ehni G. Diabetes insipidus following section of the hypophyseal stalk. J Neurosurg 1961;18:445–60.

[23] Lipsett MB, Maclean JP, West CD, et al. An analysis of the polyuria induced by hypophysectomy in man. J Clin Endocrinol Metab 1956;16(2):183–95.

[24] Adams JR, Blevins LS Jr, Allen GS, et al. Disorders of water metabolism following transsphenoidal pituitary surgery: a single institution's experience. Pituitary 2006;9(2):93–9.

[25] Richardson DW, Robinson AG. Desmopressin. Ann Intern Med 1985;103(2):228–39.

[26] Robertson GL. Thirst and vasopressin function in normal and disordered states of water balance. J Lab Clin Med 1983;101:351–71.

[27] Robinson AG, Verbalis JG. Diabetes insipidus. Curr Ther Endocrinol Metab 1997;6:1–7.

[28] Flear CT, Gill GV, Burn J. Hyponatraemia: mechanisms and management. Lancet 1981; 2(8236):26–31.

[29] Anderson RJ, Chung HM, Kluge R, et al. Hyponatremia: a prospective analysis of its epidemiology and the pathogenetic role of vasopressin. Ann Intern Med 1985;102(2): 164–8.

[30] Robinson AG, Verbalis JG. The posterior pituitary. In: Larsen PR, Kronenberg HM, Melmed S, et al, editors. Williams textbook of endocrinology. 10th edition. Philadelphia: Saunders; 2003. p. 281–329.

[31] Spital A. Diuretic-induced hyponatremia. Am J Nephrol 1999;19(4):447–52.

[32] Schrier RW. Pathogenesis of sodium and water retention in high-output and low-output cardiac failure, nephrotic syndrome, cirrhosis, and pregnancy (1). N Engl J Med 1988;319(16): 1065–72.

[33] Sane T, Rantakari K, Poranen A, et al. Hyponatremia after transsphenoidal surgery for pituitary tumors. J Clin Endocrinol Metab 1994;79(5):1395–8.

[34] Olson BR, Rubino D, Gumowski J, et al. Isolated hyponatremia after transsphenoidal pituitary surgery. J Clin Endocrinol Metab 1995;80(1):85–91.

[35] Ultmann MC, Hoffman GE, Nelson PB, et al. Transient hyponatremia after damage to the neurohypophyseal tracts. Neuroendocrinology 1992;56(6):803–11.

[36] Palmer BF. Hyponatremia in patients with central nervous system disease: SIADH versus CSW. Trends Endocrinol Metab 2003;14(4):182–7.

[37] Bartter FC. The syndrome of inappropriate secretion of antidiuretic hormone (SIADH). Dis Mon 1973;1–47.

[38] Peters JP, Welt LG, Sims EA, et al. A salt-wasting syndrome associated with cerebral disease. Trans Assoc Am Physicians 1950;63:57–64.

[39] Betjes MG. Hyponatremia in acute brain disease: the cerebral salt wasting syndrome. Eur J Intern Med 2002;13(1):9–14.

[40] Levin ER, Gardner DG, Samson WK. Natriuretic peptides. N Engl J Med 1998;339(5): 321–8.

[41] Berendes E, Walter M, Cullen P, et al. Secretion of brain natriuretic peptide in patients with aneurysmal subarachnoid haemorrhage. Lancet 1997;349(9047):245–9.

[42] Maesaka JK, Gupta S, Fishbane S. Cerebral salt-wasting syndrome: does it exist? Nephron 1999;82(2):100–9.

[43] Diringer MN, Wu KC, Verbalis JG, et al. Hypervolemic therapy prevents volume contraction but not hyponatremia following subarachnoid hemorrhage. Ann Neurol 1992;31(5): 543–50.

[44] Wijdicks EF, Vermeulen M, Hijdra A, et al. Hyponatremia and cerebral infarction in patients with ruptured intracranial aneurysms: is fluid restriction harmful? Ann Neurol 1985; 17(2):137–40.

[45] Halperin ML, Bohn D. Clinical approach to disorders of salt and water balance. Emphasis on integrative physiology. Crit Care Clin 2002;18(2):249–72.

[46] Steele A, Gowrishankar M, Abrahamson S, et al. Postoperative hyponatremia despite near-isotonic saline infusion: a phenomenon of desalination. Ann Intern Med 1997; 126(1):20–5.

[47] Reeder RF, Harbaugh RE. Administration of intravenous urea and normal saline for the treatment of hyponatremia in neurosurgical patients. J Neurosurg 1989;70(2):201–6.

[48] Verbalis JG. Hyponatremia treatment guidance consensus statement. Am J Med 2007; 120(Supple 1):S1–21.

[49] Verbalis JG. Control of brain volume during hypoosmolality and hyperosmolality. Adv Exp Med Biol 2006;576:113–29.

[50] Daggett P, Deanfield J, Moss F. Neurological aspects of hyponatraemia. Postgrad Med J 1982;58(686):737–40.

[51] Arieff AI, Llach F, Massry SG. Neurological manifestations and morbidity of hyponatremia: correlation with brain water and electrolytes. Medicine (Baltimore) 1976;55(2):121–9.

[52] Soupart A, Decaux G. Therapeutic recommendations for management of severe hyponatremia: current concepts on pathogenesis and prevention of neurologic complications. Clin Nephrol 1996;46(3):149–69.

[53] Sterns RH, Silver SM. Brain volume regulation in response to hypo-osmolality and its correction. Am J Med 2006;119(7 Suppl 1):S12–6.

[54] Oh MS, Kim HJ, Carroll HJ. Recommendations for treatment of symptomatic hyponatremia. Nephron 1995;70(2):143–50.

[55] Tomlinson BE, Pierides AM, Bradley WG. Central pontine myelinolysis. Two cases with associated electrolyte disturbance. Q J Med 1976;45(179):373–86.

[56] Norenberg MD, Leslie KO, Robertson AS. Association between rise in serum sodium and central pontine myelinolysis. Ann Neurol 1982;11(2):128–35.

[57] Verbalis JG. Vasopressin V2 receptor antagonists. J Mol Endocrinol 2002;29(1):1–9.

[58] Greenberg A, Verbalis JG. Vasopressin receptor antagonists. Kidney Int 2006;69(12): 2124–30.

[59] Lee CR, Watkins ML, Patterson JH, et al. Vasopressin: a new target for the treatment of heart failure. Am Heart J 2003;146(1):9–18.

[60] Arai Y, Fujimori A, Sudoh K, et al. Vasopressin receptor antagonists: potential indications and clinical results. Curr Opin Pharmacol 2007;7(2):124–9.

[61] Vaprisol prescribing information–Astellas Pharma Inc., February 2006. Available at: http:// www.astellas.us/docs/vaprisol.pdf.

[62] Verbalis JG. Vaptans for the treatment of hyponatremia: how, who, when, and why. Nephrology Self-Assessment Program 2007;199–209.

ENDOCRINOLOGY
AND METABOLISM
CLINICS
OF NORTH AMERICA

ELSEVIER
SAUNDERS

Endocrinol Metab Clin N Am
37 (2008) 235–261

Hypopituitarism: Clinical Features, Diagnosis, and Management

Andrew A. Toogood, MD, FRCP[a],*,
Paul M. Stewart, FRCP, FMedSci[b]

[a]University Hospital Birmingham NHS Foundation Trust, Edgbaston,
Birmingham, B15 2TH, UK
[b]University of Birmingham, Edgbaston, Birmingham, B15 2TT, UK

The pituitary gland consists of anterior and posterior lobes and is found in the pituitary fossa of the sphenoid bone. The gland is in communication with the hypothalamus via the pituitary stalk, which consists of neurones and portal blood vessels. Hormones produced in the hypothalamus pass down these structures and regulate the release of hormones from anterior pituitary gland or are released directly into the circulation. The anterior pituitary gland produces follicle-stimulating hormone (FSH) and luteinizing hormone (LH) (known collectively as the gonadotropins), growth hormone (GH), corticotropin, thyrotropin, and prolactin. The posterior lobe is responsible for the release of two hormones, vasopressin (or antidiuretic hormone) and oxytocin, which are important primarily for the regulation of water balance and parturition, respectively.

The term, hypopituitarism, describes the deficiency of one or more of the hormones of the anterior or posterior pituitary gland. Panhypopituitarism indicates the loss of all the pituitary hormones but often is used in clinical practice to describe patients deficient in GH, gonadotropins, corticotropin, and thyrotropin in whom posterior pituitary function remains intact. This article discusses anterior pituitary dysfunction; the posterior pituitary is addressed in the article by Loh and Verbalis elsewhere in this issue.

Hypopituitarism is a rare condition estimated by one population study from Spain as having an annual incidence rate of 4.2 cases per 100,000 of the population, with a prevalence rate of 45.5 per 100,000 [1]. There are many identified causes of hypopituitarism, but recent recognition that other conditions, such as head injury and cranial radiotherapy, can cause

---

* Corresponding author.
E-mail address: andrew.toogood@uhb.nhs.uk (A.A. Toogood).

hypopituitarism will result in more cases being diagnosed and, consequently, an increase in prevalence. The clinical impact of hypopituitarism can be variable and is determined by the age at which the condition occurs, its rapidity of onset, the gender of the patient, the underlying cause, and the pattern of hormone deficiencies.

Clinical features of hypopituitarism

The general features of hypopituitarism are nonspecific and often evolve insidiously before a diagnosis is made, resulting from the local effects of the underlying pathology or the developing endocrinopathy, related to specific hormone deficits in isolation or in combination. Deficits of anterior pituitary hormones may be secondary to hormone excess caused by functional pituitary tumors, for example, suppression of gonadotropins in hyperprolactinemia or GH deficiency caused by cortisol excess in Cushing's syndrome [2]. In these situations, the deficits may recover when the underlying endocrinopathy is treated. Nonspecific symptoms include a feeling of general ill health, being abnormally tired, increased lethargy, feeling cold, weight loss, reduced appetite, and abdominal pain. Symptoms attributed to the local effects of any underlying tumor include headaches, visual disturbance (typically a bitemporal hemianopia), or cerebrospinal fluid rhinorrhea.

Growth hormone deficiency

GH deficiency causes a variety of signs and symptoms determined by the age at which patients present.

A neonate who has congenital GH deficiency or hypopituitarism resulting from birth trauma presents most frequently in the first 24 hours of life with severe hypoglycemia often associated with convulsions. Other features of GH deficiency during the neonatal period are prolonged conjugated hyperbilirubinemia, hypothermia, and, in boys, possibly a micropenis [3]. Patients who have midline birth defects should be considered at risk for isolated or multiple pituitary hormone deficiencies. Older babies who escape early diagnosis may present with failure to thrive and poor weight gain.

Older children who have GH deficiency present with short stature and reduced growth velocity for their age. Those who have severe GH deficiency develop a characteristic appearance with a prominent forehead and depressed midface development caused by the lack of GH effect on endochondrial growth at the base of the skull, occiput, and sphenoid. Dentition may be delayed. Other features may be present that are attributable to the underlying etiology of the GH deficiency.

Multiple symptoms and pathophysiologic changes that affect a variety of biologic systems are attributed to GH deficiency in adult life [4]. Despite the wide-ranging nature of these changes, none is pathognomonic for the condition. Patients who have GH deficiency have impaired quality of life, complaining of tiredness, lack of energy, emotional lability, and reduced sleep quality [5,6]. It is suggested that up to 30% of patients have a degree of disability consistent with psychiatric illness requiring treatment [7]. Patients who have childhood-onset GH deficiency do not seem to suffer the same degree of impairment in quality of life as those who have adult-onset GH deficiency [8].

Patients who have GH deficiency exhibit abnormalities of protein, fat, and carbohydrate metabolism, which contribute to abnormal body composition [9]. Lean mass is reduced and fat mass is increased with a propensity to central obesity and increased intra-abdominal or visceral fat deposition [10,11]. In contrast to GH-deficient neonates who present with hypoglycemia, adults are insulin resistant and the serum lipid profile is abnormal, with elevated total and low-density lipoprotein (LDL) cholesterol and triglyceride levels [12]. Serum levels of high-density lipoprotein (HDL) cholesterol are reported as unchanged [13,14] or decreased [15–17]. Other markers of cardiovascular risk, including carotid intima media thickness, serum C-reactive protein, and interleukin 6, also are abnormal [18–20]. The adverse cardiovascular risk profile attributed to GH deficiency almost certainly contributes to the twofold increase in cardiovascular mortality observed in adults who have hypopituitarism [21–24]; however, other anterior pituitary hormone deficits and the replacement strategies used for them also may have a role [25].

GH-deficient patients have bone mineral density (BMD) that is reduced compared with healthy controls [26]. These changes are age dependent and evident particularly in young adults in whom GH has an important role in bone accrual. Early in adult life, GH is required to optimize BMD and later may have a role maintaining skeletal health. Patients who develop GH deficiency during childhood have more severe osteopenia than those who become GH deficient in adult life [27], and as the age at diagnosis increases, the decrement in bone mass falls, such that adults over age 60 have similar BMD to their age- and gender-matched healthy peers [28,29]. Fracture risk is increased in GH-deficient adults [30,31], suggesting that the observed degree of osteopenia is clinically significant in this patient cohort. Rosen and colleagues [30] demonstrated a threefold increase in fractures overall. In a study using the KIMS database, a postmarketing surveillance study, the relative risk for fracture in GH-deficient patients was 2.66 [31].

Gonadotropin deficiency

The clinical features of gonadotropin deficiency are determined by the gender and age at which the condition develops. Male infants who have congenital hypogonadotropic hypogonadism may have a combination of unilateral or bilateral cryptorchidism and a microphallus caused by the relative androgen deficiency that occurs during the third trimester. Later, in adolescence, pubertal development can fail to initiate or be abnormal with failure to progress normally. Testicular volumes can vary between those seen in prepubertal boys (<4 cm^3) and normal adult size. Pubic hair may be present, mediated by testicular or adrenal androgens, but is unlikely to be normal. Gonadotropin deficiency in girls usually becomes apparent in teenage years with delayed breast development and primary amenorrhea.

When gonadotropin deficiency is present in isolation, growth is normal during childhood and seems to slow during adolescence when the growth spurt fails to occur. Despite this, the epiphyses fail to fuse at the usual age and the long bones continue to grow, ultimately resulting in tall stature and a eunuchoid habitus.

Men who acquire gonadotropin deficiency during adult life usually achieve a normal height with proportionate growth. Adult secondary sexual characteristics are present, although the testes may become soft and reduced in size, because the FSH deficiency causes atrophy of the seminiferous tubules. Men may notice a slowing of beard growth and a need to shave less frequently. Body hair may be lost, and if the hypogonadotropism is severe and prolonged, the skin becomes thin and fine wrinkles develop. Libido may be reduced and the ability to achieve and maintain an erection may be compromised. Testosterone deficiency can lead to nonspecific symptoms, such as tiredness, reduced muscle bulk, and reduced exercise capacity. There is a fall in BMD with a risk for osteopenia or osteoporosis and increased fractures. Azoospermia usually is present in prolonged gonadotropin deficiency, although there are exceptions.

Because the symptoms of hypogonadotropism in men are nonspecific, they may not become evident for many years, particularly if fertility is not an issue. Conversely, in women, secondary gonadotropin deficiency often is diagnosed quickly when oligomenorrhea or amenorhea develops. In addition, women report symptoms of estrogen deficiency: vaginal dryness, dyspareunia, hot flashes, and breast atrophy. Pubic and axillary hair remains unless there is coexistant corticotropin deficiency with adrenal androgen deficiency.

Adrenocorticotropin deficiency

Deficiency of corticotropin results in secondary hypoadrenalism and is the most serious of anterior pituitary hormone deficits. During an intercurrent illness, an adrenal crisis with severe hyponatremia and hypovolemic shock may develop and can result in death if not diagnosed and treated appropriately. Patients who have hypopituitarism are protected somewhat from developing severe, acute hypoadrenalism compared with patients who have primary adrenal failure, as the angiotensin-aldosterone axis remains intact. Decompensation and shock occur during periods of illness or physical stress, such as surgery. Other symptoms of cortisol deficiency include lethargy, fatigue, weight loss, and nonspecific abdominal pain, and, if the diagnosis is not considered, can lead to unnecessary investigations in pursuit of intra-abdominal pathology. Hypoglycemia may be present, causing feelings of hunger, light-headedness, and sweating. Patients also may have hypotension and complain of postural symptoms. The pigmentation associated with primary adrenal failure is not present in patients who have corticotropin deficiency; the skin may be pale with an alabaster-like appearance [32].

Thyrotropin deficiency

The symptoms and signs associated with thyrotropin deficiency are similar to those of primary hypothyroidism but usually are less severe, as there often is some residual thyrotropin secretion. Tiredness, cold intolerance, weight gain, constipation, dry skin, and hair are common features. With the exception of traumatic brain injury (TBI), thyrotropin deficiency usually occurs late in the evolution of hypopituitarism and often is seen with other anterior pituitary hormone deficits. In children, secondary hypothyroidism contributes to poor growth, delayed bone age, and failure of secondary dentition.

Prolactin deficiency

Prolactin is inhibited predominately by dopamine; as a consequence, prolactin levels frequently are raised in the presence of hypothalamic-pituitary disease because of compression or transection of the pituitary stalk. Hypoprolactinemia is found in patients who have mutations of the transcription factors, PIT1 and PROP1, but in patients who have structural pituitary disease, it is a marker of severe pituitary damage [33,34]. In women, prolactin deficiency can cause failure of lactation in the postpartum period. Although prolactin is an important hormone in the animal world with multiple identified roles in growth, water homeostasis, reproduction, behavior, and growth and immune modulation [35], a phenotype attributable to prolactin deficiency in man has yet to be established.

Causes of hypopituitarism

Congenital hypopituitarism

Increased understanding of the molecular biology of pituitary development, hormone production, and hormone action has resulted in the characterization of conditions described previously as congenital or idiopathic. Increasingly, patients who have a variety of genetic causes of hypopituitarism can be recognized by the pattern of hormone deficits present alongside other clinical features. Mutations in transcription factors, such as POU1F1 or PROP-1 [36], which are required for hormone synthesis, produce multiple pituitary hormone deficits, whereas mutations in other genes may result in single hormone deficits, for example, isolated GH deficiency in patients who have GH1 mutations [37], or corticotropin deficiency caused by a mutation in the POMC gene [38]. For a comprehensive list of genetic causes of hypopituitarism, see Table 1.

Pituitary tumors

Pituitary tumors are the most common intracranial neoplasm accounting for 10.7% of primary central nervous system tumors. They are classified by size (microadenomas <10 mm and macroadenomas >10 mm) according to their ability to produce hormones (functioning and nonfunctioning adenomas). Prevalence studies suggest pituitary adenomas are common in the normal population and were present in between 1% and 35% of pituitaries studied at autopsy and in 1% to 40% of patients undergoing an MRI scan for reasons other than to assess the hypothalamic-pituitary axis. The majority of these lesions were microadenomas and not clinically significant, although prolactin staining was reported in 25% to 41% of those tumors studied. The prevalence of macroadenomas was estimated to be 0.16% to 0.20% [56].

Prolactin-secreting tumors and nonfunctioning tumors account for the majority of pituitary adenomas. Large published series indicate that 27.4% to 57.3% of patients have nonfunctioning lesions, whereas prolactinomas account for 9.3% to 39.0% of lesions. The disparity is caused by the nature of the study and the inclusion criteria used.

Suprasellar tumors

Craniopharyngiomas are the most common suprasellar tumor arising from the craniopharyngeal duct, although they are rare in the general population, with an incidence of 0.13 per 100,000 person years [57]. Other lesions that occur in the suprasellar region and can be difficult to distinguish from craniopharyngioma include cystic lesions, such as Rathke's cleft cyst; dermoid, epidermoid, and arachnoid cysts; germinoma; hamartoma; meningioma; and suprasellar aneurysm. In addition to these astrocytomas, optic nerve giomas and metastatic disease all may present as suprasellar mass lesions.

Radiation

Radiotherapy used to treat a variety of intracranial tumors can cause neuroendocrine dysfunction if the radiation fields have an impact on the hypothalamic-pituitary axis. Patients treated with radiotherapy for pituitary adenomas [58], suprasellar lesions, primary brain tumors [59], nasopharyngeal tumors [60], head and neck tumors, bone tumors affecting the skull, or acute lymphoblastic leukemia (ALL) [61] are at risk for developing pituitary hormone deficiencies.

The impact of radiotherapy on pituitary function is determined by the biologic effective dose the hypothalamic-pituitary axis is exposed to and the presence of primary pituitary disease. The GH axis is most vulnerable to the effects of radiotherapy; doses as low as 18 Gy used in the management of ALL in children have caused GH deficiency, which may not develop until many years after treatment. As the radiation dose increases, the risk for developing other anterior pituitary hormone deficits and the rate at which they develop increase. Gonadotropin deficiency usually occurs after GH deficiency followed by corticotropin and thyrotropin deficiencies (Fig. 1) [62].

Controversially, it is suggested that thyrotropin deficiency is more frequent than previously believed and may occur in isolation before GH deficiency has developed [63]. Detailed studies of the hypothalamic pituitary thyroid axis clearly demonstrate, however, that this is not the case [64]. If thyroxine treatment is commenced in a patient in whom corticotropin deficiency is present, it has the potential to precipitate an adrenal crisis.

The presence of primary pituitary pathology before irradiation increases the risk for subsequent hypopituitarism. Littley and colleagues [58] studied adults treated with radiotherapy for pituitary adenoma. In those who had normal pituitary function before treatment, 100% had GH deficiency within 5 years of treatment, and gonadotropin deficiency, corticotropin deficiency, and thyrotropin deficiency developed in 57%, 61%, and 27.5%, respectively (see Fig. 1). In patients who had nasopharyngeal carcinoma (who received a higher total radiation dose), GH deficiency was present in 63.5%, gonadotropin deficiency in 31%, corticotropin deficiency in 27%, and thyrotropin deficiency in 15% 5 years after treatment [60].

In prepubertal children, cranial irradiation can result in early or precocious puberty and, paradoxically, gonadotropin deficiency. The low-radiation doses used prophylactically during the management of ALL increase the frequency of precocious puberty in girls but not in boys. At higher radiation doses used to treat solid brain tumors (24 to 50 Gy), early or precocious puberty may occur in both genders, the risk being greater the younger the child when treated [65]. Paradoxically, patients who develop early or precocious puberty after radiation doses in excess of 30 Gy have a significant risk for developing gonadotropin deficiency during adolescence, when it causes pubertal arrest, or as young adults. Children treated with radiation doses in excess of 50 Gy are more likely to develop gonadotropin deficiency and may have a delayed onset of puberty [66]. Given the complexity of the endocrinology in children, it is recommended that any child who receives cranial irradiation must undergo assessment of growth and pubertal status every 6 months. If a decline in height velocity or evidence of precocious puberty is observed, the child should be referred to an endocrinologist so that formal assessment of pituitary function can be undertaken.

Traumatic brain injury

The observation that hypopituitarism is associated with TBI was first made almost a century ago. In industrialized countries, TBI is common,

Table 1
Genetic causes of multiple and isolated pituitary hormone deficiencies

Affected gene	Gene function	Hormone deficiencies	Inheritance	Phenotype/comments
Mutations causing multiple pituitary hormone deficits				
POU1F1 [39] (PIT-1)	Pituitary specific transcription factor expressed late in pituitary development, required for normal somatotroph, lactotroph, and thyrotroph development	GH, thyrotropin, prolactin	AD, AR	Hormone deficiencies are severe. Thyrotropin secretion may be normal initially, but secondary hypothyroidism is inevitable. Variable pituitary size.
PROP1 [40]	Pituitary specific paired-like homeodomain transcription factor required for the expression of Pou1f1.	GH, thyrotropin, LH, FSH, prolactin	AR	Deficiencies tend to be milder than in POU1F1 mutations. Corticotropin deficiency may evolve with increasing age. Pituitary size variable. Can be associated with a mass lesion [41].
HESX1 [42]	A member of the paired-like class of homeobox genes, expressed early in pituitary development, a transcriptional repressor	Range from isolated GH deficiency to panhypopituitarism, including DI	AD, AR	Associated with septo-optic dysplasia, mutations result in a variable phenotype: pituitary hypoplasia, ectopic posterior pituitary, midline forebrain abnormalities. Environmental factors, such as drugs and alcohol, are implicated.
LHX3 [43]	Member of the LIM family of homeobox genes, expressed early in Rathke's pouch; it also is present in adult pituitary. It activates the α-GSU promoter and acts synergistically with POU1F1 to activate thyrotropin-β and prolactin promoters and the POU1F1 enhancer. Expression is important for development of different cell types in the anterior pituitary.	GH, thyrotropin, LH, FSH, prolactin	AR	Patients have elevated and anteverted shoulders giving the appearance of a stubby neck with limited rotation of the head. Anterior pituitary hypoplasia is present. Corticotropin secretion is preserved.

Gene	Description	Inheritance	Hormone deficiency	Clinical features
LHX4 [44]	Closely related to LHX3	AD	GH, thyrotropin, corticotropin	MRI demonstrates small sella, persistent craniopharyngeal canal, hypoplastic anterior pituitary and ectopic posterior pituitary. The cerebellar tonsils are pointed.

Mutations causing isolated pituitary hormone deficiencies

Gene	Description	Inheritance	Hormone deficiency	Clinical features
TBX19 [45] (TPIT)	Member of the T-box family of transcription factors. Highly specific expression in POMC-expressing cells in the anterior and intermediate lobes of the pituitary.	AR	Corticotropin	Presentation in neonatal period with severe hypoglycemia and prolonged cholestatic jaundice. Undetectable corticotropin and cortisol levels. Failure to respond to corticotropin-releasing hormone. High incidence of neonatal death in affected families.
SOX2 [46]	Member of the SRY-related high mobility group box family. Homozygous mutations are lethal early in embryonic development.	De novo mutations reported.	Hypogonadotrophic hypogodanism	Associated with anophthalmia or microphthalmia, learning difficulties, developmental delay, genital abnormalities, esophageal atresia, sensorineural hearing loss.
GHRHr [47]	Encodes the GHRH receptor, a seven-transmembrane domain G-protein linked receptor of the glucagon family. Expressed on somatotrophs.	AR	GH	Short stature, proportionate growth, anterior pituitary hypoplasia
GH1 [48]	Encodes the GH peptide within the somatotroph.	AR	GH	Short stature, abnormal facies. Respond to exogenous GH treatment, but may develop antibodies.
KAL-1 [49,50]	Encodes the protein anosmin-1, a putative cell adhesion molecule. Mutations result in failure of migration of olfactory neurones and GnRH neurones.	X-linked	GnRH, FSH, LH	Presents with failed or arrested puberty. Associated with anosmia, synkinesis, unilateral renal agenisis.
FGFR-1 [51] (KAL-2)	Encodes the fibroblast growth factor receptor.	AD	GnRH, FSH, LH	Presents with failed or arrested puberty.

(continued on next page)

Table 1 (*continued*)

Affected gene	Gene function	Hormone deficiencies	Inheritance	Phenotype/comments
GNRHR1 [52]	Encodes the GnRH receptor expressed in the gonadotrophs.	FSH, LH	AR	Variable phenotype determined by the sensitivity of the mutant receptor to GnRH.
DAX1 [53]	Dosage-sensitive sex reversal, adrenal hypoplasia congenital, critical region on the X chromosome, gene 1. Encodes an orphan nuclear receptor	FSH, LH	AR or X-linked	Presents initially with severe neonatal hypoadrenalism. Subsequently, patients fail to enter puberty or suffer delayed or arrested puberty
GPR54 [54]	Encodes the G protein–coupled receptor 54	FSH, LH	AR	Presents with absent or delayed puberty.
POMC [38]	Encodes pro-opiomelanocortin peptide	Corticotropin	AR	Clinical triad of early-onset obesity, adrenal hypoplasia, cortisol deficiency.
Thyrotropin-β [55]	Encodes the β subunit of the thyrotropin molecule	Thyrotropin	AR	Causes severe congenital hypothyroidism if not detected and treated early on.

Abbreviations: AD, autosomal dominant; AR, autosomal recessive; DI, diabetes insipidus; GnRH, gonadotropin releasing hormone; GSU, glycoprotein subunit; POMC, pro-opiomelanocortin.

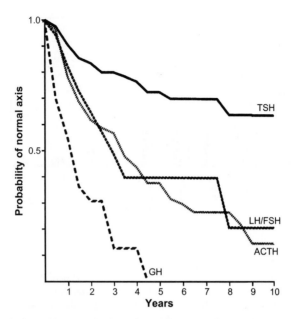

Fig. 1. The evolution of hypopituitarism after radiotherapy for pituitary disease in patients who had intact pituitary function before irradiation. (*From* Littley MD, Shalet SM, Beardwell CG, et al. Hypopituitarism following external radiotherapy for pituitary tumours in adults. Q J Med 1989;70:145–60; with permission.)

with an annual incidence of 180 to 250 per 100,000 of the population, with men below age 35 at greatest risk. The cause of posttraumatic hypopituitarism is believed to be infarction, found at post mortem in 26% to 86% of patients who died after TBI. Putative mechanisms for this include compression of the pituitary gland caused by changes in intracranial pressure resulting from cerebral edema, hemorrhage or skull fracture, hypoxia, or direct damage to the gland itself [67]. A recent study of 102 patients treated for significant TBI in a single center over a 2-year period assessed anterior pituitary function at least 6 months after the index event. The study demonstrated that 28.4% of patients had one or more anterior pituitary hormone deficits; 22.5% had isolated deficits and 5.9% had multiple hormone deficits. Severe GH deficiency, gonadotropin, and corticotropin and thyrotropin deficiency were present in 7.8%, 11.8%, 12.8%, and 1% respectively. Only one patient was found who had panhypopituitarism (Fig. 2). The presence of pituitary dysfunction was not associated with Glasgow Coma Scale scores, CT scan appearance, presence of cerebral edema, or a history of operative mass evacuation. Hyperprolactinemia was present in 11.8% of patients and not predicted by any of the factors discussed previously [68].

The pattern of hormone deficits changes with time after TBI. Abnormal axes during the acute phase may recover and additional hormone deficits evolve between the acute phase and 6 months after injury. Of particular

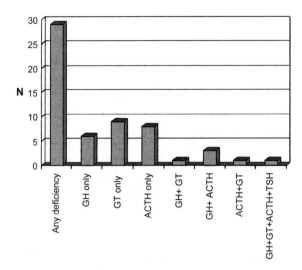

Fig. 2. The pattern of pituitary hormone deficits present in 102 patients who had TBI. (*From* Agha A, Rogers B, Sherlock M, et al. Anterior pituitary dysfunction in survivors of traumatic brain injury. J Clin Endocrinol Metab 2004;89(10):4929–36; with permission.)

importance is the observation that 10% of patients developed corticotropin deficiency during this period. It is suggested, therefore, that all patients sustaining moderate or severe head injury undergo assessment of anterior pituitary function during the acute phase and at 6 months. If pituitary function is normal at 6 months, then no further action is required, but if hormone deficits are detected, then appropriate replacement therapy should be instigated and patients retested if delayed recovery is suspected [69].

Infiltration

Lymphocytic hypophysitis is a rare condition, affecting women more frequently than men, often presenting during pregnancy as a pituitary mass with signs of local pressure, such as headache and visual disturbance. The estimated incidence of lymphocytic hypophysitis is 1 per 9 million. Other causes of hypophyseal infiltration include sarcoidosis, tuberculosis, Wegener's granulomatosis, Langerhans' cell histiocytosis, and syphyllis [70].

Diagnosis of hypopituitarism

A high level of suspicion should be maintained and a diagnosis of hypopituitarism considered in patients who have nonspecific symptoms of lethargy. A careful clinical history and examination can elicit features that support the diagnosis; for example, early menopause in women or declining libido in men should raise the possibility of the diagnosis. Ultimately, the diagnosis of hypopituitarism is confirmed biochemically using a combination of basal hormone measurements and dynamic function tests in patients known to have hypothalamic-pituitary disease or who are at risk for pituitary dysfunction after radiotherapy.

Growth hormone deficiency

The definition of GH deficiency in adulthood differs from that in childhood. In children, the diagnosis of GH deficiency is made in the presence of a reduced growth velocity. In adults, the clinical features attributed to GH deficiency are numerous and nonspecific; there is no single pathognomonic feature that alerts clinicians to the diagnosis. In a consensus statement, the Growth Hormone Research Society made it clear that the diagnosis of GH deficiency should be considered only in adults who have a history of pituitary disease, secondary to neoplastic disease, surgery, or cranial radiation or in those who have had a history of treatment with GH during childhood and adolescence [71]. Recent studies in patients after significant TBI indicate that they also should be added to the list of patients at risk for GH deficiency. One must be wary of diagnosing GH deficiency in patients who do not fulfill these criteria, as the results of dynamic tests of GH status are affected by obesity (all stimuli) [72] and age [73] and could lead to an inappropriate diagnosis.

The insulin tolerance test (ITT) is considered the gold standard used to diagnose GH deficiency in adults, using a diagnostic threshold of 3 µg/L. The ITT is not suitable for use in all patients and is contraindicated in patients who have a history of seizures or ischemic heart disease. Consequently, the majority of endocrinologists do not use the ITT in patients over 65 in case undiagnosed heart disease is present.

Although there are many agents that can be used to stimulate GH release, the majority of clinicians develop expertise using two or three tests. The behavior of the tests varies in children and adults. In children, different stimuli produce GH responses of similar magnitude and seem to produce interchangeable results [74]; this is not the case in adults. Rahim and colleagues [75] studied the GH response to a variety of stimuli in young adult men and observed that the ITT produced the greatest response, followed by the glucagon stimulation test and the arginine stimulation test. In this cohort, clonidine was no more effective than placebo at eliciting a GH response. Subsequent studies using a combination of growth hormone–releasing hormone (GHRH) plus arginine showed that this was a more exuberant stimulus of GH release, producing a significantly greater GH response than the ITT [76]. The diagnostic threshold for the GHRH plus arginine test is 9 µg/L, significantly higher than that used for the ITT. Whichever test is used, however, an appropriate threshold must be applied. It is recommended strongly that clonidine not be used to diagnose GH deficiency in adults.

Given the complexity, the need for medical supervision, and the potential risk for dynamic tests of GH status, a simple marker of GH status has been sought. Insulin-like growth factor (IGF)-I is a GH-dependent peptide, although the level of dependence seems to diminish with increasing age. In adults who have severe GH deficiency the relationship between serum IGF-I and age seems to be lost, but as age increases, the distinction between normal and severe GH deficiency becomes blurred [77]. In young adults who have childhood-onset GH deficiency, 95% [78] have serum IGF-I below the normal range, whereas 82% of GH-deficient patients over 60 years old have a normal IGF-I [73]. Serum IGF-I may be used as a marker of GH deficiency, particularly in young adults who have childhood-onset GH deficiency, but it must be done with knowledge of age-specific normal data and with the understanding that a normal level does not exclude the diagnosis, particularly in older adults.

Gonadotropin deficiency

The diagnosis of gonadotropin deficiency in women is straightforward. In women of a postmenopausal age, low or undetectable levels of FSH and LH are sufficient to make a diagnosis. In younger women, amenorrhoea with low estradiol levels and low or normal gonadotropins is consistent with the diagnosis of gonadotropin deficiency. In addition to these serum markers, failure to induce a withdrawal bleed after a progesterone challenge confirms the presence of a hypoestrogenic state.

In men, gonadotropin deficiency is diagnosed in the presence of low or normal serum gonadotropin levels and a low serum testosterone. The latter displays a diurnal rhythm; ideally it should be measured at 9:00 AM. Semen analysis is useful when considering fertility and may demonstrate oligospermia or azoospermia.

Adrenocorticotropin deficiency

The activity of the hypothalamic-pituitary-adrenal (HPA) axis exhibits a diurnal rhythm; serum cortisol levels often are undetectable at midnight during sleep rising and peak at approximately 5:00 AM, declining gradually over the course of the day. As a consequence of this diurnal variation, it often is necessary to undertake a dynamic test to assess the integrity of the HPA axis, although this may not be necessary in the presence of a 09.00 h cortisol in excess of 20 µg/dL (500 nmol/L) or less than 4 µg/dL (100 nmol/L), which usually confirms sufficiency or deficiency, respectively [79]. The ITT has been regarded as the gold standard for assessing the HPA axis since the late 1960s, when it was demonstrated that it predicted a good cortisol response to major abdominal surgery [80]. A peak response to hypoglycemia (blood glucose <2.2 mmol/L) of greater than 20 µg/dL is considered a normal response [81,82]. The ITT tests the integrity of the whole HPA axis and has the advantage of simultaneously assessing the GH status of patients. The ITT, however, does have limitations (discussed previously) and, consequently, alternative tests of the HPA are sought.

The test used most frequently as an alternative to the ITT is the short Synacthen test (SST) [83], which measures the serum cortisol response after an intramuscular injection of cosyntropin (Synacthen) (250 μg) [79,84,85]. The SST is based on the premise that corticotropin deficiency results in atrophy of the adrenal cortex and subsequently becomes unresponsive to a single pulse of corticotropin. A serum cortisol value of 22 μg/dL (550 nmol/L) or higher 30 minutes after administration of Synacthen is consistent with normal corticotropin reserve. This has been shown to correlate well with the peak cortisol level during the ITT [86]. Although it is a simple investigation that can be performed in an outpatient clinic, there are limitations to the test, in particular the risk for a false negative result (a perception that patients have normal corticotropin reserve). In situations when the onset of corticotropin deficiency is acute, for example, as a result of pituitary apoplexy or after pituitary surgery, the SST is unreliable and may give false reassurance, as the cortex remains responsive to exogenous corticotropin while it atrophies gradually, a process that takes several weeks [87–89]. It is recommended, therefore, that the SST should not be performed until at least 6 weeks after surgery or an apoplectic event.

The standard SST uses a pharmacologic dose of Synacthen, which has led some investigators to question its ability to detect subtle abnormalities of corticotropin secretion and suggest the use of a 1-μg dose of Synacthen or low-dose SST (LDSST) [90]. A recent meta-analysis of studies using the SST and the LDSST has demonstrated that both tests are of similar efficacy and there is no advantage in using the LDSST [91]. As Synacthen is available only in a 250-μg vial, there are considerable difficulties making the necessary dilution and it generally is recommended that the standard SST be used in routine clinical practice.

Thyroid-stimulating hormone deficiency

Thyrotropin deficiency is diagnosed in the presence of a low or normal serum thyrotopin measurement with a low serum free thyroxine (fT_4) level. Measurement of serum fT_3 is not required but may be low or normal. In patients treated with radiotherapy, sequential falls in the serum fT_4 toward the lower end of the normal range associated with evolving symptoms of hypothyroidism may be sufficient to warrant instigation of levothyroxine. The thyrotopin response to thyrotropin-releasing hormone is used less frequently since the introduction of sensitive thyrotropin assays.

Pituitary hormone replacement therapy

Growth hormone replacement

GH replacement in children who have GH deficiency results in an increase in linear growth and its use for that purpose is accepted universally.

Recombinant human GH has allowed GH replacement to be used in adults. Since then, many studies have evaluated the impact of GH replacement on multiple parameters, including quality of life, body composition, bone density, and cardiovascular risk factors, such as total cholesterol and carotid intima media thickness [92]. Overall, the results suggest beneficial effects, but the quality and extent of robust clinical trials is poor, leading to different approaches to provision of GH replacement in different countries. In some, the presence of severe GH deficiency is sufficient to warrant replacement based on the argument that cardiovascular risk profile will be improved [93]. Other countries restrict the use of GH treatment to adults who demonstrate specific criteria. In the United Kingdom, GH replacement is available to two groups of adults: those who have a demonstrable deficit and subsequent improvement in quality of life and young adults under age 25, to optimize bone mass [94].

Optimization of the benefit of GH treatment requires careful consideration of each individual case. Once the indication has been determined, diagnosis confirmed, and the decision to treat made, careful monitoring of patients is required to keep side effects to a minimum. The usual starting dose of GH is between 0.2 and 0.4 mg, determined by the age and gender of a patient. The dose of GH is in increments of 0.1 mg every 2 to 4 weeks until the serum IGF-I level is in the upper part of the normal range. Young adults require a higher dose than older adults and women tend to be GH resistant compared with men, in particular those receiving estrogens by mouth [95]. This measured approach in carefully selected patients minimizes risks for side effects and ensures that those receiving GH obtain the greatest benefit from it [96].

In the event of side effects (peripheral edema, arthralgia, and headaches) during the titration phase, the dose of GH should be reduced or, if severe, treatment should be withdrawn. As GH antagonizes the action of insulin, glycemic control should be monitored by determining blood glucose and glycosylated hemoglobin concentrations at baseline and after 6 months of treatment. Although concerns about the risk for tumor recurrence, particularly in patients treated for primary brain tumors, have not been realized [97], such patients should undergo surveillance scans at baseline and 12 months. Thereafter, the frequency of scans should be determined by the local protocol for surveillance or clinical symptoms [98]. In addition to these safety parameters, patients on GH replacement should be assessed on a 6-months' basis for general health, side effects, and the continued efficacy of the treatment. Serum IGF-I should be monitored at each visit to ensure it remains stable and to identify compliance issues should they arise [4].

Sex steroid and gonadotropin replacement

The aim of androgen replacement in men is to maintain secondary sexual characteristics, restore a sense of well-being, prevent loss of and optimize bone mass, and improve sexual function [99]. Until recently, testosterone replacement was limited to oral testosterone undecanoate (Restandol) (not available in the United States), 2- to 4-weekly depot injections of testosterone esters or pellets inserted every 6 months. Restandol is administered in 2 to 3 daily doses with meals. Absorbed through the lymphatic system, there is significant variability in the serum levels attained within and between individual patients. Consequently, it is used infrequently in men who have hypopituitarism. Depot testosterone esters have provided the mainstay of androgen replacement for many years in many endocrine units. They produce significant swings in serum testosterone levels, which can be supraphysiologic immediately after administration and become subtherapeutic before the next injection is due. As a consequence, patients may complain of symptoms of androgen deficiency, which can be alleviated by increasing the frequency of the injections. Testosterone pellets provide a stable physiologic testosterone level over a 6-month period. They do require a minor surgical procedure, which can leave the abdomen scarred, particularly in younger men who require two procedures a year. There also is the risk for the pellet falling out and, occasionally, infection.

More recently, there have been several new systems introduced for testosterone delivery; patches [100] and gels [101] applied to the skin and buccal bioadhesive tablets [102]. These preparations provide reliable noninvasive testosterone replacement, which normalizes testosterone levels rapidly and maintains them in the normal range. These preparations have the advantage of being able to be withdrawn immediately should patients experience any short-term adverse effects, such as psychologic disturbance, peripheral edema, or hypertension. The depot preparations of testosterone are joined by a longer-acting preparation of testosterone undecanoate, administered as an intramuscular injection every 3 months [103].

The efficacy of testosterone is determined clinically, the goal of treatment being the resolution of symptoms of hypogonadism. Side effects that may occur over the longer term with testosterone include prostate abnormalities, gynecomastia, polycythemia, liver dysfunction (including cholestatic jaundice), and, rarely, tumors. Concerns of the risk for prostate disease, benign and malignant, are addressed in recent guidelines published by the Endocrine Society [99]. At annual visits, patients should be assessed for prostatic symptoms, have a serum prostate specific antigen measured, and undergo a digital rectal examination. Referral to a urologist is required if patients have significant prostatic symptoms, a serum prostate specific antigen that is elevated or has increased by more than 1.4 ng/mL over 12 months, or if an abnormality is detected on digital rectal examination. The hematocrit also should be assessed. If polycythemia is present, testosterone should be withdrawn until the hematocrit returns to normal before treatment is reinstated at a lower dose.

Women who have gonadotropin deficiency require sex steroid replacement to alleviate the symptoms of estrogen deficiency and to optimize bone health. The effects of estrogen on cardiovascular risk remain a matter for debate. All women who have an intact uterus must receive cyclical replacement with regular withdrawal bleeds. Sex steroid replacement therapy should be continued until ages 50 to 55, when menopause occurs naturally.

Induction of puberty should be undertaken by a pediatric endocrinologist experienced in the management of hypopituitarism in children. In boys, monthly injections of testosterone esters (using a low initial dose of 25 to 50 mg) optimizes compliance and growth potential. The dose is increased gradually every 6 to 12 months to achieve an adult dose after 3 years [104]. In girls, conjugated estrogens or ethinyl estradiol can be used. Again, the initial dose should be low to optimize growth and prevent abnormal breast development. The dose of estrogen is increased every 6 to 12 months until an adult dose is reached. Once young women have been taking this for 6 months, or if breakthrough bleeding occurs, cyclical progesterone should be added [105].

Induction of fertility can be achieved in men and women using exogenous gonadotropins. In men, human chorionic gonadotropin can be used initially (in doses of 2000 IU twice weekly) to stimulate spermatogenesis [106]. The dose is titrated against testicular volume and serum testosterone. Most patients also require FSH, either recombinant or purified human menopausal gonadotropin (in starting doses of 75 IU 3 times per week). Spermatogenesis usually is obtained within 6 to 9 months, but treatment for many months may be needed for spontaneous conception. Semen should be cryopreserved for future use.

In women, ovulation induction is initiated with FSH or human menopausal gonadotropin. Careful ultrasound monitoring of follicular recruitment should be undertaken to ensure that only one or two follicles develop, to prevent superstimulation and prevent multiple pregnancies. Once a follicle has matured, a single dose of human chorionic gonadotropin is administered to stimulate ovulation, which occurs within 36 to 48 hours. Using exogenous gonadotropins, conception occurs in 5% to 15% of cycles [107].

Adrenocorticosteroid replacement

Cortisol

Hydrocortisone is the glucocorticoid of choice for patients who have secondary adrenal insufficiency, administered 2 to 3 times per day with a higher dose first thing in the morning and a lower dose in the evening in an attempt to mimic the normal diurnal variability of cortisol secretion. Occasionally, patients may require an additional dose of hydrocortisone in the middle of the day to alleviate tiredness, which can be associated with nadir cortisol levels. Hydrocortisone is favored over cortisone acetate, which undergoes first pass metabolism to cortisol by hepatic 11β-hydroxysteroid dehydrogenase and produces more variable serum cortisol levels. Other glucocorticoid preparations (prednisolone or dexamethasone) occasionally are used in some patients who have adrenal insufficiency, but their longer duration of action increases the likelihood of overtreatment and they now are used rarely in patients who have pituitary disease.

Optimizing glucocorticoid replacement therapy. Early studies of cortisol production in healthy individuals suggested that hydrocortisone requirements were approximately 30 mg per day. Subsequent studies suggested this figure was lower and most endocrinologists now use hydrocortisone doses of 15 to 25 mg a day [108]. The dose of hydrocortisone required by a patient is determined primarily by the symptoms and signs of cortisol deficiency. The dose should be sufficient to prevent a patient developing symptoms of cortisol deficiency or an adrenal crisis while avoiding the potential detrimental effects of glucocorticoid excess (weight gain, glucose intolerance, and low BMD).

Glucocorticoid requirements increase during times of stress caused by injury, surgery, or dental treatment or during intercurrent illness. Patients must be educated to inform all medical and dental personnel that they are on long-term steroid replacement therapy whenever they require treatment. They should be advised to increase their daily glucocorticoid dose during these times, usually by doubling the dose they normally take, until they have recovered. Patients should carry a card at all times that details the steroid replacement they are taking and the contact details of their physician. Patients also should be encouraged to wear a bracelet or necklace (eg, SOS Talisman, Glasgow, United Kingdom), which identifies them as requiring steroid replacement in case of accident. If patients cannot take their steroids because of vomiting or because they have undergone surgery, then parenteral steroids should be given. If patients show signs of an acute adrenal crisis hydrocortisone, 100 mg should be administered intravenously followed by 50 mg intravenously or intramuscularly 3 times daily [32].

There is a potential interaction with GH replacement. GH deficiency results in reduced cortisol clearance because of enhanced cortisone to cortisol conversion mediated by 11β-hydroxysteroid dehydrogenase type 1 [109]. (It is for this reason that the authors use a lower daily hydrocortisone replacement dose for patients who have hypopituitarism than they do for those who have primary adrenal failure). When starting GH replacement, cortisol clearance increases and patients may need a slight increase in hydrocortisone dose (on average 5 mg per day).

Hydrocortisone doses also should be increased during pregnancy by approximately 50% commencing in late second or early third trimesters [32].

Monitoring glucocorticoid replacement therapy. Patients taking hydrocortisone replacement should be assessed regularly to ensure that they do not have symptoms or signs of steroid deficiency or excess. There are no specific markers that allow endocrinologists to determine the appropriateness of patients' steroid dose. Measurement of 24-hour urine free cortisol levels has been suggested but is unreliable. Cortisol day curves are advocated by some to determine peak and nadir cortisol levels in the serum, but a paucity of normal data and the need to tailor doses to individuals makes day curves difficult to interpret. They often are reserved for patients in whom symptoms persist despite increased doses to demonstrate the hydrocortisone is being absorbed appropriately. The authors advocate assessment based on clinical parameters only (well-being, supine and erect blood pressure, weight, glucose, and lipids). Such patients have an intact renin-angiotensin axis and do not require mineralocorticoid replacement.

Dehydroepiandrosterone

In addition to cortisol, the adrenal cortex produces androgens regulated by corticotropin; thus, patients who have corticotropin deficiency also are deficient in dehydroepiandrosterone (DHEA) [110]. Studies of patients on conventional hormone replacement therapy regimens, including GH, demonstrate that treatment with DHEA (25–50 mg per day) improves quality of life and measures of sexuality in women who have adrenal failure secondary to hypopituitarism [110–112]. The effects of DHEA in men and women are variable [113] and not all patients respond. Side effects of DHEA include androgenic effects in women (greasy skin, acne, increased body hair growth, and, rarely, hair loss), which may be transient or can persist. In patients receiving GH replacement, DHEA can augment the IGF-I response, leading to a reduction in GH dose [114].

Thyroxine replacement

Patients who have thyrotopin deficiency should receive replacement therapy with levothyroxine. In young patients who have no evidence of ischemic heart disease, a starting dose of 100 μg should be used. In older patients or patients known to have cardiovascular disease, caution should be used with an initial dose of 25 to 50 μg. In secondary hypothyroidism, the serum thyrotopin level cannot be used to determine the patients dose of thyroxine, so the aim of replacement is to place the fT_4 in the normal range. Without the ability to normalize the serum thyrotropin, it is not possible to determine individuals' precise levothyroxine requirements. Care must be taken not to overtreat, as a suppressed serum thyrotropin in the normal population, indicative of subclinical thyrotoxicosis, is associated with increased risk for cardiac arrythmias, particularly atrial fibrillation. It is not known whether or not replacing thyroxine to achieve serum fT_4 levels in the upper part of the normal range, rather than the lower part, confers additional benefit in terms of quality of life and cardiovascular risk. A pragmatic approach is to aim for a serum fT_4 level in the upper half of the normal range.

Long-term consequences of hypopituitarism

Patients who have hypothalamic-pituitary disease and are receiving a combination of sex steroids, glucocorticoids, and thyroxine, but not GH replacement, for a range of anterior pituitary hormone deficiencies have an approximately twofold increase in mortality compared with the general population [21–23]. In the largest study to date, there was an increase in deaths from cardiovascular, cerebrovascular, and respiratory disease [22]. There is considerable debate among endocrinologists as to whether or not the increased mortality is caused by hormone replacement strategies that are nonphysiologic untreated GH deficiency, or a combination of both [25]. GH replacement therapy improves several markers of cardiovascular disease: serum total and LDL cholesterol are reduced [12] (HDL cholesterol is unchanged [9,13] or increased slightly [15]), and carotid intima media thickness [115] is reduced as are other markers of cardiovascular risk, such as C-reactive protein and interleukin 6 [116]. These observations demonstrate that GH replacement therapy improves individual cardiovascular risk profiles. Long-term postmarketing surveillance studies of patients receiving GH indicate that in the short term, mortality is not increased compared with the normal population, but the duration of treatment is short [117]. It will be some time before the true impact of GH on mortality is known.

Long-term follow-up of patients who have hypopituitarism

Hypopituitarism is a rare chronic disease associated with considerable morbidity, a reduction in life span, and the need for long-term replacement regimes that require specific monitoring and modification during various phases of life. Patients who have hypopituitarism require continued follow-up under the care of a physician who has expertise in the field. Once hormone replacement treatments are optimized, patients should be assessed on an annual basis to determine their cardiovascular risk. Particular attention should be paid to blood pressure and cholesterol levels and treatment with antihypertensives and cholesterol lowering agents instigated as appropriate. To optimize the long-term outcome for patients, they should remain under the supervision of an endocrinologist.

References

[1] Regal M, Paramo C, Sierra SM, et al. Prevalence and incidence of hypopituitarism in an adult Caucasian population in northwestern Spain. Clin Endocrinol (Oxf) 2001;55(6):735–40.
[2] Hughes NR, Lissett CA, Shalet SM. Growth hormone status following treatment for Cushing's syndrome. Clin Endocrinol (Oxf) 1999;51(1):61–6.
[3] Ogilvy-Stuart AL. Growth hormone deficiency (GHD) from birth to 2 years of age: diagnostic specifics of GHD during the early phase of life. Horm Res 2003;60(Suppl 1):2–9.
[4] Molitch ME, Clemmons DR, Malozowski S, et al. Evaluation and treatment of adult growth hormone deficiency: an Endocrine Society Clinical Practice Guideline. J Clin Endocrinol Metab 2006;91(5):1621–34.
[5] Burman P, Broman JE, Hetta J, et al. Quality of life in adults with growth hormone (GH) deficiency: response to treatment with recombinant human GH in a placebo-controlled 21-month trial. J Clin Endocrinol Metab 1995;80(12):3585–90.

[6] Holmes SJ, Shalet SM. Characteristics of adults who wish to enter a trial of growth hormone replacement. Clin Endocrinol (Oxf) 1995;42:613–8.

[7] McGauley GA, Cuneo RC, Salomon F, et al. Psychological well-being before and after growth hormone treatment in adults with growth hormone deficiency. Horm Res 1990; 33(Suppl 4):52–4.

[8] Attanasio AF, Lamberts SWJ, Matranga AMC, et al. Adult growth hormone deficient patients demonstrate heterogeneity between childhood onset and adult onset before and during human GH treatment. J Clin Endocrinol Metab 1997;82:82–8.

[9] Beshyah SA, Henderson A, Niththyanathan R, et al. Metabolic abnormalities in growth hormone deficient adults: carbohydrate tolerance and lipid metabolism. Endocrinol Metab 1994;1:173–80.

[10] Beshyah SA, Freemantle C, Thomas E, et al. Abnormal body composition and reduced bone mass in growth hormone deficient hypopituitary adults. Clin Endocrinol (Oxf) 1995;42:179–89.

[11] Lonn L, Kvist, Grangärd U, et al. CT-determined body composition changes with recombinant human growth hormone treatment to adults with growth hormone deficiency. Basic Life Sci 1993;60:229–31.

[12] Beshyah SA, Johnston DG. Cardiovascular disease and risk factors in adults with hypopituitarism. Clin Endocrinol (Oxf) 1999;50(1):1–15.

[13] de Boer H, Blok GJ, Voerman HJ, et al. Serum lipid levels in growth hormone deficient men. Metabolism 1994;43:199–203.

[14] Vahl N, Jorgensen JO, Hansen TB, et al. The favourable effects of growth hormone (GH) substitution on hypercholesterolaemia in GH-deficient adults are not associated with concomitant reductions in adiposity. A 12 month placebo-controlled study. Int J Obes Relat Metab Disord 1998;22(6):529–36.

[15] Cuneo RC, Salomon F, Watts GF, et al. Growth hormone treatment improves serum lipids and lipoproteins in adults with growth hormone deficiency. Metabolism 1993;42(12): 1519–23.

[16] Rosen T, Eden S, Larson G, et al. Cardiovascular risk factors in adult patients with growth hormone deficiency. Acta Endocrinol (Copenh) 1993;129:195–200.

[17] Sanmarti A, Lucas A, Hawkins F, et al. Observational study in adult hypopituitary patients with untreated growth hormone deficiency (ODA study). Socio-economic impact and health status. Collaborative ODA (Observational GH Deficiency in Adults) Group. Eur J Endocrinol 1999;141(5):481–9.

[18] Klibanski A. Growth hormone and cardiovascular risk markers. Growth Horm IGF Res 2003;13(Suppl):S109–15.

[19] Leonsson M, Hulthe J, Johannsson G, et al. Increased Interleukin-6 levels in pituitary-deficient patients are independently related to their carotid intima-media thickness. Clin Endocrinol (Oxf) 2003;59(2):242–50.

[20] Pfeifer M, Verhovec R, Zizek B, et al. Growth hormone (GH) treatment reverses early atherosclerotic changes in GH-deficient adults. J Clin Endocrinol Metab 1999;84(2):453–7.

[21] Rosen T, Bengtsson B. Premature mortality due to cardiovascular disease in hypopituitarism. Lancet 1990;336:285–8.

[22] Tomlinson JW, Holden N, Hills RK, et al. Association between premature mortality and hypopituitarism. West Midlands Prospective Hypopituitary Study Group. Lancet 2001; 357(9254):425–31.

[23] Bates AS, Van't Hoff W, Jones PJ, et al. The effect of hypopituitarism on life expectancy. J Clin Endocrinol Metab 1996;81(3):1169–72.

[24] Bulow B, Hagmar L, Mikoczy Z, et al. Increased cerebrovascular mortality in patients with hypopituitarism. Clin Endocrinol (Oxf) 1997;46(1):75–81.

[25] Toogood AA. Cardiovascular risk and mortality in patients with growth hormone deficiency. In: Abs R, Feldt-Rasmussen U, editors. Growth hormone deficiency in adults: 10 years of KIMS. 1st edition. Oxford (UK): Oxford Pharmagenesis; 2004. p. 63–74.

[26] Holmes SJ, Economou G, Whitehouse RW, et al. Reduced bone mineral density in patients with adult onset growth hormone deficiency. J Clin Endocrinol Metab 1994;78: 669–74.

[27] Attanasio AF, Howell S, Bates PC, et al. Body composition, IGF-I and IGFBP-3 concentrations as outcome measures in severely GH-deficient (GHD) patients after childhood GH treatment: a comparison with adult onset GHD patients. J Clin Endocrinol Metab 2002; 87(7):3368–72.

[28] Murray RD, Columb B, Adams JE, et al. Low bone mass is an infrequent feature of the adult growth hormone deficiency syndrome in middle-age adults and the elderly. J Clin Endocrinol Metab 2004;89(3):1124–30.

[29] Toogood AA, Adams JE, O'Neill PA, et al. Elderly patients with adult onset growth hormone deficiency are not osteopenic. J Clin Endocrinol Metab 1997;82:1462–6.

[30] Rosen T, Wilhelmsen L, Landin-Wilhelmsen K, et al. Increased fracture frequency in adult patients with hypopituitarism and GH deficiency. Eur J Endocrinol 1997;137:240–5.

[31] Wüster C, Abs R, Bengtsson BA, et al. The influence of growth hormone deficiency, growth hormone replacement therapy, and other aspects of hypopituitarism on fracture rate and bone mineral density. J Bone Miner Res 2001;16(2):398–405.

[32] Arlt W, Allolio B. Adrenal insufficiency. Lancet 2003;361(9372):1881–93.

[33] Mukherjee A, Murray RD, Columb B, et al. Acquired prolactin deficiency indicates severe hypopituitarism in patients with disease of the hypothalamic-pituitary axis. Clin Endocrinol (Oxf) 2003;59(6):743–8.

[34] Toledano Y, Lubetsky A, Shimon I. Acquired prolactin deficiency in patients with disorders of the hypothalamic-pituitary axis. J Endocrinol Invest 2007;30(4):268–73.

[35] Bole-Feysot C, Goffin V, Edery M, et al. Prolactin (PRL) and its receptor: actions, signal transduction pathways and phenotypes observed in PRL receptor knockout mice. Endocr Rev 1998;19(3):225–68.

[36] Dattani MT. Growth hormone deficiency and combined pituitary hormone deficiency: does the genotype matter? Clin Endocrinol (Oxf) 2005;63(2):121–30.

[37] Vnencak-Jones CL, Phillips JA 3rd, Chen EY, et al. Molecular basis of human growth hormone gene deletions. Proc Natl Acad Sci U S A 1988;85(15):5615–9.

[38] Krude H, Biebermann H, Luck W, et al. Severe early-onset obesity, adrenal insufficiency and red hair pigmentation caused by POMC mutations in humans. Nat Genet 1998; 19(2):155–7.

[39] Andersen B, Rosenfeld MG. POU domain factors in the neuroendocrine system: lessons from developmental biology provide insights into human disease. Endocr Rev 2001; 22(1):2–35.

[40] Sornson MW, Wu W, Dasen JS, et al. Pituitary lineage determination by the Prophet of Pit-1 homeodomain factor defective in Ames dwarfism. Nature 1996;384(6607):327–33.

[41] Turton JP, Mehta A, Raza J, et al. Mutations within the transcription factor PROP1 are rare in a cohort of patients with sporadic combined pituitary hormone deficiency (CPHD). Clin Endocrinol (Oxf) 2005;63(1):10–8.

[42] Dattani MT, Martinez-Barbera JP, Thomas PQ, et al. Mutations in the homeobox gene HESX1/Hesx1 associated with septo-optic dysplasia in human and mouse. Nat Genet Jun 1998;19(2):125–33.

[43] Netchine I, Sobrier ML, Krude H, et al. Mutations in LHX3 result in a new syndrome revealed by combined pituitary hormone deficiency. Nat Genet 2000;25(2):182–6.

[44] Machinis K, Pantel J, Netchine I, et al. Syndromic short stature in patients with a germline mutation in the LIM homeobox LHX4. Am J Hum Genet 2001;69(5):961–8.

[45] Pulichino AM, Vallette-Kasic S, Couture C, et al. Human and mouse TPIT gene mutations cause early onset pituitary ACTH deficiency. Genes Dev 2003;17(6):711–6.

[46] Kelberman D, Rizzoti K, Avilion A, et al. Mutations within Sox2/SOX2 are associated with abnormalities in the hypothalamo-pituitary-gonadal axis in mice and humans. J Clin Invest 2006;116(9):2442–55.

[47] Maheshwari HG, Silverman BL, Dupuis J, et al. Phenotype and genetic analysis of a syndrome caused by an inactivating mutation in the growth hormone-releasing hormone receptor: Dwarfism of Sindh. J Clin Endocrinol Metab 1998;83(11):4065–74.

[48] Cogan JD, Phillips JA 3rd, Sakati N, et al. Heterogeneous growth hormone (GH) gene mutations in familial GH deficiency. J Clin Endocrinol Metab 1993;76(5):1224–8.

[49] Legouis R, Hardelin JP, Levilliers J, et al. The candidate gene for the X-linked Kallmann syndrome encodes a protein related to adhesion molecules. Cell 1991;67(2):423–35.

[50] Franco B, Guioli S, Pragliola A, et al. A gene deleted in Kallmann's syndrome shares homology with neural cell adhesion and axonal path-finding molecules. Nature 1991; 353(6344):529–36.

[51] Dode C, Levilliers J, Dupont JM, et al. Loss-of-function mutations in FGFR1 cause autosomal dominant Kallmann syndrome. Nat Genet 2003;33(4):463–5.

[52] Beranova M, Oliveira LM, Bedecarrats GY, et al. Prevalence, phenotypic spectrum, and modes of inheritance of gonadotropin-releasing hormone receptor mutations in idiopathic hypogonadotropic hypogonadism. J Clin Endocrinol Metab 2001;86(4):1580–8.

[53] Lin L, Gu WX, Ozisik G, et al. Analysis of DAX1 (NR0B1) and steroidogenic factor-1 (NR5A1) in children and adults with primary adrenal failure: ten years' experience. J Clin Endocrinol Metab 2006;91(8):3048–54.

[54] de Roux N, Genin E, Carel JC, et al. Hypogonadotropic hypogonadism due to loss of function of the KiSS1-derived peptide receptor GPR54. Proc Natl Acad Sci U S A 2003;100(19): 10972–6.

[55] Vuissoz JM, Deladoey J, Buyukgebiz A, et al. New autosomal recessive mutation of the TSH-beta subunit gene causing central isolated hypothyroidism. J Clin Endocrinol Metab 2001;86(9):4468–71.

[56] Ezzat S, Asa SL, Couldwell WT, et al. The prevalence of pituitary adenomas: a systematic review. Cancer 2004;101(3):613–9.

[57] Karavitaki N, Cudlip S, Adams CB, et al. Craniopharyngiomas. Endocr Rev 2006;27(4): 371–97.

[58] Littley MD, Shalet SM, Beardwell CG, et al. Hypopituitarism following external radiotherapy for pituitary tumours in adults. Q J Med 1989;70:145–60.

[59] Agha A, Sherlock M, Brennan S, et al. Hypothalamic-pituitary dysfunction after irradiation of nonpituitary brain tumors in adults. J Clin Endocrinol Metab 2005;90(12):6355–60.

[60] Lam KSL, Wang C, Yeung RTT, et al. Hypothalamic hypopituitarism following cranial irradiation for nasopharyngeal carcinoma. Clin Endocrinol (Oxf) 1986;24:643–51.

[61] Brennan BM, Rahim A, Mackie EM, et al. Growth hormone status in adults treated for acute lymphoblastic leukaemia in childhood. Clin Endocrinol (Oxf) 1998;48(6):777–83.

[62] Toogood AA. Endocrine consequences of brain irradiation. Growth Horm IGF Res 2004; 14(Suppl A):S118–24.

[63] Rose SR, Lustig RH, Pitukcheewanont P, et al. Diagnosis of hidden central hypothyroidism in survivors of childhood cancer. J Clin Endocrinol Metab 1999;84(12):4472–9.

[64] Darzy KH, Shalet SM. Circadian and stimulated thyrotropin secretion in cranially irradiated adult cancer survivors. J Clin Endocrinol Metab 2005;90(12):6490–7.

[65] Ogilvy-Stuart AL, Clayton PE, Shalet SM. Cranial irradiation and early puberty. J Clin Endocrinol Metab 1994;78:1282–6.

[66] Ogilvy-Stuart AL, Shalet SM. Growth and puberty after growth hormone treatment after irradiation for brain tumours. Arch Dis Child 1995;73:141–6.

[67] Agha A, Thompson CJ. Anterior pituitary dysfunction following traumatic brain injury (TBI). Clin Endocrinol (Oxf) 2006;64(5):481–8.

[68] Agha A, Rogers B, Sherlock M, et al. Anterior pituitary dysfunction in survivors of traumatic brain injury. J Clin Endocrinol Metab 2004;89(10):4929–36.

[69] Agha A, Phillips J, O'Kelly P, et al. The natural history of post-traumatic hypopituitarism: implications for assessment and treatment. Am J Med 2005;118(12):1416.e1–1416.e7.

[70] Caturegli P, Newschaffer C, Olivi A, et al. Autoimmune hypophysitis. Endocr Rev 2005; 26(5):599–614.

[71] Growth Hormone Research Society. Consensus guidelines for the diagnosis and treatment of adults with growth hormone deficiency: summary statement of the Growth Hormone Research Society workshop on adult growth hormone deficiency. J Clin Endocrinol Metab 1998;83:379–81.

[72] Shalet S, Toogood A, Rahim A, et al. The diagnosis of growth hormone deficiency in children and adults. Endocr Rev 1998;19:203–23.

[73] Toogood A, Jones J, O'Neill P, et al. The diagnosis of severe growth hormone deficiency in elderly patients with hypothalamic-pituitary disease. Clin Endocrinol (Oxf) 1998;48: 569–76.

[74] Ghigo E, Bellone J, Aimaretti G, et al. Reliability of provocative tests to assess growth hormone secretory status. Study in 472 normally growing children. J Clin Endocrinol Metab 1996;81(9):3323–7.

[75] Rahim A, Toogood AA, Shalet SM. The assessment of growth hormone status in normal young adult males using a variety of provocative tests. Clin Endocrinol (Oxf) 1996;45: 557–62.

[76] Aimaretti G, Corneli G, Razzore P, et al. Comparison between insulin-induced hypoglycemia and growth hormone (GH)-releasing hormone + arginine as provocative tests for the diagnosis of GH deficiency in adults. J Clin Endocrinol Metab 1998;83(5):1615–8.

[77] Ghigo E, Aimaretti G, Gianotti L, et al. New approach to the diagnosis of growth hormone deficiency in adults. Eur J Endocrinol 1996;134:352–6.

[78] de Boer H, Blok G-J, Popp-Snijders C, et al. Diagnosis of growth hormone deficiency in adults (letter). Lancet 1994;343:1645–6.

[79] Stewart PM, Corrie J, Seckl JR, et al. A rational approach for assessing the hypothalamo-pituitary-adrenal axis. Lancet 1988;1(8596):1208–10.

[80] Plumpton FS, Besser GM. The adrenocortical response to surgery and insulin-induced hypoglycaemia in corticosteroid-treated and normal subjects. Br J Surg 1969;56(3): 216–9.

[81] Tuchelt H, Dekker K, Bahr V, et al. Dose-response relationship between plasma ACTH and serum cortisol in the insulin-hypoglycaemia test in 25 healthy subjects and 109 patients with pituitary disease. Clin Endocrinol (Oxf) 2000;53(3):301–7.

[82] Nelson JC, Tindall DJ Jr. A comparison of the adrenal responses to hypoglycemia, metyrapone and ACTH. Am J Med Sci 1978;275(2):165–72.

[83] Reynolds RM, Stewart PM, Seckl JR, et al. Assessing the HPA axis in patients with pituitary disease: a UK survey. Clin Endocrinol (Oxf) 2006;64(1):82–5.

[84] Clayton RN. Short Synacthen test versus insulin stress test for assessment of the hypothalamo [correction of hypothalmo]-pituitary–adrenal axis: controversy revisited. Clin Endocrinol (Oxf) 1996;44(2):147–9.

[85] Kane KF, Emery P, Sheppard MC, et al. Assessing the hypothalamo-pituitary-adrenal axis in patients on long-term glucocorticoid therapy: the short synacthen versus the insulin tolerance test. QJM 1995;88(4):263–7.

[86] Hurel SJ, Thompson CJ, Watson MJ, et al. The short Synacthen and insulin stress tests in the assessment of the hypothalamic-pituitary-adrenal axis. Clin Endocrinol (Oxf) 1996; 44(2):141–6.

[87] Watts NB, Tindall GT. Rapid assessment of corticotropin reserve after pituitary surgery. JAMA 1988;259(5):708–11.

[88] Auchus RJ, Shewbridge RK, Shepherd MD. Which patients benefit from provocative adrenal testing after transsphenoidal pituitary surgery? Clin Endocrinol (Oxf) 1997;46(1): 21–7.

[89] Mukherjee JJ, de Castro JJ, Kaltsas G, et al. A comparison of the insulin tolerance/glucagon test with the short ACTH stimulation test in the assessment of the

hypothalamo-pituitary-adrenal axis in the early post-operative period after hypophysectomy. Clin Endocrinol (Oxf) 1997;47(1):51–60.

[90] Abdu TA, Elhadd TA, Neary R, et al. Comparison of the low dose short synacthen test (1 microg), the conventional dose short synacthen test (250 microg), and the insulin tolerance test for assessment of the hypothalamo-pituitary-adrenal axis in patients with pituitary disease. J Clin Endocrinol Metab 1999;84(3):838–43.

[91] Dorin RI, Qualls CR, Crapo LM. Diagnosis of adrenal insufficiency. Ann Intern Med 2003; 139(3):194–204.

[92] Toogood A. Safety and efficacy of growth hormone replacement therapy in adults. Expert Opin Drug Saf 2005;4(6):1069–82.

[93] Bengtsson BA, Johannsson G, Shalet SM, et al. Treatment of growth hormone deficiency in adults. J Clin Endocrinol Metab 2000;85(3):933–42.

[94] Human growth hormone (somatropin) in adults with growth hormone deficiency. National Institute for Clinical Excellence; August 2003. Available at: http://www.nice.org.uk/guidance/index.jsp?action=download&o=32665. Accessed December 11, 2007.

[95] Drake WM, Howell SJ, Monson JP, et al. Optimizing GH therapy in adults and children. Endocr Rev 2001;22(4):425–50.

[96] Drake WM, Coyte D, Camacho-Hubner C, et al. Optimizing growth hormone replacement therapy by dose titration in hypopituitary adults. J Clin Endocrinol Metab 1998;83(11): 3913–9.

[97] Swerdlow AJ, Reddingius RE, Higgins CD, et al. Growth hormone treatment of children with brain tumors and risk of tumor recurrence. J Clin Endocrinol Metab 2000;85(12):4444–9.

[98] Chung TT, Drake WM, Evanson J, et al. Tumour surveillance imaging in patients with extrapituitary tumours receiving growth hormone replacement. Clin Endocrinol (Oxf) 2005; 63(3):274–9.

[99] Bhasin S, Cunningham GR, Hayes FJ, et al. Testosterone therapy in adult men with androgen deficiency syndromes: an Endocrine Society clinical practice guideline. J Clin Endocrinol Metab 2006;91(6):1995–2010.

[100] Arver S, Dobs AS, Meikle AW, et al. Long-term efficacy and safety of a permeation-enhanced testosterone transdermal system in hypogonadal men. Clin Endocrinol (Oxf) 1997;47(6):727–37.

[101] Swerdloff RS, Wang C, Cunningham G, et al. Long-term pharmacokinetics of transdermal testosterone gel in hypogonadal men. J Clin Endocrinol Metab 2000;85(12):4500–10.

[102] Wang C, Swerdloff R, Kipnes M, et al. New testosterone buccal system (Striant) delivers physiological testosterone levels: pharmacokinetics study in hypogonadal men. J Clin Endocrinol Metab 2004;89(8):3821–9.

[103] Harle L, Basaria S, Dobs AS. Nebido: a long-acting injectable testosterone for the treatment of male hypogonadism. Expert Opin Pharmacother 2005;6(10):1751–9.

[104] Schneider HJ, Aimaretti G, Kreitschmann-Andermahr I, et al. Hypopituitarism. Lancet 2007;369(9571):1461–70.

[105] Kiess W, Conway G, Ritzen M, et al. Induction of puberty in the hypogonadal girl—practices and attitudes of pediatric endocrinologists in Europe. Horm Res 2002; 57(1–2):66–71.

[106] Vicari E, Mongioi A, Calogero AE, et al. Therapy with human chorionic gonadotrophin alone induces spermatogenesis in men with isolated hypogonadotrophic hypogonadism—long-term follow-up. Int J Androl 1992;15(4):320–9.

[107] Ascoli P, Cavagnini F. Hypopituitarism. Pituitary 2006;9(4):335–42.

[108] Esteban NV, Loughlin T, Yergey AL, et al. Daily cortisol production rate in man determined by stable isotope dilution/mass spectrometry. J Clin Endocrinol Metab 1991; 72(1):39–45.

[109] Moore JS, Monson JP, Kaltsas G, et al. Modulation of 11 beta-hydroxysteroid dehydrogenase isozymes by growth hormone and insulin-like growth factor: In vivo and in vitro studies. J Clin Endocrinol Metab 1999;84(11):4172–7.

[110] Arlt W, Callies F, van Vlijmen JC, et al. Dehydroepiandrosterone replacement in women with adrenal insufficiency. N Engl J Med 1999;341(14):1013–20.

[111] Johannsson G, Burman P, Wiren L, et al. Low dose dehydroepiandrosterone affects behavior in hypopituitary androgen-deficient women: a placebo-controlled trial. J Clin Endocrinol Metab 2002;87(5):2046–52.

[112] Brooke AM, Kalingag LA, Miraki-Moud F, et al. Dehydroepiandrosterone improves psychological well-being in male and female hypopituitary patients on maintenance growth hormone replacement. J Clin Endocrinol Metab 2006;91(10):3773–9.

[113] van Thiel SW, Romijn JA, Pereira AM, et al. Effects of dehydroepiandrostenedione, superimposed on growth hormone substitution, on quality of life and insulin-like growth factor I in patients with secondary adrenal insufficiency: a randomized, placebo-controlled, crossover trial. J Clin Endocrinol Metab 2005;90(6):3295–303.

[114] Brooke AM, Kalingag LA, Miraki-Moud F, et al. Dehydroepiandrosterone (DHEA) replacement reduces growth hormone (GH) dose requirement in female hypopituitary patients on GH replacement. Clin Endocrinol (Oxf) 2006;65(5):673–80.

[115] Gibney J, Wallace JD, Spinks T, et al. The effects of 10 years of recombinant human growth hormone (GH) in adult GH-deficient patients. J Clin Endocrinol Metab 1999;84(8): 2596–602.

[116] Sesmilo G, Biller BM, Llevadot J, et al. Effects of growth hormone administration on inflammatory and other cardiovascular risk markers in men with growth hormone deficiency. A randomized, controlled clinical trial. Ann Intern Med 2000;133(2):111–22.

[117] Bengtsson BA, Koppeschaar HP, Abs R, et al. Growth hormone replacement therapy is not associated with any increase in mortality. J Clin Endocrinol Metab 1999;84(11):4291–2.

ELSEVIER
SAUNDERS

Endocrinol Metab Clin N Am
37 (2008) 263–275

ENDOCRINOLOGY
AND METABOLISM
CLINICS
OF NORTH AMERICA

Radiotherapy for Pituitary Adenomas

Michael Brada, BSc, FRCP, FRCR[a,b,*], Petra Jankowska, MRCP, FRCR[b]

[a]*Academic Unit of Radiotherapy and Oncology, The Institute of Cancer Research,
Downs Road, Sutton, Surrey SM2 5PT, UK*
[b]*Neuro-Oncology Unit, The Royal Marsden NHS Foundation Trust,
London and Sutton, UK*

External beam radiotherapy (RT) is generally used in patients with pituitary adenoma as second-line treatment after failure of surgery and medical therapy. In patients who have secreting tumors, it normalizes elevated serum hormone concentrations, albeit with delay, and in patients who have unresectable progressive and recurrent nonfunctioning tumors, it achieves excellent long-term tumor control. Hypothalamic-pituitary insufficiency is the most frequent late complication of treatment, although serious late effects are uncommon. Modern techniques of high-precision conformal and stereotactic RT delivery treat less normal tissue to high radiation doses than conventional RT, with the aim of reducing late morbidity even further, although demonstrating such benefit requires large long-term studies.

Radiotherapy techniques

Conventional radiotherapy

Conventional external beam RT for pituitary adenoma is given with photons using a linear accelerator. Practical steps in the preparation for treatment include patient immobilization, CT, and MRI imaging for accurate

This work was supported in part by the Neuro-Oncology Research fund, The Royal Marsden NHS Trust, and Cancer Research UK. The work was undertaken by the Royal Marsden NHS Trust, which received a proportion of its funding from the NHS Executive; the views expressed are those of the authors and not necessarily those of the NHS Executive.

Petra Jankowska, MRCP, FRCR, is currently in the Heamatology and Oncology Unit, Taunton & Somerset NHS Trust Foundation, Musgrove Park, Taunton, Somerset TA1 5DA, UK.

* Corresponding author. The Institute of Cancer Research and The Royal Marsden NHS Foundation Trust, Downs Road, Sutton, Surrey SM2 5PT, United Kingdom.

E-mail address: michael.brada@icr.ac.uk (M. Brada).

localization of the tumor and computerized 3-D planning to achieve local-ized delivery of radiation conforming to the shape of the tumor.

The precision of the treatment is aided by the use of immobilization devices. The device used most frequently is an individually molded, closely fitting plastic mask with a relocation accuracy of 2 to 5 mm.

Imaging for treatment planning is performed in the treatment position (supine) in the immobilization device using CT and MRI, which should be coregistered. The MRI visible mass and possible residual disease based on preoperative images and surgical notes are delineated; this is defined as the gross tumor volume (GTV). Based on the known technical uncertainty of planning, immobilization, and treatment delivery, a 3-D margin is added to the GTV; this is defined as the planning target volume (PTV). The margin should be based on the actual measurement of uncertainty specific to the RT center and for conventional RT is in the region of 5 to 10 mm. The aim of conventional RT planning is to achieve a homogeneous dose to the PTV with the least dose to the surrounding normal tissue.

Conventional RT generally uses three fixed radiation fields—an anterior oblique field aimed at the pituitary through the forehead and two lateral opposing beams traversing through the temporal regions. Beams are shaped using a multileaf collimator (MLC) to conform to the shape of the tumor and to shield out normal structures; this is described as conformal RT.

MLC leaves may also be used to alter the intensity of radiation across the target; this is described as intensity-modulated RT. Currently there is no advantage of intensity-modulated RT over conformal RT in the treatment of pituitary adenomas [1].

Radiosurgery and stereotactic conformal radiotherapy

Stereotactic technique enables more precise localization of a tumor and adjacent critical neural structures and more precise treatment delivery, and is a refinement of conformal RT. Stereotactic irradiation can be given as single-fraction radiosurgery (SRS), using either a multiheaded cobalt unit (gamma knife [GK]) or a linear accelerator, or as fractionated stereo-tactic conformal RT (SCRT), delivered as fractionated treatment on a linear accelerator.

Immobilization for SRS traditionally is with invasive neurosurgical-type frames. For fractionated SCRT, immobilization is achieved with relocatable frames [2,3], with a relocation accuracy of 1 to 2 mm and more precisely fitting mask systems [4], with accuracy of 2 to 3 mm allowing for a smaller margin around the GTV.

Pituitary adenoma is delineated as for conventional RT on MRI, which is accurately coregistered with CT. The position of the tumor is defined using 3-D coordinates with the aid of external fiducial markers or fixed internal anatomic structures. Accurate identification of all parts of a tumor before treatment is essential for any modern RT technique, and image interpretation is the cornerstone of successful treatment with any high-precision delivery techniques using small safety margins.

Linear accelerator beams are shaped with a narrow-leaf MLC of 3 mm (micro-MLC) or 5 mm (mini-MLC) leaf width. The leaves are positioned automatically to predefined shapes based on information transferred directly from a planning computer. The use of four to six rather than three beams improves the dose differential between a tumor and normal tissue and leads to further normal tissue sparing. There is no clear therapeutic gain using a larger number of fixed beams [5].

In SRS, beams from multiple fixed cobalt sources of a multiheaded cobalt unit (GK) are collimated through a collimator helmet to produce small spherical high-dose volumes ranging from 6 mm to 18 mm in diameter. Larger or nonspherical tumors, such as the majority of pituitary adenomas, are treated with a combination of several spheres, described as a multiple isocenter technique. Computerized 3-D planning determines the optimum number and distribution of isocenters and this can be aided by selective occlusion of GK collimator apertures.

Comparison of conformal radiosurgery techniques

The only published comparison of GK multiple isocenter technique and linear accelerator multiple fixed-field treatment [6] shows no clear advantage of either technique in terms of sparing of normal tissue receiving high radiation doses with excellent conformity achieved with GK and linear accelerator fixed-field treatments. The wide hemispheric distribution of multiple cobalt sources from GK increases the volume of normal brain receiving low radiation doses. Although the clinical significance is at present uncertain, low-dose whole brain irradiation may increase the risk for radiation-induced second malignancies.

Linear accelerator SCRT delivers a homogenous dose to the tumor, whereas overlapping radiation spheres of multiple isocenters lead to inhomogeneous dose distribution in the target with small high-dose regions (hot spots). In the absence of normal neural structures within the target, this is unlikely to be of clinical importance in terms of toxicity. Multiple isocenter treatment of tumors involving the cavernous sinus or the optic apparatus, however, may produce hot spots within cranial nerves with a risk for late radiation damage.

In the early days of stereotactic RT, linear accelerators were adapted with fixed circular collimators to mimic GK dose distribution using the technique of multiple arc rotation. Four to six conformal, fixed-field SCRT technique produces superior dose distribution within and outside the target [7] and largely has superseded the multiple-arc multiple isocenter technique.

In summary, GK SRS and linear accelerator SCRT treat similar volumes of normal brain to high radiation doses. GK SRS produces dose inhomogeneity within the target and increases the volume of normal brain receiving low radiation doses (1%–5%), whereas linear accelerator SCRT achieves homogenous target dose and tends to treat larger volumes of normal brain to medium to low doses (20%–30%). The claimed benefit of GK SRS over linear accelerator SCRT is precision of relocation and patient convenience of a single treatment albeit with the added risk of single-fraction radiation toxicity. This compares to the small inaccuracy of relocation of an immobilization device and inconvenience of multiple treatments, although with lesser risk for morbidity. Whether or not such technical differences likely translate to different clinical outcomes is not clear.

The initial rationale for SRS was based on the perception of single high radiation dose as a surgical tool causing tissue destruction. Although a large single dose of radiation results in a higher cell kill than the same dose given in a number of small fractions, it is more toxic to normal tissues, in particular neural structures. The comparative benefit of different treatments is assessed appropriately by the differential effect on a tumor and normal tissue, described as the therapeutic ratio.

Dose fractionation

The majority of pituitary adenomas requiring additional treatment with radiation lie in close proximity to the optic apparatus and the nerves of the cavernous sinus. The early enthusiastic use of high-dose SRS for large adenomas containing the optic apparatus led to an unacceptably high incidence of optic radiation neuropathy [8]. As the risk for radiation optic neuropathy after SRS is dose dependent [9,10], current practice aims to avoid irradiating the optic apparatus beyond single doses of 8 to 10 Gy. Consequently, radiosurgery is limited to small adenomas away from the optic apparatus (usually ≥5 mm) and to radiation doses that do not cause tissue ablation.

Fractionated SCRT, as conventional RT, is given in doses of 45 to 50 Gy at less than 2 Gy per fraction, which is below the tolerance dose of the central nervous system with minimal risk for structural radiation damage (<1%). The perceived benefit of SRS over SCRT for pituitary adenoma is based on radiobiologic formalism defining equivalent doses and fractionation schemes through mathematically derived models [11,12]. Such models are not validated for single-fraction treatments for benign tumors, and theoretic claims for a benefit of SRS over fractionated irradiation [13] are based on constants not derived from experimental data and are therefore potentially misleading. Currently, there is no clear basis for claims of improved therapeutic ratio of SRS over SCRT.

Clinical evidence

The efficacy of radiation treatment of pituitary adenoma should be assessed in terms of survival, actuarial tumor control (progression-free survival [PFS]), and quality of life. Information on the effect of different treatments on survival and quality of life is limited, and the principal efficacy endpoints reported in patients who have nonfunctioning pituitary adenoma are PFS and late morbidity. In patients who have secreting tumors, the principal endpoints used are the normalization of elevated hormone concentrations, long-term tumor control, and morbidity. As the delay in achieving normal hormonal status is largely related to pretreatment hormone levels, assessment of the rate of decline is made best in relation to the initial level, with one appropriate measure the time to reach 50% of initial hormone level. "Control rate," without indication of time and duration of follow-up, and the proportion of patients achieving normal hormone levels without a clear relationship to pretreatment values may at first glance seem appealing, but they do not provide the appropriate measures of efficacy and are potentially misleading.

The reporting of outcome of different treatment techniques is affected by selection bias. Fractionated SCRT in doses of 45 to 50 Gy in 25 to 30 fractions, which are below the conventional radiation tolerance of surrounding normal structures, including the optic chiasm, allows for the treatment of pituitary adenomas of all sizes, including large tumors with suprasellar extension frequently encasing or in close proximity to the optic apparatus. The damaging effect of large single doses of radiation to critical normal structures dictates that patients treated with SRS have small tumors well away from the optic chiasm. The outcome data after GK SRS, therefore, represent results in patients who have small adenomas generally after radical surgery.

Efficacy and toxicity of conventional radiotherapy

Tumor control

The 10-year PFS reported in seven large series of conventional external beam RT for pituitary adenoma is 80% to 94% [14–23]. In the largest series of 411 patients, the 10-year PFS was 94% at 10 years and 89% at 20 years [14].

Hormone control

Acromegaly. The rate of reduction of growth hormone (GH) after conventional therapy is reported as a 50% drop in 27 (±5) months [24]. The rate of reduction of insulin-like growth factor I is slower, with normalization in 60% of patients 5 to 10 years after treatment [24].

Cushing's disease. Fifty percent to 100% of patients treated with conventional radiation achieve normalization of plasma and urinary cortisol, with the majority normalizing in the first 2 years after treatment [25].

Prolactinoma. As RT is rarely used as the sole treatment for prolactinoma, information about the rate of decline of prolactin is limited. It is used occasionally in patients who fail surgery and medical therapy.

Toxicity

The toxicity of fractionated external beam RT is low, with a 1.5% risk of radiation-induced optic neuropathy [14,26] and 0.2% risk of necrosis of normal brain structures [27]. Although radiation is implicated in late cognitive impairment, there is no clear evidence that small-volume fractionated irradiation affects cognitive function in adults beyond the deleterious effect of surgery and the tumor itself [28–30]. The most frequent late morbidity of radiation is hypopituitarism likely to be primarily the result of hypothalamic injury, although direct effect on the pituitary gland cannot be excluded. In patients who have normal pituitary function around the time of RT, hormone replacement therapy is required in 20% to 40% at 10 years.

Cranial irradiation is associated with an increased risk for developing a radiation-induced brain tumor and is described in children receiving prophylactic cranial irradiation for acute lymphoblastic leukemia [31,32] and in children treated with scalp irradiation for tinea capitis [33]. The reported incidence of gliomas and meningiomas after RT for pituitary adenoma is approximately of 2% at 10 to 20 years [34–37]. Although there is an increased incidence of cerebrovascular accidents and excess cerebrovascular mortality in patients who have pituitary adenoma treated with radiation, the influence of radiation on its frequency is not defined [38–41].

Efficacy and toxicity of gamma knife single-fraction radiosurgery

A systematic review of outcome of radiosurgery has been published previously [42] and is summarized, with the addition of new studies. Between 1985 and 2006, 42 studies involving 1877 patients treated with GK radiosurgery were reported. The primary clinical outcomes assessed were PFS, hormonal normalization for secretory tumors, and the frequency of adverse events.

Hormone control

Acromegaly. Although SRS data for 713 patients are reported in 25 studies, actuarial outcome data are limited (updated results from [42]). Overall, normalization of serum GH concentrations was reported in 164 (23%) patients and a decrease in 210 patients. No information on hormonal response was reported in more than half of the patients and the reliability of the data is not clear. Studies where the rate of GH decline is related to pretreatment serum GH report a time to reaching 50% of initial level of approximately 2 years [43,44], which is similar to the rate of decline after fractionated irradiation.

Cushing's disease. The updated results of SRS for 269 patients in 21 studies report normalization of hormone level in 165 patients (61%), a decrease in 40 (15%), and no information on response in 50 patients. At a corrected median follow-up of 55 months, 61% of patients had normalization of elevated hormone level [42]. There is no data to demonstrate faster decline in elevated cortisol levels than achieved after conventional RT. Latest results in 90 patients with Cushing's disease report 54% (49/90) remission rate; of these, 20% (10/49) subsequently relapsed, suggesting poor efficacy of GK SRS [45].

Prolactinoma. SRS was reported in 375 patients who had prolactinoma in 19 studies. Although the serum prolactin concentrations normalized in 96 (26%) and decreased in 206 (55%), the results are difficult to disentangle from the effect of other interventions. The reported time to hormonal response (normalization or decrease) was 5 to 41 months after SRS. If follow-up time reported is assumed to represent the median follow-up, 26% of patients had normalization of prolactin level at a corrected median follow-up of 25 months [42]. The rate of decline of prolactin and comparison to conventional RT is not assessable from the available studies.

Tumor control in nonfunctioning pituitary adenoma

The results of SRS are reported for 617 patients in 19 studies (updated results from [42]). Five reported a "control rate" of more than 90% (weighted mean 96%) without specifying the length of follow-up or time of assessment [46–50]. More recent studies report a 5-year PFS of 88% to 96% [51–53] and 3 years' PFS of 94% to 95% [54,55]. The corrected (weighted) 5-year PFS is 92% [42], which is well below the results reported for conventional RT.

Toxicity of single-fraction radiosurgery

Hypopituitarism remains a frequent complication of SRS and has been reported in 4% to 66% of patients at an overall corrected median follow-up of 64 months [54,56–62]. Although many studies do not record complications, 10% of 90 patients (nine cases) who had Cushing's disease developed cranial nerve deficit; five had ophthalmoplegia resulting from third or sixth nerve palsies and four a decrease in visual acuity presumed to represent optic radiation neuropathy [45]. Similarly, 10% patients who had prolactinoma developed cranial nerve deficit after SRS [63].

Summary of gamma knife radiosurgery

Currently there is no evidence of faster decline of elevated hormone concentrations after GK SRS than that reported after conventional therapy. Studies that take into account individual hormone concentrations show similar rate of decline as seen after fractionated irradiation [42,44,64]. The majority of reports do not provide appropriate information to assess the efficacy of GK radiosurgery in terms of tumor control in secretory or nonfunctioning pituitary adenomas. Based on the limited evidence available, the actuarial tumor control of small adenomas suitable for GK SRS seems inferior to the control rate achieved with fractionated irradiation given to adenomas of all sizes. The available information on comparative morbidity of SRS suggests a disturbingly high complication rate not seen with fractionated irradiation.

Efficacy and toxicity of linear accelerator single-fraction radiosurgery

Systematic review of linear accelerator stereotactic cranial irradiation has been reported previously [65]. In the largest of five published studies of SRS, where 175 patients who had pituitary adenomas were treated with a single fraction of 20 Gy and followed for a minimum of 12 months (mean ±SD, 82 ± 37 months), the local "tumor control" rate was reported as 96% (at an unspecified time). The mean time from treatment to hormone normalization was 36 ± 24 months, with an overall probability of normalization of 34% at 3 years and 51% at 5 years. The results were not related to pretreatment hormone levels. The reported side effects at a short follow-up included anterior pituitary dysfunction (12%), radiation-induced tissue damage (3%), and radiation-induced neuropathy (1%). Four further studies contain fewer than 30 patients and provide little information to assess the efficacy of treatment. The overall results of linear accelerator SRS are broadly comparable to GK SRS, although the follow-up is short and the endpoints in individual studies not appropriate for providing meaningful comparative information on long-term tumor control and treatment-related toxicity.

Efficacy and toxicity of linear accelerator stereotactic
conformal radiotherapy

Five studies of SCRT have been reviewed previously [65]. Since then, an update of GH-secreting adenoma subgroup from a previous study has been reported [66], and the authors published the results from the Royal Marsden Hospital [67]. Local control in secretory and nonsecretory macroadenomas ranged from 85% to 100% [66–71]. Twenty percent of patients needed new hormone replacement [66,68]. Although studies report the proportion of patients who normalized their GH levels, this is not related to pretreatment values and the rate of decline of elevated hormone levels cannot be assessed.

The PFS in 92 patients treated at the Royal Marsden Hospital at a median follow-up of 32 months was 98% at 3 and 5 years and respective survival 98%. In patients who had acromegaly, 50% of baseline GH level was achieved in less than 2 years [67]. The late toxicity seen most frequently was hypopituitarism, with 22% of patients experiencing deterioration in pituitary function [67].

In summary, the early results of linear accelerator SCRT are within the range reported for conventional RT and it is not possible to claim that either disease control or survival are significantly improved. The technical advantage of high-precision stereotactic RT aims at reducing the amount of normal brain receiving high radiation doses. It is hoped this will translate into further reduction in long-term toxicity. Improvement in late morbidity is not yet demonstrated, however, and will require many years of follow-up and large cohorts of patients to obtain statistically meaningful results.

Treatment of recurrent pituitary adenoma

A small proportion of patients with pituitary adenoma progresses after RT. Re-irradiation is considered too risky because of the presumed cumulative damaging effect of radiation on normal brain, in particular the optic chiasm and cranial nerves. Primate spinal cord studies suggest that provided initial radiation is given to doses below conventional radiation tolerance, considerable recovery of latent radiation damage is seen 2 or more years after treatment [72]. Re-irradiation using conventional techniques to repeat of initial radiation doses resulted in only a small risk for radiation optic neuropathy [73,74]. Stereotactic techniques can further reduce the radiation dose to sensitive surrounding structures, provided they are not in close proximity to the tumor. Eleven patients who had recurrent tumors treated with SCRT at the Royal Marsden Hospital so far have remained without late radiation optic neuropathy (Brada and colleagues, unpublished data, 2006). SRS for recurrent pituitary adenoma has to be restricted to tumors away from the optic chiasm and nerves. In patients who had persistent hormone elevation, SRS resulted in a decline of elevated hormone levels similar to that seen after SRS as primary therapy, so far with no reported radiation optic neuropathy [75].

The available data do not provide sufficient information on long-term tumor or hormonal control after re-irradiation with SRS or SCRT. Reported evidence from conventional fractionated treatment suggests that fractionated treatment has acceptable efficacy and toxicity [73,74].

Summary

RT remains an effective treatment in patients with progressive pituitary adenomas not cured by surgery or medical therapy, achieving excellent long-term tumor and endocrine control. Hypopituitarism represents the late complication of RT reported most commonly with low incidence of other late effects.

There is much debate about the relative efficacy of SRS and SCRT. The efficacy of SCRT in terms of local tumor control is comparable to the results of conventional external beam RT. Currently reported results suggest that SRS achieves worse tumor control than fractionated treatment. The rate of decline of elevated hormone levels is no faster after single treatment compared with fractionated irradiation. The reported neurologic toxicity of SRS is considerably higher than that seen with fractionated irradiation at a short follow-up.

Treating less normal brain to high radiation doses with stereotactic irradiation is a clear technical improvement of modern RT that may in the future translate into clinical benefit as a reduction in the incidence of late effects of radiation. The short follow-up, however, requires caution in interpretation until more mature and reliable results are available in terms of efficacy and late radiation–induced toxicity.

A single-fraction treatment may represent a convenient approach for pituitary adenomas, but the technique is suitable only for small residual tumors well away from the optic chiasm. On the basis of the available evidence, there is little justification for its use, as it is associated with worse morbidity, inferior tumor control, and, in secreting tumors, no faster hormone decline than that seen with fractionated treatment. SRS, therefore, cannot be recommended as the appropriate treatment of nonfunctioning adenomas of any size and its use in patients who have hormone secreting tumors remains questionable. Prospective studies comparing SRS with fractionated stereotactic RT may be of value in helping to define the comparative long-term efficacy and toxicity of the techniques. The strongly held views about the relative merits of each technique, however, largely based on local availability of the equipment, make it unlikely that such studies will be performed in the foreseeable future.

Acknowledgments

The authors wish to acknowledge the contributions of Dr. Thankama Ajithkumar and Dr. Giuseppe Minniti to the initial systematic review.

References

[1] Khoo VS, Oldham M, Adams EJ, et al. Comparison of intensity-modulated tomotherapy with stereotactically guided conformal radiotherapy for brain tumors. Int J Radiat Oncol Biol Phys 1999;45(2):415–25.

[2] Gill SS, Thomas DG, Warrington AP, et al. Relocatable frame for stereotactic external beam radiotherapy. Int J Radiat Oncol Biol Phys 1991;20(3):599–603.

[3] Graham JD, Warrington AP, Gill SS, et al. A non-invasive, relocatable stereotactic frame for fractionated radiotherapy and multiple imaging. Radiother Oncol 1991;21(1):60–2.

[4] Karger CP, Jakel O, Debus J, et al. Three-dimensional accuracy and interfractional reproducibility of patient fixation and positioning using a stereotactic head mask system. Int J Radiat Oncol Biol Phys 2001;49(5):1493–504.

[5] Perks JR, Jalali R, Cosgrove VP, et al. Optimization of stereotactically-guided conformal treatment planning of sellar and parasellar tumors, based on normal brain dose volume histograms. Int J Radiat Oncol Biol Phys 1999;45(2):507–13.

[6] Yu C, Luxton G, Jozsef G, et al. Dosimetric comparison of three photon radiosurgery techniques for an elongated ellipsoid target. Int J Radiat Oncol Biol Phys 1999;45(3):817–26.

[7] Laing RW, Bentley RE, Nahum AE, et al. Stereotactic radiotherapy of irregular targets: a comparison between static conformal beams and non-coplanar arcs. Radiother Oncol 1993;28(3):241–6.

[8] Rocher FP, Sentenac I, Berger C, et al. Stereotactic radiosurgery: the Lyon experience. Acta Neurochir Wien 1995;63:109–14.

[9] Tishler RB, Loeffler JS, Lunsford D, et al. Tolerance of cranial nerves of the cavernous sinus to radiosurgery. Int J Radiat Oncol Biol Phys 1993;27:215–21.

[10] Leber KA, Bergloff J, Pendl G. Dose-response tolerance of the visual pathways and cranial nerves of the cavernous sinus to stereotactic radiosurgery. J Neurosurg 1998;88(1):43–50.

[11] Gutin PH, Leibel SA, Sheline GA. Radiation injury to the nervous system. New York: Raven Press; 1991.

[12] Steel GG, editor. Basic clinical radiobiology. 3rd edition. London: Edward Arnold; 2002.

[13] Larson DA, Flickinger JC, Loeffler JS. The radiobiology of radiosurgery. Int J Radiat Oncol Biol Phys 1993;25(3):557–61.

[14] Brada M, Rajan B, Traish D, et al. The long term efficacy of conservative surgery and radiotherapy in the control of pituitary adenomas. Clin Endocrinol (Oxf) 1993;38(6):571–8.

[15] Sheline G. Pituitary tumours: radiation therapy. In: Beardwell C, Robertson G, editors. Clinical endocrinology 1: the pituitary. London: Butterworths; 1987. p. 106–39.

[16] Sheline GE. Role of conventional radiation thrapy in treatment of functional pituitary tumours. In: Linfott JA, editor. Recent advances in the diagnosis and tratment of pituitary tumours. New York: Raven Press; 1979. p. 289–313.

[17] Erlichman C, Meakin JW, Simpson WJ. Review of 154 patients with non functioning pituitary tumors. Int J Radiat Oncol Biol Phys 1979;5:1981–6.

[18] Halberg FE, Sheline GE. Radiotherapy of pituitary tumors. Endocrinol Metab Clin North Am 1987;16(3):667–84.

[19] Flickinger JC, Nelson PB, Martinez AJ, et al. Radiotherapy of nonfunctional adenomas of the pituitary gland. Results with long-term follow-up. Cancer 1989;63(12):2409–14.

[20] Tsang RW, Brierley JD, Panzarella T, et al. Role of radiation therapy in clinical hormonally-active pituitary adenomas. Radiother Oncol 1996;41(1):45–53.

[21] Breen P, Flickinger JC, Kondziolka D, et al. Radiotherapy for nonfunctional pituitary adenoma: analysis of long-term tumor control. J Neurosurg 1998;89(6):933–8.

[22] Grigsby P, Stokes S, Marks J, et al. Prognostic factors and results of radiotherapy alone in the management of pituitary adenoma. Int J Radiat Oncol Biol Phys 1988;15:1103–10.

[23] Gittoes NJ, Bates AS, Tse W, et al. Radiotherapy for non-function pituitary tumours. Clin Endocrinol (Oxf) 1998;48(3):331–7.

[24] Biermasz NR, Dulken HV, Roelfsema F. Postoperative radiotherapy in acromegaly is effective in reducing GH concentration to safe levels. Clin Endocrinol (Oxf) 2000;53(3):321–7.

[25] Estrada J, Boronat M, Mielgo M, et al. The long-term outcome of pituitary irradiation after unsuccessful transsphenoidal surgery in Cushing's disease [see comments]. N Engl J Med 1997;336(3):172–7.

[26] Tsang RW, Brierley JD, Panzarella T, et al. Radiation therapy for pituitary adenoma: treatment outcome and prognostic factors. Int J Radiat Oncol Biol Phys 1994;30(3):557–65.

[27] Becker G, Kocher M, Kortmann RD, et al. Radiation therapy in the multimodal treatment approach of pituitary adenoma. Strahlenther Onkol 2002;178(4):173–86.

[28] Grattan Smith PJ, Morris JG, Shores EA, et al. Neuropsychological abnormalities in patients with pituitary tumours. Acta Neurol Scand 1992;86(6):626–31.

[29] Peace KA, Orme SM, Sebastian JP, et al. The effect of treatment variables on mood and social adjustment in adult patients with pituitary disease. Clin Endocrinol (Oxf) 1997;46(4):445–50.

[30] van Beek AP, van den Bergh AC, van den Berg LM, et al. Radiotherapy is not associated with reduced quality of life and cognitive function in patients treated for nonfunctioning pituitary adenoma. Int J Radiat Oncol Biol Phys 2007;68(4):986–91.

[31] Neglia JP, Meadows AT, Robison LL, et al. Second neoplasms after acute lymphoblastic leukemia in childhood. N Engl J Med 1991;325(19):1330–6.

[32] Walter AW, Hancock ML, Pui CH, et al. Secondary brain tumors in children treated for acute lymphoblastic leukemia at St Jude Children's Research Hospital. J Clin Oncol 1998; 16(12):3761–7.

[33] Ron E, Modan B, Boice JD Jr, et al. Tumors of the brain and nervous system after radiotherapy in childhood. N Engl J Med 1988;319(16):1033–9.

[34] Brada M, Ford D, Ashley S, et al. Risk of second brain tumour after conservative surgery and radiotherapy for pituitary adenoma. Br Med J 1992;304(6838):1343–6.

[35] Minniti G, Traish D, Ashley S, et al. Risk of second brain tumor after conservative surgery and radiotherapy for pituitary adenoma: update after an additional 10 years. J Clin Endocrinol Metab 2005;90(2):800–4.

[36] Tsang R, Laperriere N, Simpson W, et al. Glioma arising after radiation therapy for pituitary adenoma: a report of four patients and estimation of risk. Cancer 1993;72:2227–33.

[37] Erfurth EM, Bulow B, Mikoczy Z, et al. Incidence of a second tumor in hypopituitary patients operated for pituitary tumors. J Clin Endocrinol Metab 2001;86(2):659–62.

[38] Brada M, Ashley S, Ford D, et al. Cerebrovascular mortality in patients with pituitary adenoma. Clin Endocrinol (Oxf) 2002;57(6):713–7.

[39] Brada M, Burchell L, Ashley S, et al. The incidence of cerebrovascular accidents in patients with pituitary adenoma. Int J Radiat Oncol Biol Phys 1999;45(3):693–8.

[40] Tomlinson JW, Holden N, Hills RK, et al. Association between premature mortality and hypopituitarism. West Midlands Prospective Hypopituitary Study Group. Lancet 2001; 357(9254):425–31.

[41] Erfurth EM, Bulow B, Hagmar LE. Is vascular mortality increased in hypopituitarism? Pituitary 2000;3(2):77–81.

[42] Brada M, Ajithkumar TV, Minniti G. Radiosurgery for pituitary adenomas. Clin Endocrinol (Oxf) 2004;61(5):531–43.

[43] Attanasio R, Barausse M, Cozzi R. GH/IGF-I normalization and tumor shrinkage during long-term treatment of acromegaly by lanreotide. J Endocrinol Invest 2001;24(4):209–16.

[44] Castinetti F, Taieb D, Kuhn JM, et al. Outcome of gamma knife radiosurgery in 82 patients with acromegaly: correlation with initial hypersecretion. J Clin Endocrinol Metab 2005; 90(8):4483–8.

[45] Jagannathan J, Sheehan JP, Pouratian N, et al. Gamma Knife surgery for Cushing's disease. J Neurosurg 2007;106(6):980–7.

[46] Izawa M, Hayashi M, Nakaya K, et al. Gamma knife radiosurgery for pituitary adenomas. J Neurosurg 2000;93(Suppl 3):19–22.

[47] Mokry M, Ramschak-Schwarzer S, Simbrunner J, et al. A six year experience with the postoperative radiosurgical management of pituitary adenomas. Stereotact Funct Neurosurg 1999;72(Suppl 1):88–100.

[48] Pan L, Zhang N, Wang E, et al. Pituitary adenomas: the effect of gamma knife radiosurgery on tumor growth and endocrinopathies. Stereotact Funct Neurosurg 1998;70(Suppl 1): 119–26.

[49] Sheehan JP, Kondziolka D, Flickinger J, et al. Radiosurgery for residual or recurrent nonfunctioning pituitary adenoma. J Neurosurg 2002;97(Suppl 5):408–14.

[50] Wowra B, Stummer W. Efficacy of gamma knife radiosurgery for nonfunctioning pituitary adenomas: a quantitative follow up with magnetic resonance imaging-based volumetric analysis. J Neurosurg 2002;97(Suppl 5):429–32.

[51] Pollock BE, Carpenter PC. Stereotactic radiosurgery as an alternative to fractionated radiotherapy for patients with recurrent or residual nonfunctioning pituitary adenomas. Neurosurgery 2003;53(5):1086–91 [discussion: 91–4].

[52] Losa M, Valle M, Mortini P, et al. Gamma knife surgery for treatment of residual nonfunctioning pituitary adenomas after surgical debulking. J Neurosurg 2004;100(3):438–44.

[53] Iwai Y, Yamanaka K, Yoshioka K. Radiosurgery for nonfunctioning pituitary adenomas. Neurosurgery 2005;56(4):699–705 [discussion: 699–705].

[54] Petrovich Z, Yu C, Giannotta SL, et al. Gamma knife radiosurgery for pituitary adenoma: early results. Neurosurgery 2003;53(1):51–9 [discussion: 9–61].

[55] Muacevic A, Uhl E, Wowra B. Gamma knife radiosurgery for nonfunctioning pituitary adenomas. Acta Neurochir Suppl 2004;91:51–4.

[56] Degerblad M, Brismar K, Rahn T, et al. The hypothalamus-pituitary function after pituitary stereotactic radiosurgery: evaluation of growth hormone deficiency. J Intern Med 2003; 253(4):454–62.

[57] Degerblad M, Rahn T, Bergstrand G, et al. Long-term results of stereotactic radiosurgery to the pituitary gland in Cushing's disease. Acta Endocrinol (Copenh) 1986;112(3):310–4.

[58] Hoybye C, Grenback E, Rahn T, et al. Adrenocorticotropic hormone-producing pituitary tumors: 12- to 22-year follow-up after treatment with stereotactic radiosurgery. Neurosurgery 2001;49(2):284–91 [discussion: 91–2].

[59] Morange-Ramos I, Regis J, Dufour H, et al. Short-term endocrinological results after gamma knife surgery of pituitary adenomas. Stereotact Funct Neurosurg 1998;70(Suppl 1):127–38.

[60] Pollock BE, Nippoldt TB, Stafford SL, et al. Results of stereotactic radiosurgery in patients with hormone-producing pituitary adenomas: factors associated with endocrine normalization. J Neurosurg 2002;97(3):525–30.

[61] Pollock BE, Young WF Jr. Stereotactic radiosurgery for patients with ACTH-producing pituitary adenomas after prior adrenalectomy. Int J Radiat Oncol Biol Phys 2002;54(3): 839–41.

[62] Sheehan JM, Vance ML, Sheehan JP, et al. Radiosurgery for Cushing's disease after failed transsphenoidal surgery. J Neurosurg 2000;93(5):738–42.

[63] Pouratian N, Sheehan J, Jagannathan J, et al. Gamma knife radiosurgery for medically and surgically refractory prolactinomas. Neurosurgery 2006;59(2):255–66.

[64] Attanasio R, Epaminonda P, Motti E, et al. Gamma-knife radiosurgery in acromegaly: a 4-year follow-up study. J Clin Endocrinol Metab 2003;88(7):3105–12.

[65] Ajithkumar T, Brada M. Stereotactic linear accelerator radiotherapy for pituitary tumors. Treat Endocrinol 2004;3(4):211–6.

[66] Milker-Zabel S, Zabel A, Huber P, et al. Stereotactic conformal radiotherapy in patients with growth hormone-secreting pituitary adenoma. Int J Radiat Oncol Biol Phys 2004; 59(4):1088–96.

[67] Minniti G, Traish D, Ashley S, et al. Fractionated stereotactic conformal radiotherapy for secreting and nonsecreting pituitary adenomas. Clin Endocrinol (Oxf) 2006;64(5):542–8.

[68] Mitsumori M, Shrieve D, Alexander E, et al. Initial clinical results of LINAC-based stereotactic radiosurgery and stereotactic radiotherapy for pituitary adenomas. Int J Radiat Oncol Biol Phys 1998;42(3):573–80.

[69] Selch MT, Gorgulho A, Lee SP, et al. Stereotactic radiotherapy for the treatment of pituitary adenomas. Minim Invasive Neurosurg 2006;49(3):150–5.

[70] Milker-Zabel S, Debus J, Thilmann C, et al. Fractionated stereotactically guided radiotherapy and radiosurgery in the treatment of functional and nonfunctional adenomas of the pituitary gland. Int J Radiat Oncol Biol Phys 2001;50(5):1279–86.

[71] Coke C, Andrews DW, Corn BW, et al. Multiple fractionated stereotactic radiotherapy of residual pituitary macroadenomas: initial experience. Stereotact Funct Neurosurg 1997; 69(1–4 Pt 2):183–90.

[72] Ang KK, Price RE, Stephens LC, et al. The tolerance of primate spinal cord to re irradiation. Int J Radiat Oncol Biol Phys 1993;25:459–64.

[73] Flickinger JC, Deutsch M, Lunsford LD. Repeat megavoltage irradiation of pituitary and suprasellar tumors. Int J Radiat Oncol Biol Phys 1989;17(1):171–5.

[74] Schoenthaler R, Albright NW, Wara WM, et al. Re-irradiation of pituitary adenoma. Int J Radiat Oncol Biol Phys 1992;24(2):307–14.

[75] Swords FM, Allan CA, Plowman PN, et al. Stereotactic radiosurgery XVI: a treatment for previously irradiated pituitary adenomas. J Clin Endocrinol Metab 2003;88(11):5334–40.

ELSEVIER
SAUNDERS

Endocrinol Metab Clin N Am
37 (2008) 277–296

ENDOCRINOLOGY
AND METABOLISM
CLINICS
OF NORTH AMERICA

Index

Note: Page numbers of article titles are in **boldface** type.

A

Abscess(es), pituitary, primary sellar, 196, 205–206

Acromegaly, **101–122**
  diagnosis of, 102–106
    biochemical markers in, 105–106, 114–115
    imaging in, 106
    signs and symptoms in, 102–105
  follow-up monitoring of, 114–115
  isolated familial, pituitary adenomas associated with, 37–38
  mortality ratio of, 104–105, 107
  pathogenesis of, 101–102
  pituitary adenoma prevalence in, 24
  radiotherapy and, in pituitary adenomas, 267–268
  screening for, 155
  treatment of, 106–115
    approach to, 113–115
      algorithm for, 114
    dopamine analogs in, 112
      results of, 108–109
    goals of, 106, 108–109
    growth hormone receptor antagonist in, 111–112
      results of, 108–109
    pharmacotherapy in, 107, 111–114
      results of, 108–109
    radiotherapy in, 112–113
      results of, 107–109
    somatostatin receptor ligands in, 107, 111
      results of, 108–109
    surgery as, 106–107, 113
      macroadenomas and, 62–63
      results of, 107–109

ACTH-secreting adenomas, euvolemic hyponatremia and, 224

Activin, in gonadotropin regulation, 14

Actuarial tumor control, in radiotherapy, for pituitary adenomas, 266–267, 269

Acute lymphoblastic leukemia (ALL), radiotherapy for, hypopituitarism caused by, 240–241

Adamantinomatous craniopharyngioma, 174–175

Adenoma(s), ACTH-secreting, euvolemic hyponatremia and, 224
  corticotroph, clinically nonfunctioning, 155
    phenotypes of, 30–32
    prevalence of, 23
  gonadotroph, clinically nonfunctioning, 155
    prevalence of, 23–24
  pituitary, acromegaly related to, 101, 104
    radiotherapy for, 108–109, 112–113
    surgery for, 106–107, 113
      results of, 107–109
    biopsy of, gene expression profiles in, 26–27
      phenotypes revealed in, 30–32
    clinically nonfunctioning, **151–171**
      asymptomatic, 152–158
      description of, 61–62, 151–152
      symptomatic, 158–165
    diverse characteristics of, 23–24
    familial syndromes associated with, 37–38
    functional, 62–63
    growth characteristics of, 24–25
      aneuploidy and, 35
      clonal skewing and, 32–35
    incidence of, 23
    macro-. See *Macroadenoma.*
    micro-. See *Microadenoma.*
    molecular and trophic mechanisms of, **23–50**. See also *Tumorigenesis.*
    non-MEN1 and non-Carney complex isolated familial, 37–39

Moving?

Make sure your subscription moves with you!

To notify us of your new address, find your **Clinics Account Number** (located on your mailing label above your name), and contact customer service at:

E-mail: elspcs@elsevier.com

800-654-2452 (subscribers in the U.S. & Canada)
407-345-4000 (subscribers outside of the U.S. & Canada)

Fax number: 407-363-9661

Elsevier Periodicals Customer Service
6277 Sea Harbor Drive
Orlando, FL 32887-4800

*To ensure uninterrupted delivery of your subscription, please notify us at least 4 weeks in advance of move.